SELF ASSESSMENT IN RADIOLOGY

Paediatric Radiology

Dr Christopher O'Callaghan

B.Med.Sci, MB, BS, MRCP
Lecturer in Child Health
University Hospital
Nottingham

Wolfe Medical Publications Ltd

To my parents

Copyright © C. O'Callaghan, 1989
First published 1989 by Wolfe Publishing Ltd
Printed by W. S. Cowell Ltd, Ipswich, England
ISBN 0 7234 0978 1

A CIP catalogue record for this book is available from the
British Library.

Other subjects of titles in the series
Ear, Nose & Throat Radiology
Gastro-Intestinal Radiology
Mammography
Nuclear Medicine
Orthopaedics
Chest Radiology

For a full list of our other publications please write to
Wolfe Publishing Ltd,
Brook House, 2-16 Torrington Place,
London WC1E 7LT, England

Preface

Questions are based on X-rays from the Paediatric Departments of Nottingham University and Brompton Hospitals, England, and the Royal Children's Hospital, Australia, and represent a paediatrician's keyhole view of paediatric radiology.

I am indebted to the following who supplied radiographs and gave advice on the text:

Dr Alan Crispin, Dr Phillip Small, Dr Ian Kerr, Dr Geoff Narbrough, Dr John Trounce, Dr Alan Watson and Miss L. Kapila. With Dr Crispin's help it has been possible to produce a text to match the quality of the prints.

C.O'C

Foreword

So much paediatric radiology and imaging is undertaken outside specialist paediatric centres that many perceptive paediatricians realise the need to secure all the help they can obtain. This collection of pictures with an interrogative text and a comprehensive index is designed to provide insights, information and help.

The clarity of the method of presenting the images first, then posing the relevant question and then providing guidance in the answers is useful. The reason is that the method encourages observation, thought and analysis.

At the outset each picture is concerned with one dominant aspect of paediatric work. Often it has proved possible to set such individual examples into the context of wider knowledge. The result of the style and method of presentation is a text useful to paediatricians and also to radiologists.

Dr Alan Crispin
MB, FRCP, DMRD
Consultant Radiologist,
City and University Hospitals, Nottingham
Clinical Teacher, The University of Nottingham

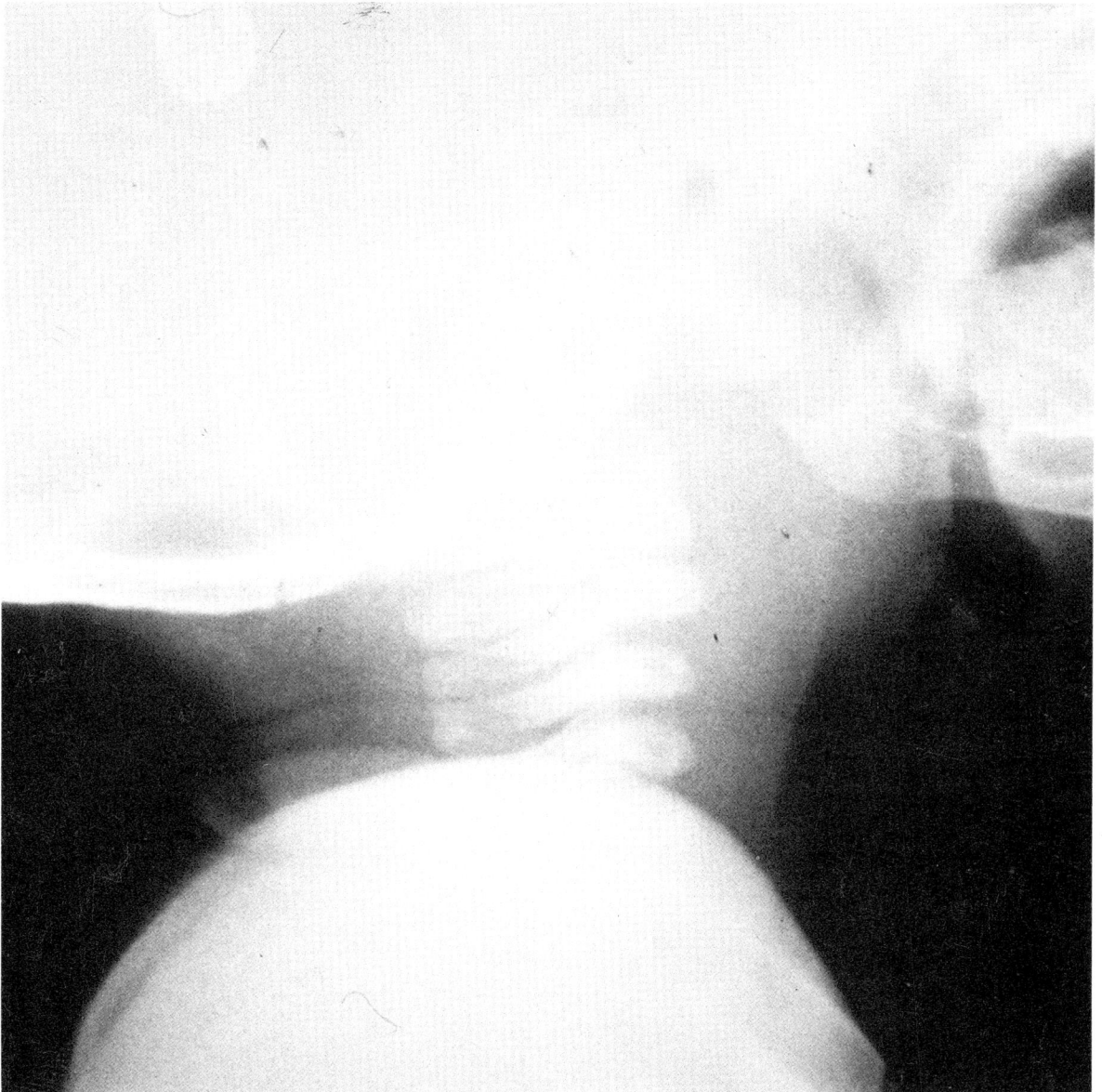

This child presented to casualty following a recent respiratory tract infection. Over the last few hours he had become pyrexial, was unable to drink and was having difficulty breathing. He was holding his head down, drooling saliva and was noted to have stridor. A lateral neck X-ray was taken.

- What is the diagnosis?
- Why would you question such a diagnosis in an 8 year old child?
- What treatment may be required?
- What are the other causes of acute inspiratory stridor in childhood?

A1

The child has a retropharyngeal abscess, which is seen radiologically as an anterior displacement of the pharynx, larynx and trachea. The normal space between the trachea and cervical spine is one vertebral body and an increase in this may be pathological. However, if the radiograph is taken in expiration an apparent increase in this space may be seen which disappears on inspiratory films.

Retropharyngeal abscesses occur in infancy and are caused by suppuration in the lymph glands of Litre. These lie on the prevertebral fascia and gradually disappear during the third year. A staphylococcal or streptococcal organism is usually responsible for the infection.

Treatment involves drainage of the abscess under anaesthesia using an endotracheal tube and packing the hypopharynx. Antibiotics are indicated. The child will feel remarkably better by the following day.

Other causes of acute inspiratory stridor in childhood include:
— croup
— epiglottitis
— acute pseudomembranous croup
— diphtheria
— foreign body
— upper airway burns
— angioneurotic oedema.

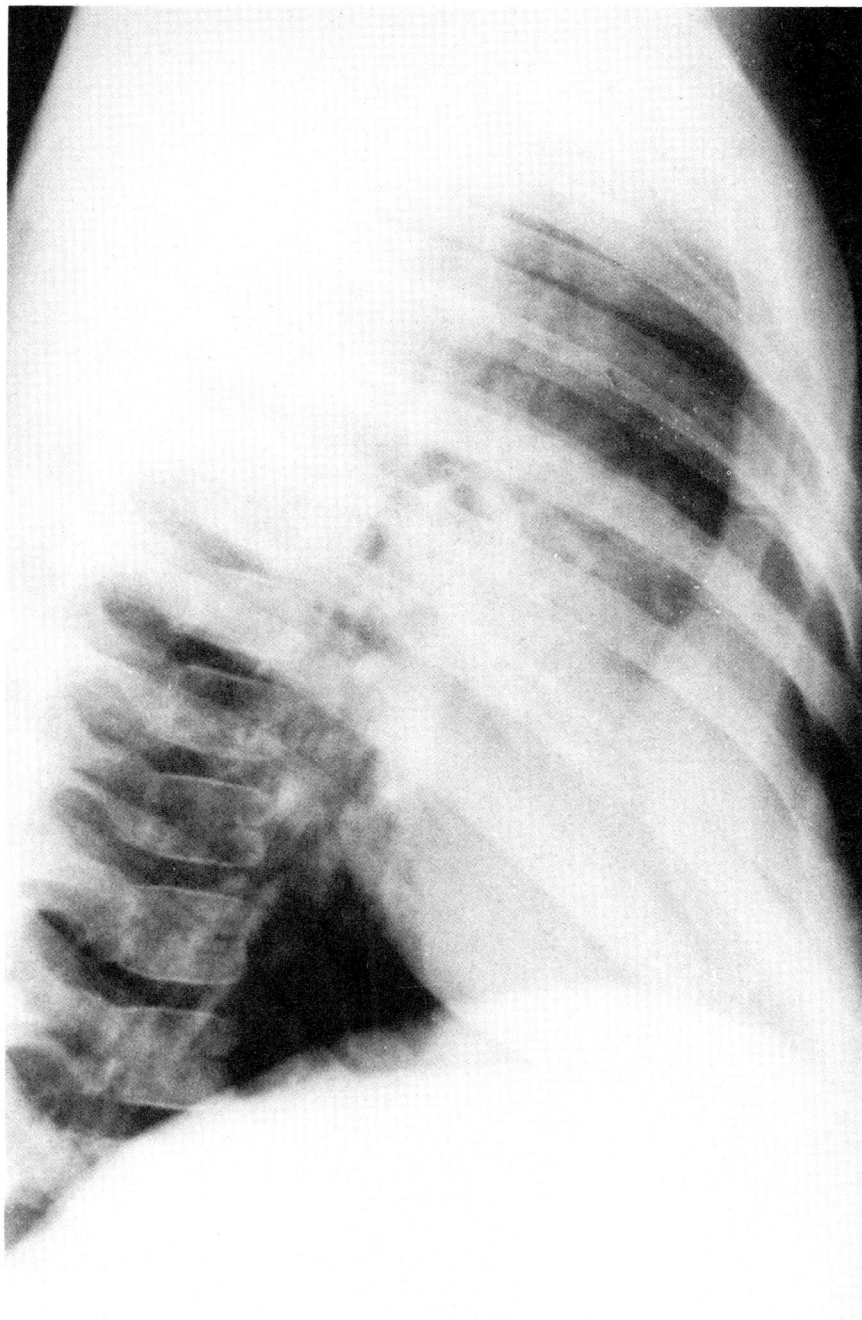

This is the chest X-ray of a young boy.

- What abnormality is seen?
- How may this alter the appearance of the AP chest X-ray?
- Is this abnormality usually acquired?

A2

There is marked sternal depression.

Sternal depression may flatten the heart, displace it to the left and elevate the apex (Film B).

Sternal depression (pectus excavatum) is usually congenital.

Although the deformity has been considered a cosmetic problem, many patients report symptoms that improve after its repair. Recent studies have shown a physiological basis for this improvement. Maximum voluntary ventilation and exercise tolerance improve post-operatively and right and left ventricular volume increase suggesting release of cardiac compression. In a substantial number of patients regional ventilatory and perfusion deficits, primarily of the lower left lung, become normal after surgery.

Film C shows contiguous transectional sections of an infant with pectus excavatum. The heart has been pushed into the left side of the thorax by the deformity. These photographs have been taken by a new form of nuclear magnetic resonance, developed in Nottingham, called Echo-Planar Imaging (EPI). The EPI procedure requires no gating since each image is a snapshot acquired within 32ms. Therefore, each image is relatively free from motion artefact due to either cardiac or respiratory movement and studies require no sedation. It follows that EPI may be used to advantage in children who have high heart and respiratory rates. 'Movie' loops may be constructed to view slices showing patterns of blood flow. Blood at standstill gives a relatively high signal and appears bright. Blood moving out of the plane of the study yields little signal and appears black. Additionally, constructions in the sagittal, coronal or any other plane may be made and transformed into a 'movie'.

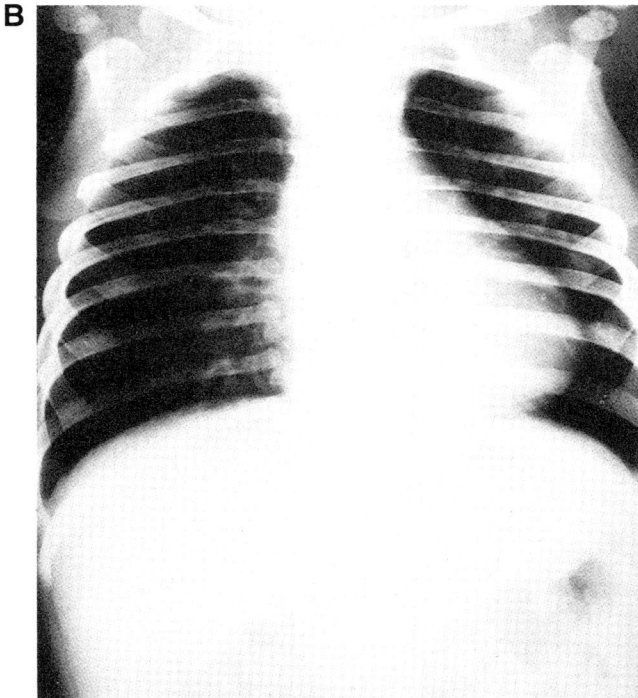

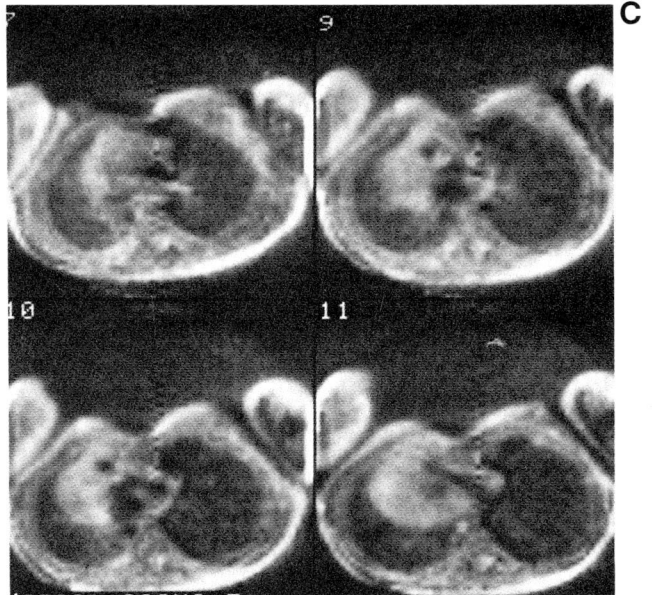

The junior house physician was concerned about a strange central translucent area on this chest X-ray (arrowed).

• What is the cause?

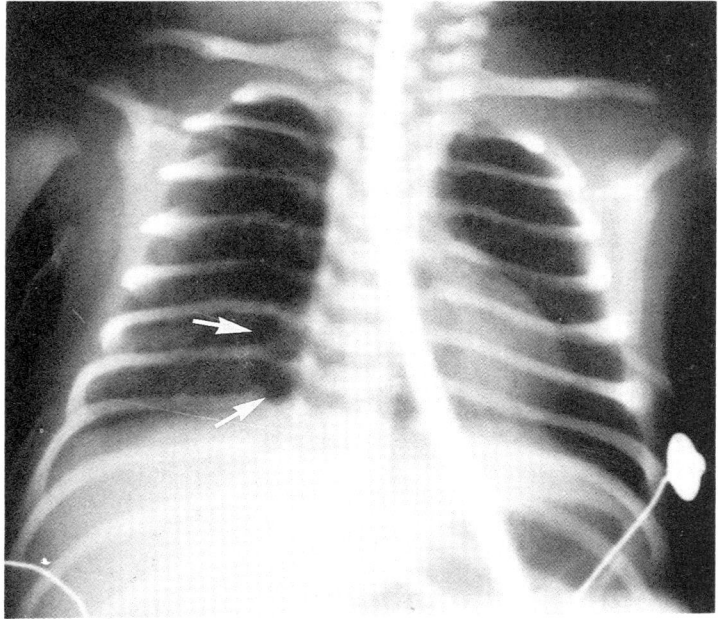

Q4

This is the chest X-ray of a healthy 12 year old girl.

• What would you find on clinical examination?

• What other radiological abnormalities may be present in this condition?

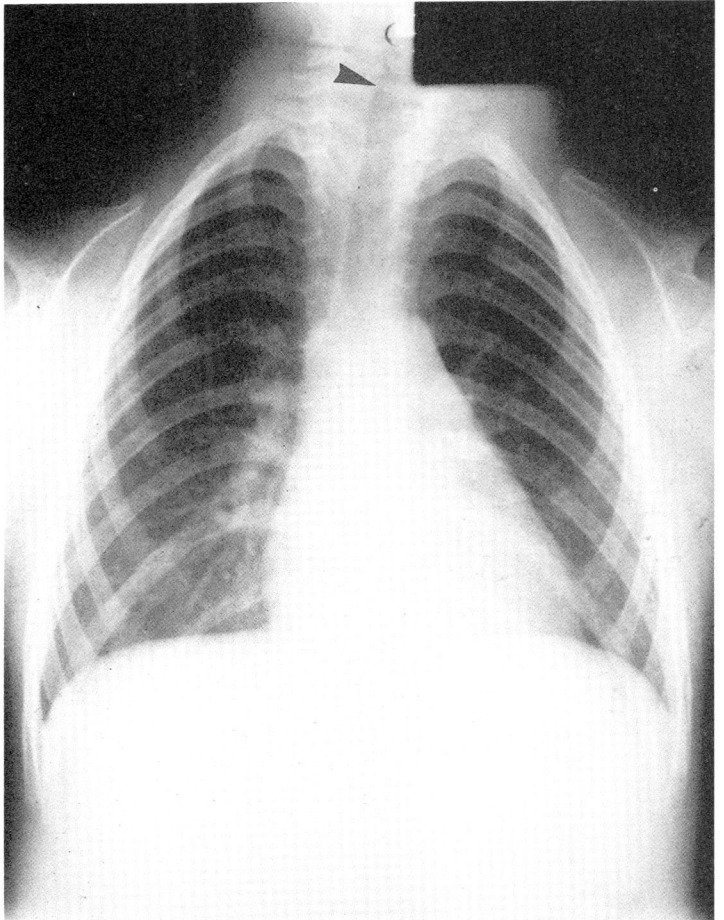

A3

It is due to the porthole in the top of the incubator.

A4

The girl has cleidocranial dysostosis. In this case her clavicles are absent, resulting in hypermobile shoulders that can be folded across the chest. The thorax is usually narrow with short ribs directed obliquely downwards. The X-ray also shows failure of fusion of the neural arches (arrowed) which is best seen at the cervical/thoracic junction.

These children tend to be small and may have a hypoplastic maxilla, hypertelorism, a high arched palate and malocclusion.

The fontanelles, if present, are often wide and wormian bones are frequently seen on skull radiographs. In the newborn mineralization of the skull may be delayed.

There is defective ossification of the symphysis pubis and this is a constant feature of this disorder. Congenital coxa vara, and elongation of the second metacarpals may occur.

Intelligence is normal. Inheritance is autosomal dominant.

This neonate presented with respiratory distress.

- What is the diagnosis?
- How do children with this condition present in the neonatal period?

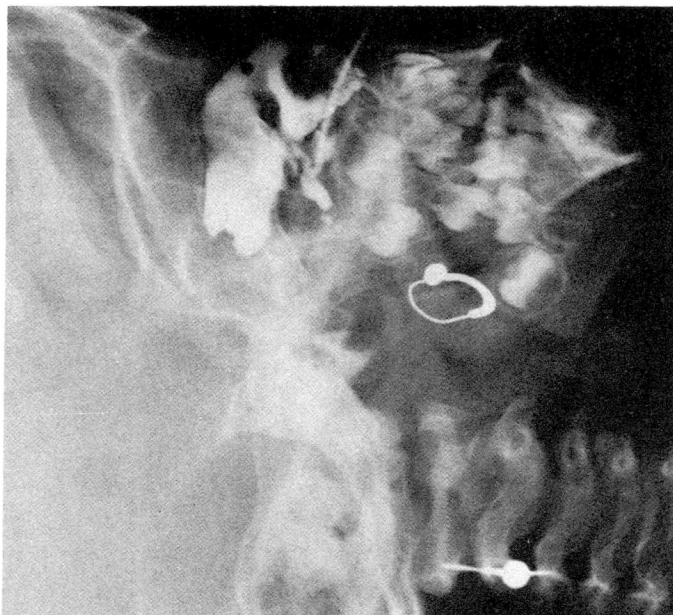

Q6

This child suffered from a persistent inspiratory and expiratory wheeze.

- What is your diagnosis?
- Name several other causes of recurrent or persistent wheezing in childhood

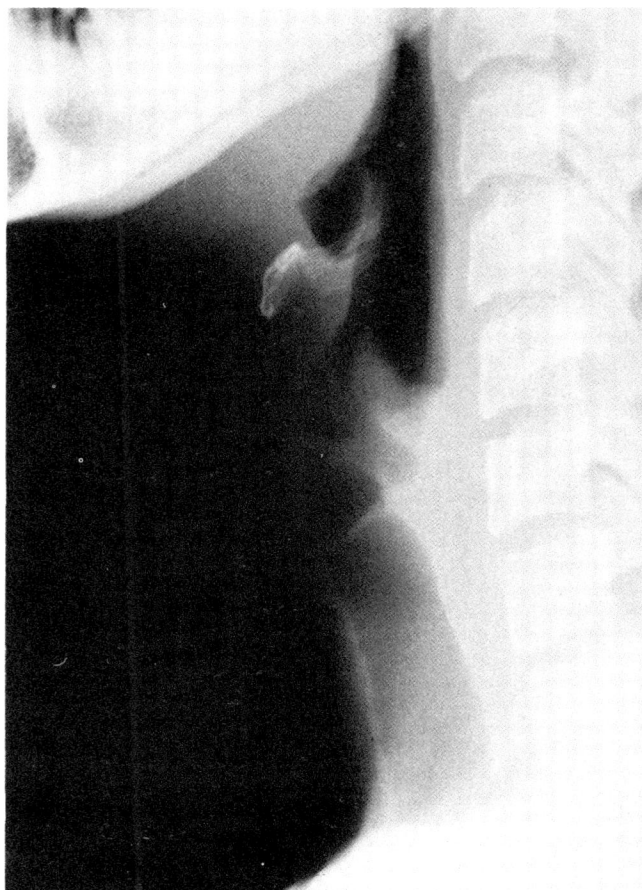

A5

This child has choanal atresia. It has been demonstrated by the hold-up of contrast medium in the nasal cavity while lying supine. Obstructions may be unilateral or bilateral and may be membranous or bony.

Until recently it was widely thought that neonatal patients were compulsive nose-breathers. If this was the case babies with bilateral choanal atresia would asphyxiate. Indeed a history of cyanosis which disappears on crying may be obtained. However, some infants can breathe through the mouth at birth. Choanal atresia has been diagnosed in patients beyond the neonatal period and as late as 6 years of age. A study has been conducted in which the nares of infants, shortly after birth and at 6 weeks of age, were occluded for a maximum of 25 seconds. In 3% of new-borns, there was no attempt to initiate oral respiration following nasal occlusion, whereas 10% struggled against the occlusion but could not achieve oral air flow within 25 seconds. All others breathed through the mouth. Surprisingly, in the 6 week group, more than 20% of infants were unable to get air to flow through the mouth within 25 seconds of acute nasal occlusion. These results and those of others indicate that many infants are not obligate nasal breathers.

Unilateral obstruction may cause breathing difficulty if the patent side is compressed. This may be missed for many years and the problem discovered at a later date because of a unilateral nasal discharge. Inheritance appears to be multi-factorial and the risk to siblings should be less than 5%. Rarely associated congenital defects may include Treacher Collins syndrome, palatal abnormalities, colobomas, tracheo-oesophageal fistulas and congenital heart disease.

A6

The child has a tracheal web. Tracheal webs and tracheal stenosis usually produce inspiratory and expiratory wheeze. Webs may occur at any site in the trachea and are very rare. Stridor has its aetiology in the large airways from the glottis to the main bronchi. Intra-thoracic obstruction is usually responsible for the combination of inspiratory stridor and expiratory wheeze.

Recurrent or persistent wheezing may be caused by obstructive lesions in the trachea or main bronchus such as:
— foreign body in the trachea, bronchus or oesophagus
— vascular rings
— tuberculous lymph glands
— mediastinal cysts and tumours
— tracheomalacia
— tracheal webs, stenosis and bronchial stenosis.

Obstructive disease of the small airways may also be responsible for wheeze:
— asthma
— aspiration
— cystic fibrosis
— bronchomalacia
— obliterative bronchiolitis
— alpha-1-antitrypsin deficiency.

This child presented with general malaise. This is his chest X-ray.

- What is the diagnosis?
- What may you find on fundo-scopy that will confirm your diagnosis?
- If the patient had a predominant cough what would you suspect?

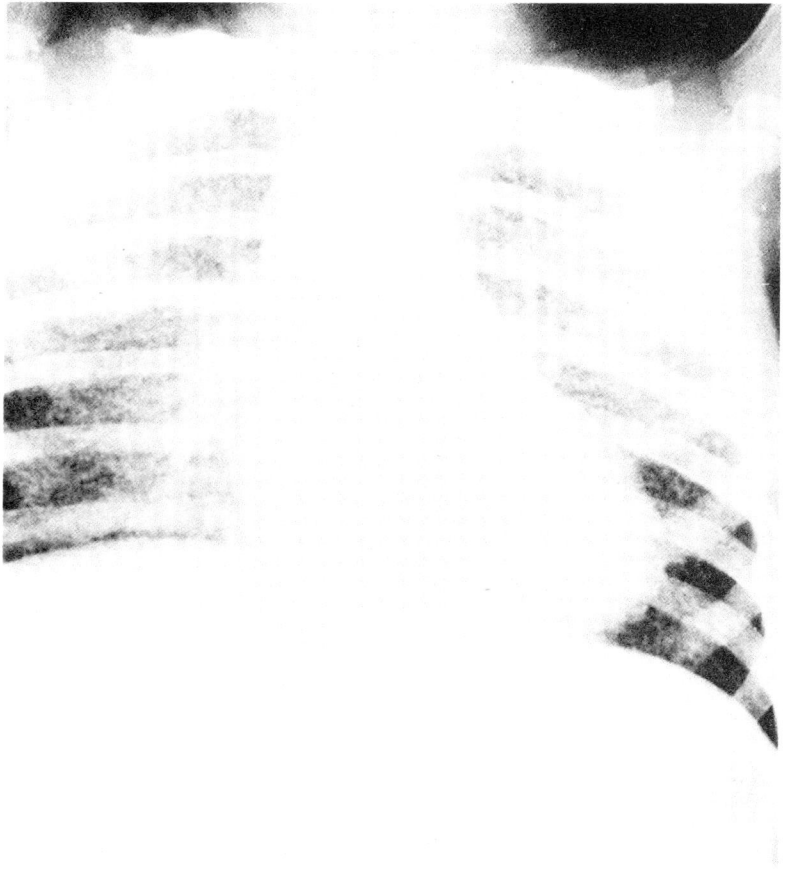

Q8

This child was asymptomatic at the time of his chest X-ray.

- What is the differential diagnosis in a patient with this radiological feature?
- What may occur at birth and produce a similar appearance?

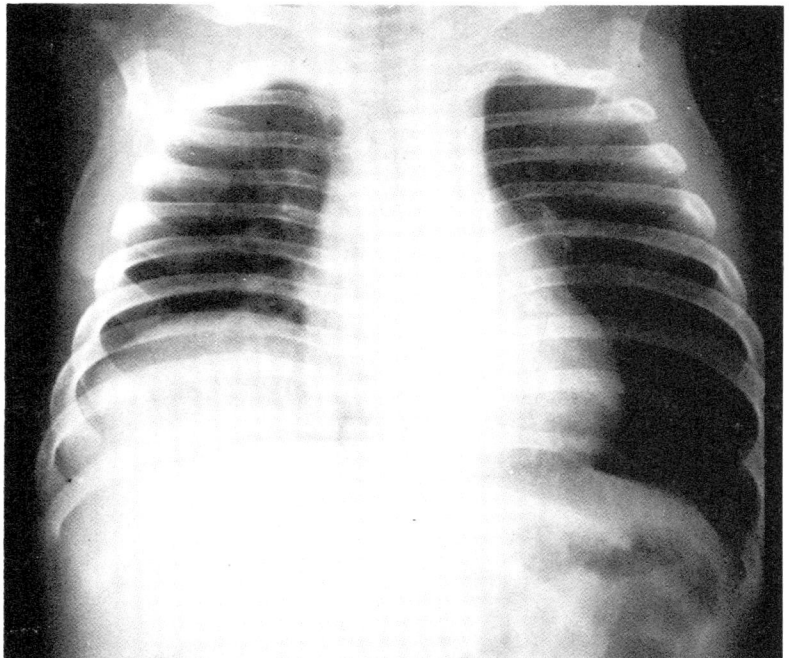

A7

The chest X-ray shows a diffuse fine mottling throughout both lung fields characteristic of miliary tuberculosis.

Fundoscopy along the vessels close to the optic disc may reveal yellow choroidal tubercles. These are diagnostic.

Chest signs are frequently absent until the disease is extensive when crepitations throughout the lung fields may be heard. A cough suggests enlarged nodes are present, causing bronchial compression.

A8

This patient has an eventration of his right diaphragm.

This is due to hypoplasia or atrophy of the diaphragm resulting in an upward displacement of contents on the poorly developed side. It is more common on the left side. Symptoms are often delayed until late childhood compared to the earlier problems encountered with diaphragmatic herniae.

The differential diagnosis of unilateral elevation of the diaphragm includes:
— Paralysis due to various causes including surgery and trauma, infection, tuberculous glands and neoplasms.
— Congenital eventration and humps.
— Subpulmonary effusions.
— Lower lobe collapse, pulmonary hypoplasia or pulmonary embolus.
— Scoliosis and rib fractures.
— Subphrenic abscess, hepatomegaly, splenomegaly, or an abdominal mass.

Brachial plexus trauma at the time of delivery may cause diaphragmatic palsy with similar radiological features.

This 12 year old girl suddenly became dyspnoeic again.

- Describe the chest X-ray.
- What is the likely diagnosis?

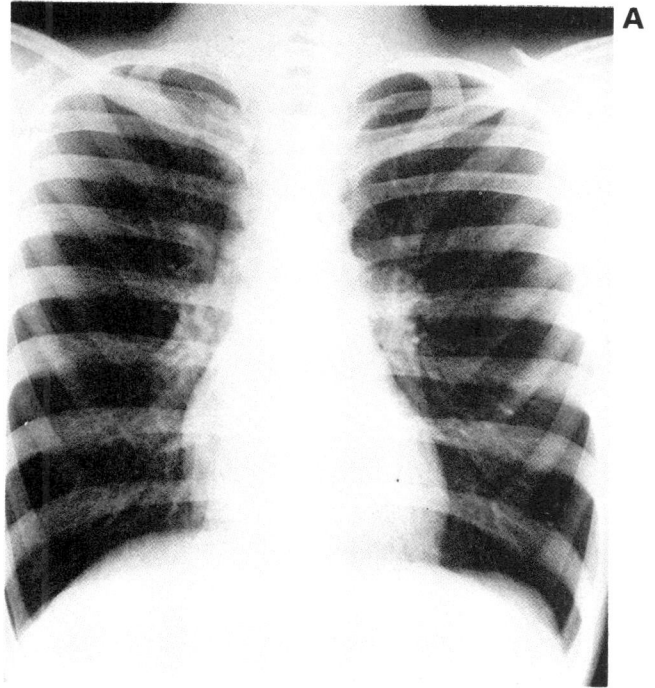

A

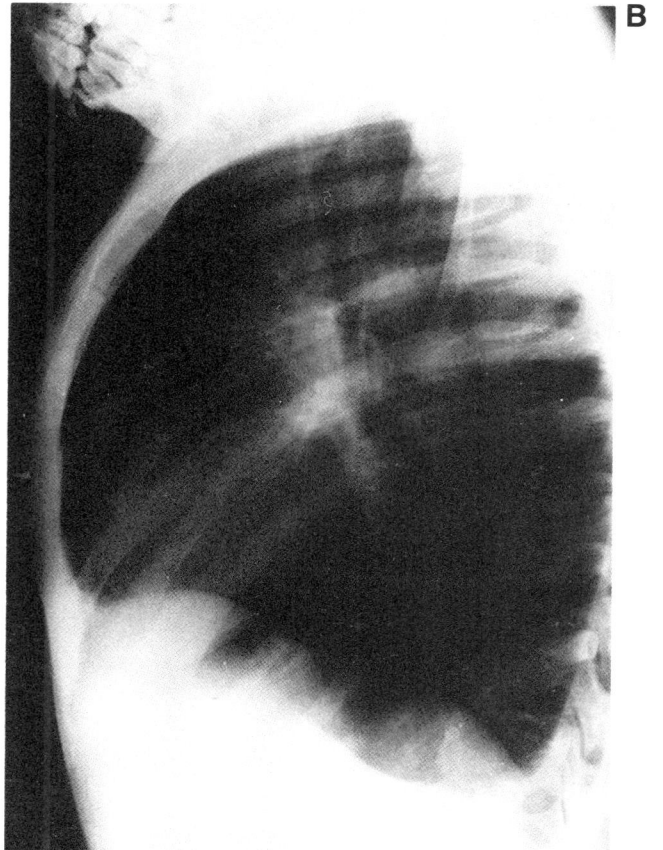

B

A9

The girl is suffering from an asthma attack. This is the typical appearance with over-inflated lungs and clearly visible vascular markings at the hila. Note the flattened diaphragm, elevated ribs and markedly increased antero-posterior diameter of the chest on the lateral film.

An asthmatic attack is the commonest cause of a small cardiac shadow.

A chest X-ray is not essential in every child with asthma. It is advisable in children with frequent or persistent wheeze and may exclude other causes of airway obstruction.

Q10

A

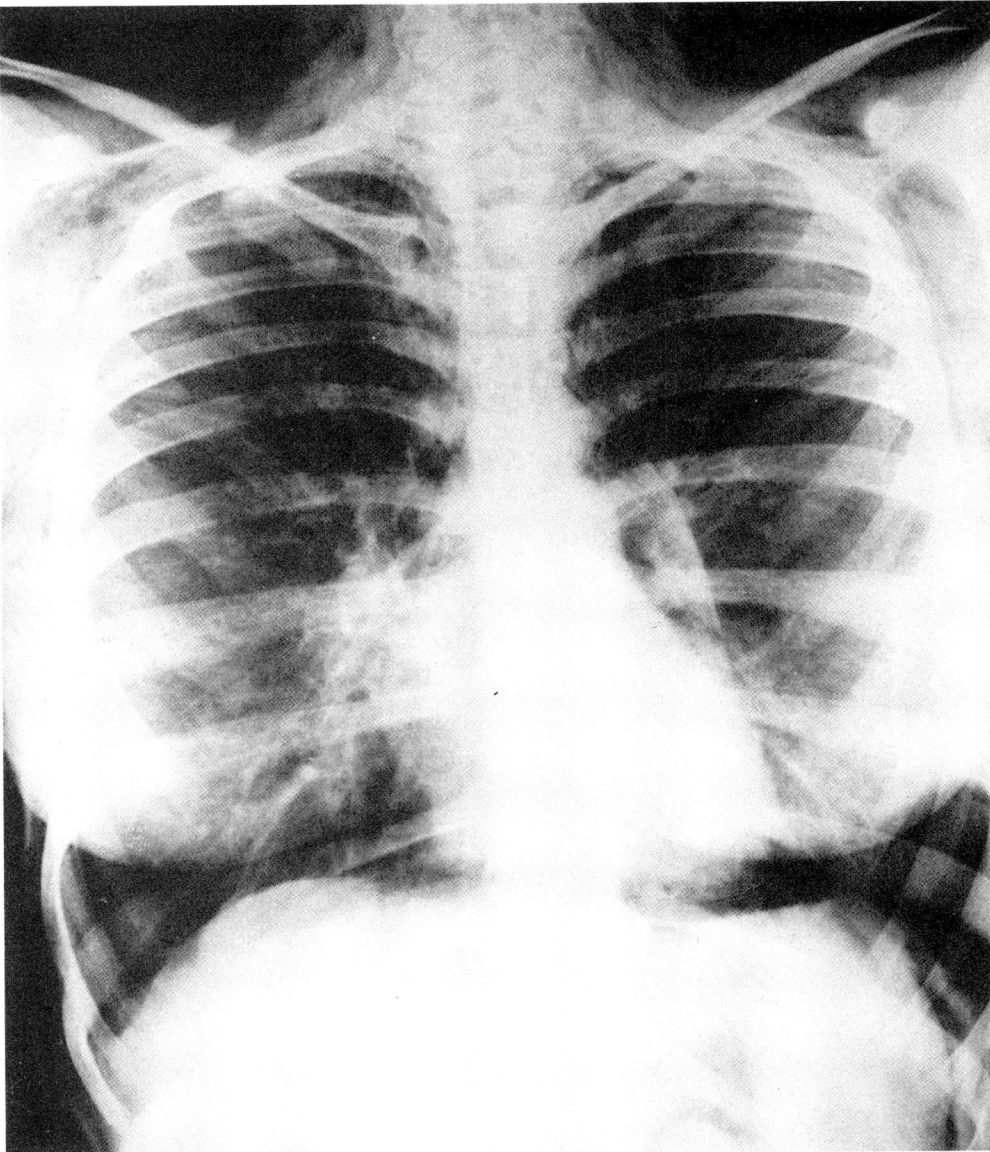

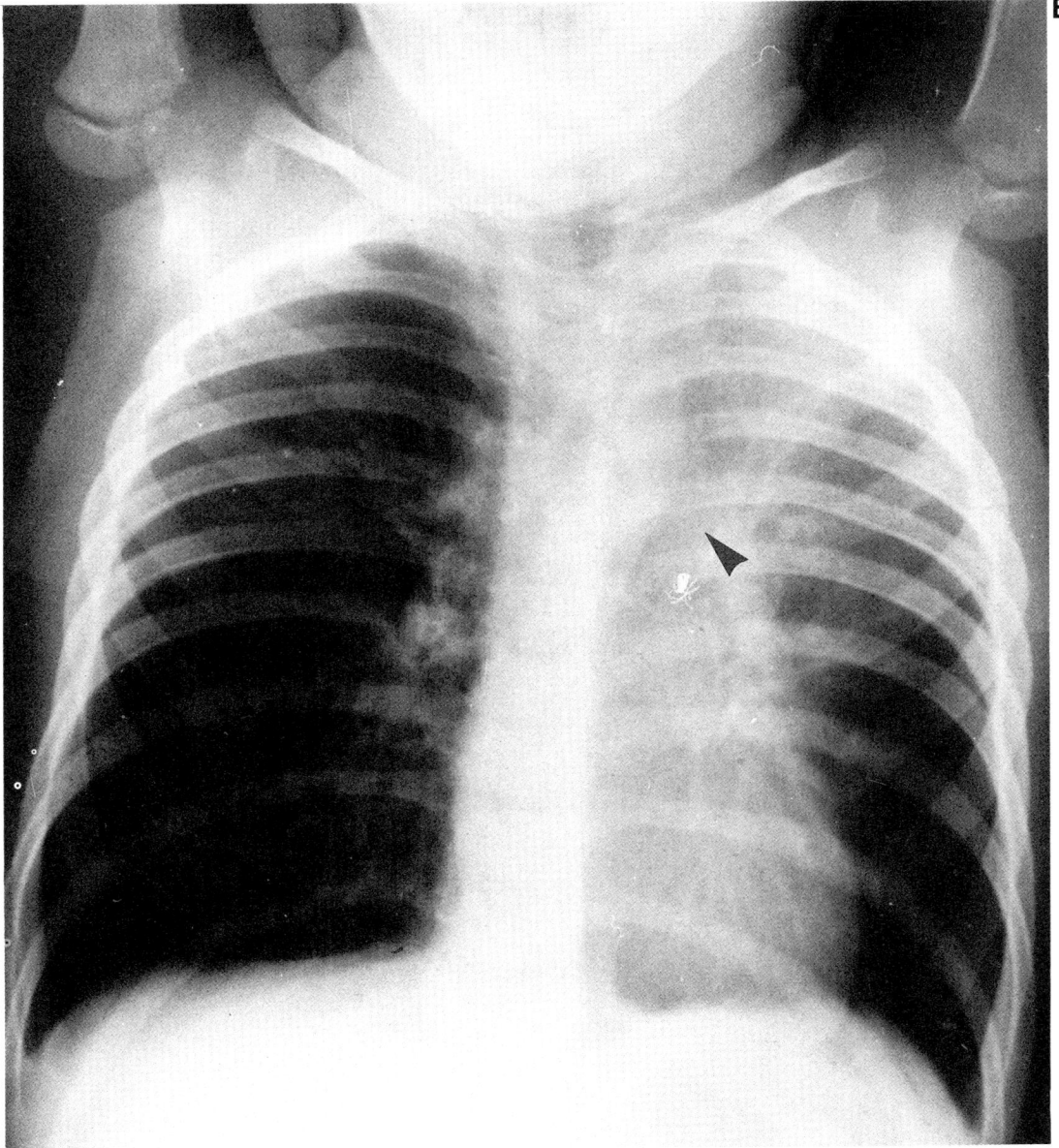

Film A is of an asthmatic patient.

- Describe the radiological features seen on this chest X-ray.
- What will clinical examination reveal?
- What treatment is required?
- Film B is also of an asthmatic child. Describe the radiological features seen in the left upper zone (arrowed).

A10

A pneumomediastinum is seen in film A. The chest X-ray shows extensive linear translucencies due to air tracking along the mediastinal borders and into the soft tissues of the neck and chest wall.

Breast shadows can be seen. The child is hyper-inflated with flattening of the diaphragm due to an asthmatic attack which was responsible for her pneumomediastinum.

The presence of gas tracking through the tissues is called surgical emphysema and it may be detected clinically as crepitus on palpation if it has reached the neck and chest wall.

Treatment is that of the underlying asthmatic attack. The emphysema is gradually absorbed.

Film B shows collapse of the left upper lobe. Note the deviation of the trachea to the left. The air seen to the left of the aortic arch is within the left lower lobe (arrowed), which has expanded to fill the gap.

Film C shows another complication of asthma. The left lung has collapsed during an asthmatic attack due to a large mucous plug. Following intubation, suction, removal of a mucous plug and anti-asthma therapy full re-expansion of the left lung occurred. In acute asthma collapse of a lung is exceptional but collapse of a lung lobe is common and often transient.

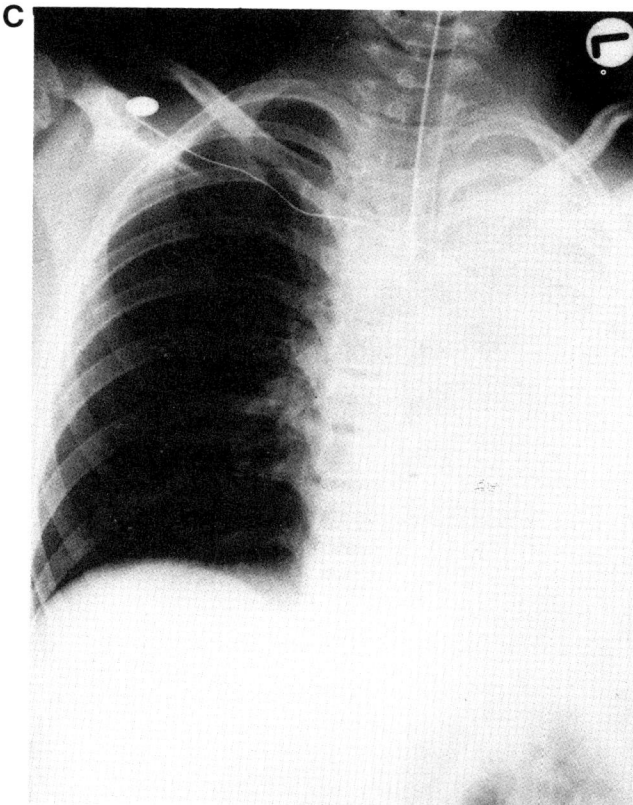

C

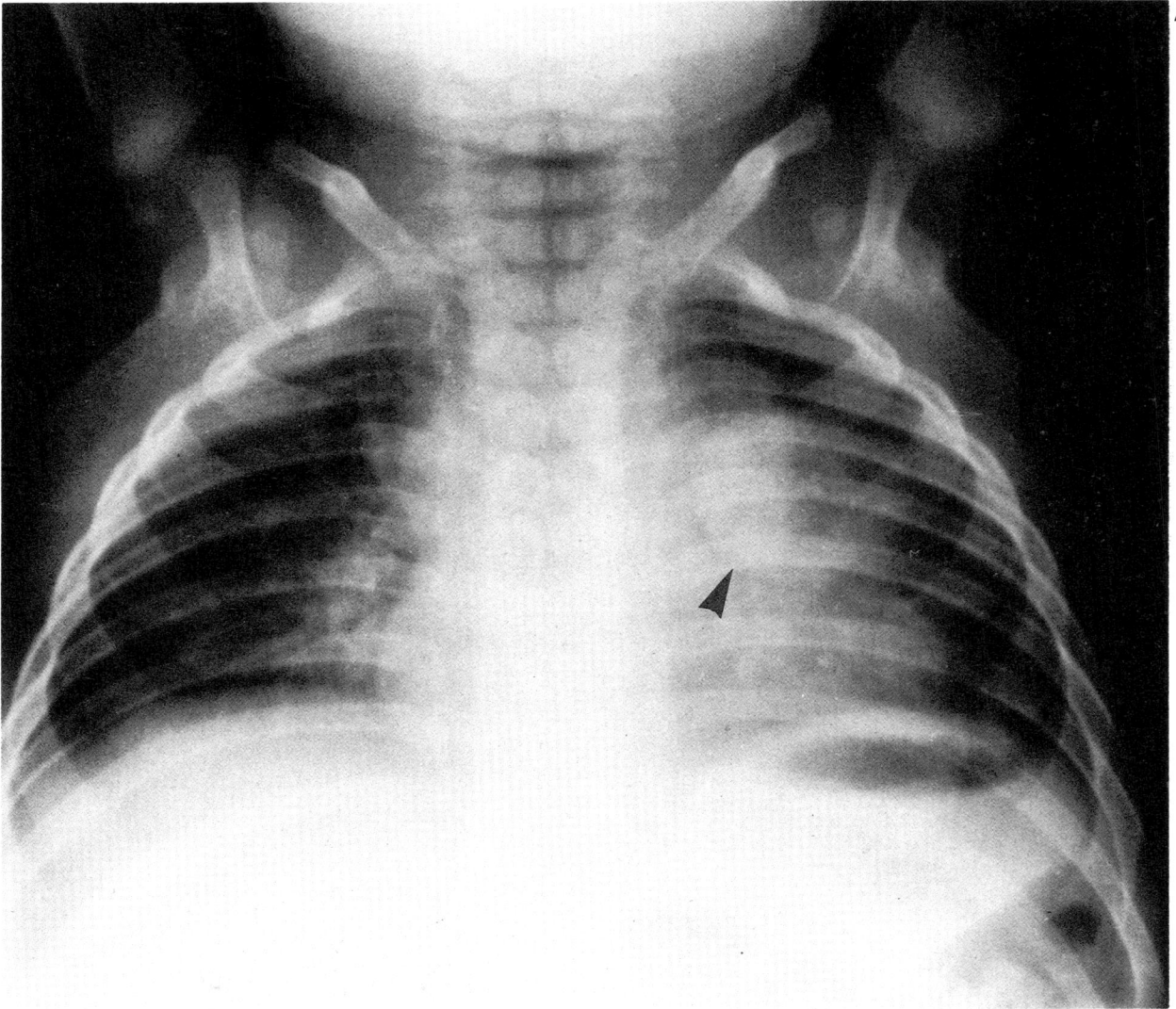

One of the doctors is concerned about the circular lesion in the left lung field seen on the chest X-ray of this patient (arrowed).

- What might you find on clinical examination?

A11

Examination of the patient revealed a large firm nodule on the patient's back. This is clearly demonstrated on the lateral chest X-ray. Nipple shadows may also cause confusion. Lesions that are extremely well defined on AP chest films should lead one to suspect an extra-pulmonary cause.

B

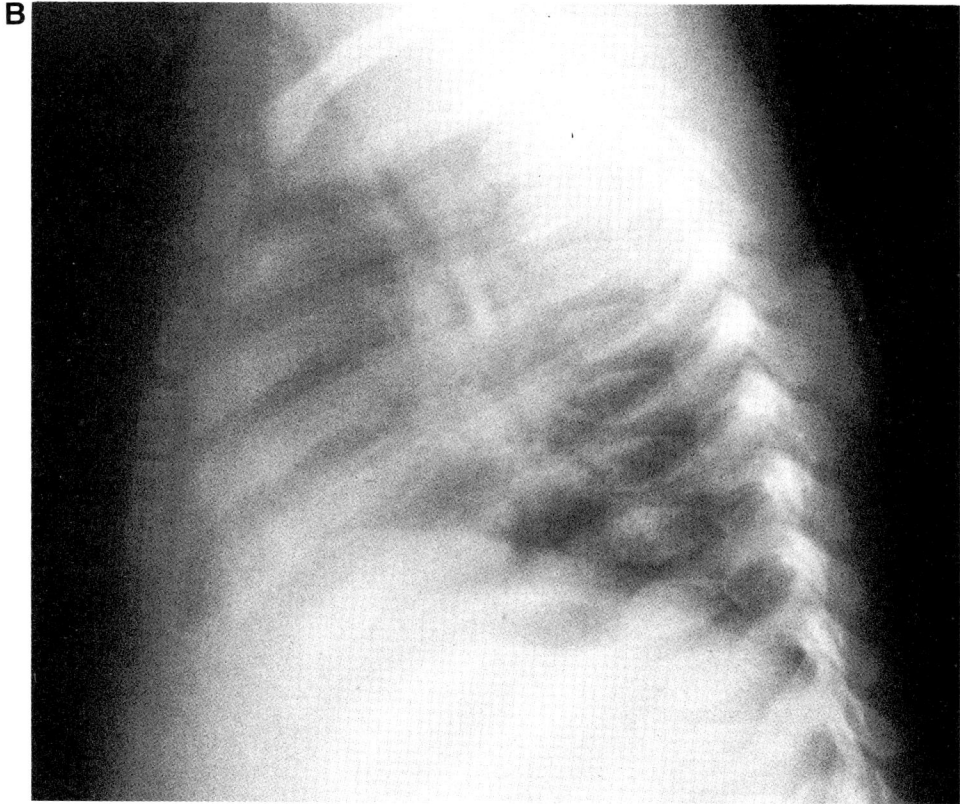

Eighteen months previously this child developed a frequent cough. Symptoms had become worse over the past 4 months with breathlessness and occasional fever. Ten months ago the child had iron deficiency anaemia which responded to oral iron. The anaemia recurred following withdrawal of iron therapy, it seemed. His Mantoux test was negative. His most recent chest films are shown.

- What is the likely diagnosis?
- Examination of macrophages from a tracheal aspirate confirmed the diagnosis. What was found?

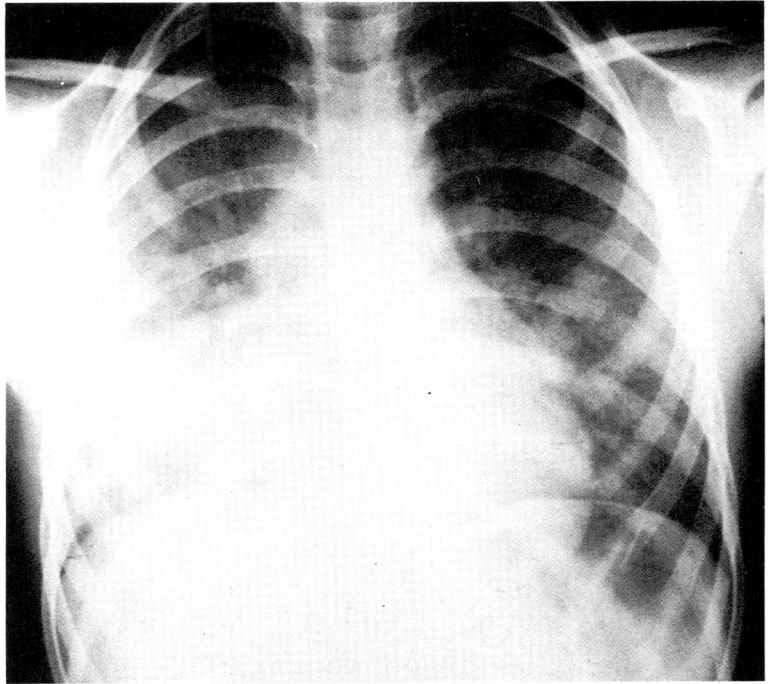

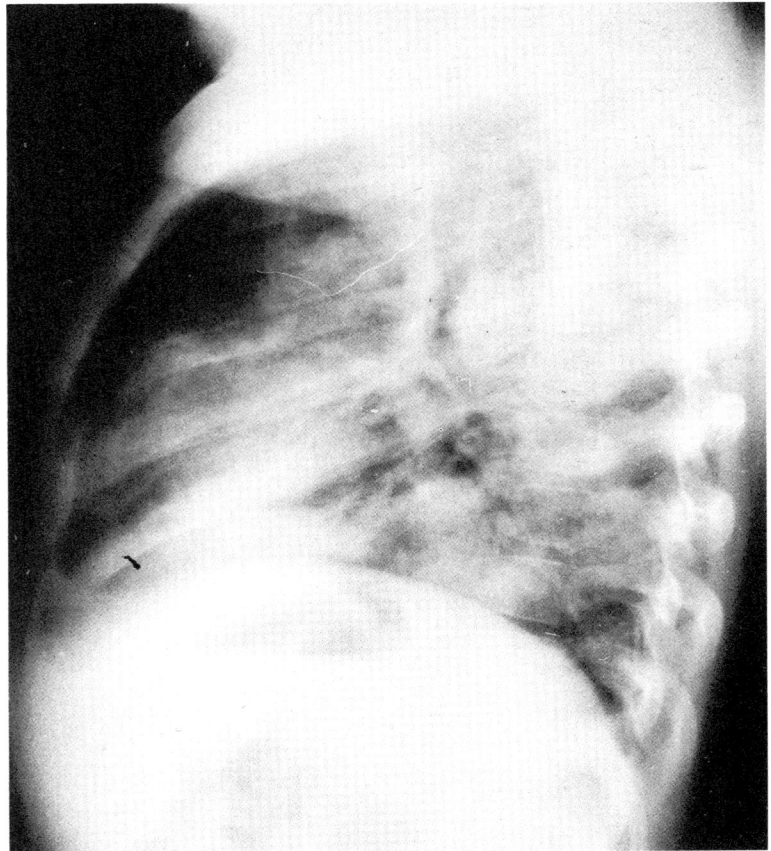

A12

The child is suffering from idiopathic pulmonary haemosiderosis which is characterized by recurrent intra-alveolar haemorrhage. This results in deposition of haemosiderin in the lung tissue and iron deficiency anaemia. It is an uncommon disease most commonly beginning in infancy and childhood.

The finding of haemosiderin-laden macrophages in sputum, tracheal aspirate, or gastric aspirate helps to confirm the diagnosis.

In the earlier stage the chest X-ray typically shows soft fluffy and mottled shadows in the lung. Diffuse speckling in the more peripheral portions of the lung field may occur later and may be mistaken for miliary tuberculosis on a radiograph.

Approximately 50% of patients die within 5 years, usually due to massive pulmonary haemorrhage producing respiratory failure. Other patients appear to go into complete remission, though radiological changes persist. Some develop cor pulmonale.

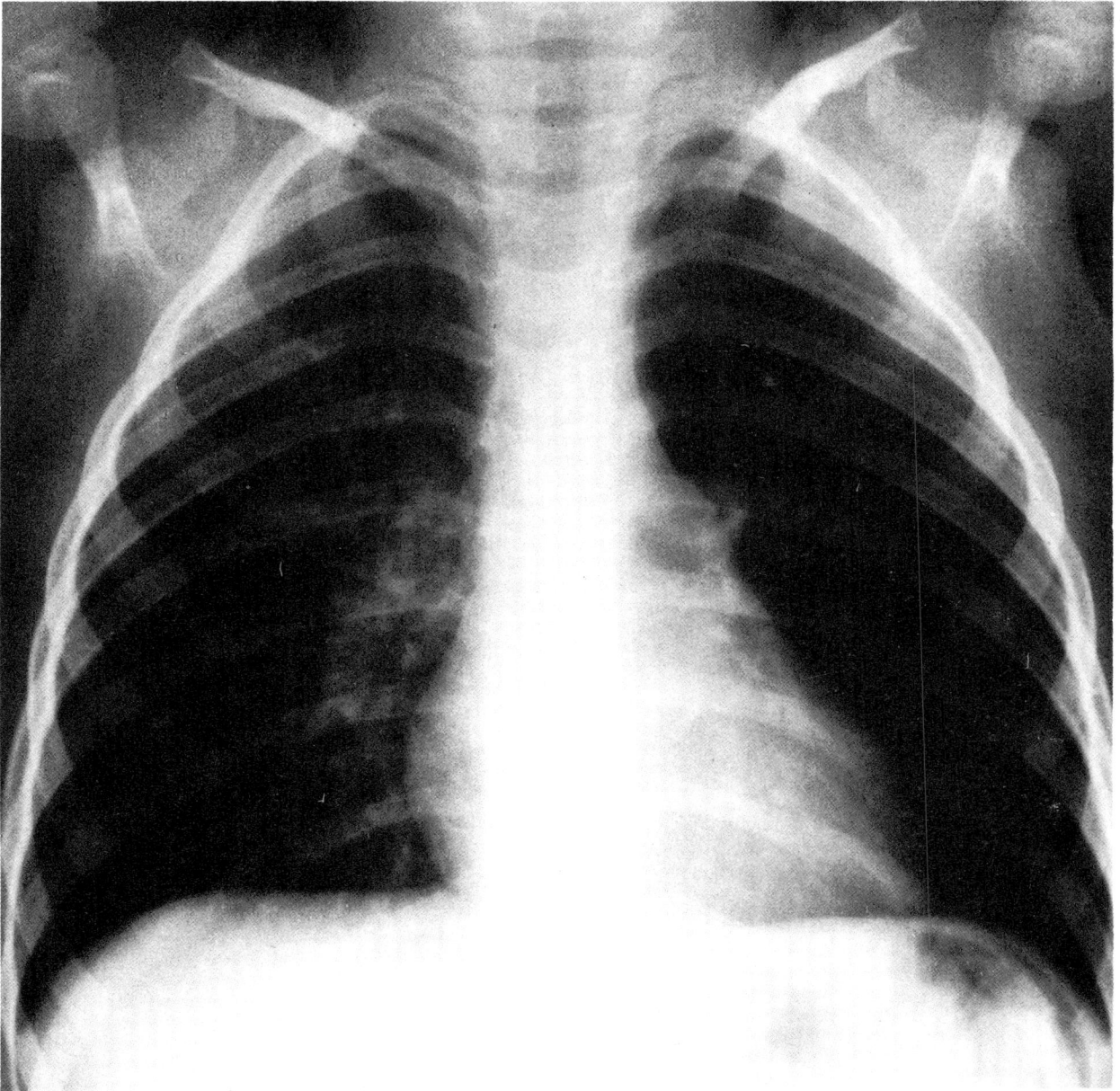

This young boy presented to casualty with sudden onset of wheeze and cough. There was no history of asthma. On auscultation wheeze was heard over the left side of his chest.

- What is your diagnosis on this film taken in full inspiration?

- How would you confirm this?

A13

The story and clinical findings are suggestive of an intra-bronchial foreign body and this should be the provisional diagnosis until proved otherwise. This film has been taken on inspiration and shows hyperinflation with flattening of the diaphragm. The diagnosis was confirmed by a film taken on expiration (Film B) demonstrating air trapping on the left side due to a peanut in the left main bronchus.

The majority of foreign bodies are not radio-opaque. Bronchial obstruction is usually suggested by hyperinflation, collapse and con-solidation, or any combination of these. Films taken on full inspiration and full expiration are essential to demonstrate the effect of ball valve obstruction. Normal radiological examination does not exclude a foreign body, for example a flat seed or a bead with a hole in it may not cause complete bronchial obstruction. Radiological fluoroscopy of the diaphragm and chest may be necessary in young children when inspiratory and expiratory films are difficult to obtain. Bronchoscopy is usually required to remove the foreign body.

Delay in diagnosis is not uncommon and is usually due to medical staff not being aware that the child's respiratory symptoms could be due to inhalation of a foreign body. The patterns of illness in patients with delayed diagnosis include:
— cough, wheeze and sometimes fever
— failed resolution of an acute respiratory infection
— chronic cough and haemoptysis
— chronic cough and lung collapse
— respiratory failure.

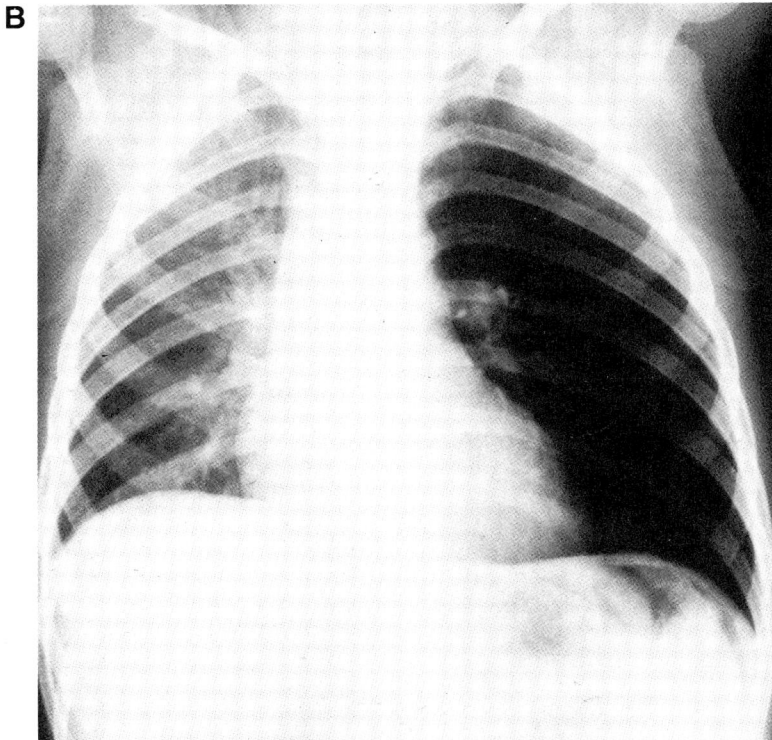

B

This is the chest X-ray of a very ill neonatal patient.

- What are the diagnoses?
- What immediate management is required?

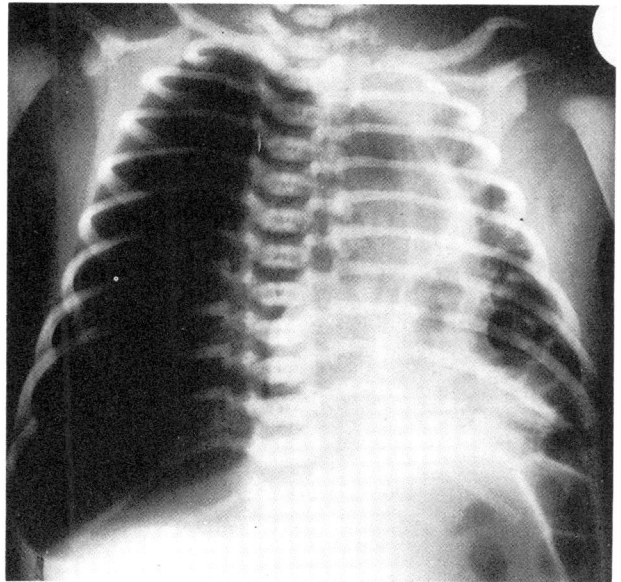

Q15

- What examination is being performed in this young child with recurrent chest infections and intolerance of fizzy cold drinks?
- What is the diagnosis?
- What method is available to make the diagnosis in a ward setting?

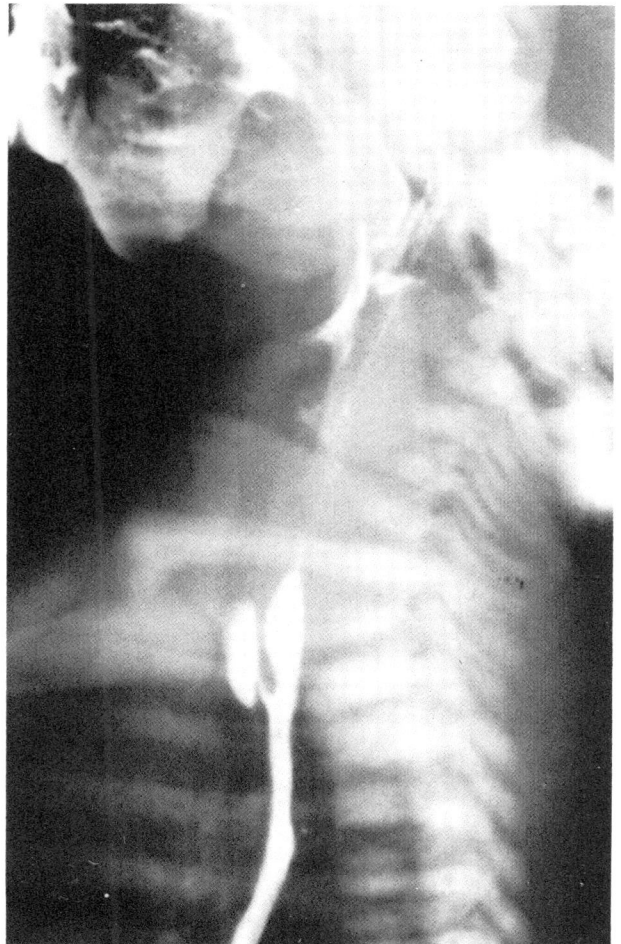

A14

This boy was born with a diaphragmatic hernia. Loops of bowel are seen in the left side of the chest. Coincidentally, he has developed a right sided tension pneumothorax. There are no lung markings on this side and the mediastinum has been pushed to the left.

A needle placed in the right side of the chest relieved the tension and a chest drain was inserted.

The patient died before surgical repair was attempted.

It is important to include the abdomen on the chest X-ray of patients suspected of having a diaphragmatic hernia so that bowel can be assessed. A cystic adenomatoid malformation of the lung or staphylococcal aerocoeles may resemble bowel loops in the chest.

A15

The child has a rare type of tracheo-oesophageal fistula (H-type) which runs obliquely upwards from the oesophagus to the trachea and is commonly situated high in the oesophagus. In this case bronchographic contrast medium has been injected through a fine catheter placed in the oesophagus and demonstrates the fistula. Poor oesophageal peristalsis is usually seen and may provide a clue to the existence of a fistula when the tract fails to fill with contrast medium. Patients are studied prone under continuous fluoroscopic control. Tracheoscopy should reveal the fistula. Following repair patients may suffer from a persistent cough (TOF cough) due to tracheomalacia.

On the ward a firm catheter may be passed down the oesophagus with the other end immersed in water. As the fistula is approached air passing through the fistula into the oesophagus will be seen to bubble out of the catheter. Although rare it is important to be mindful of tracheo-oesophageal fistula as an isolated finding.

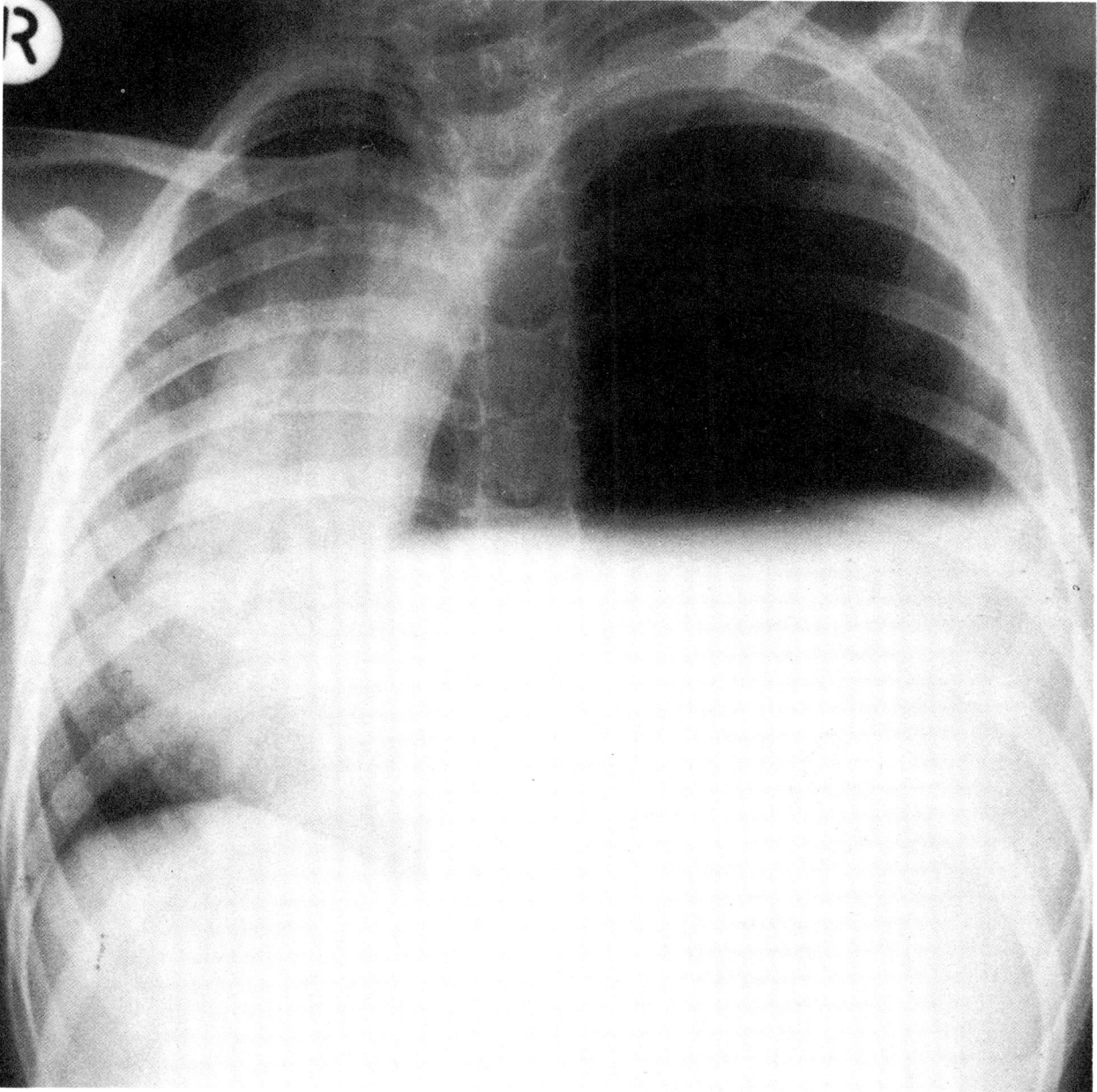

This child presented in casualty following a road traffic accident. She was suffering from surprisingly little respiratory distress.

- What does the X-ray show?
- The resident doctor made the diagnosis of a pneumothorax and inserted a chest drain. How would you have managed this patient?

A16

The casualty officer attending this patient thought that the X-ray showed a pneumothorax, and inserted a chest drain. However, on this film, gas does not reach the apex of the pleural cavity. Film B shows that contrast medium injected through a nasogastric tube defines the stomach. The cause is a traumatic diaphragmatic hernia in the thorax.

Decompression via the nasogastric tube and ventilation were required prior to successful repair of the diaphragm.

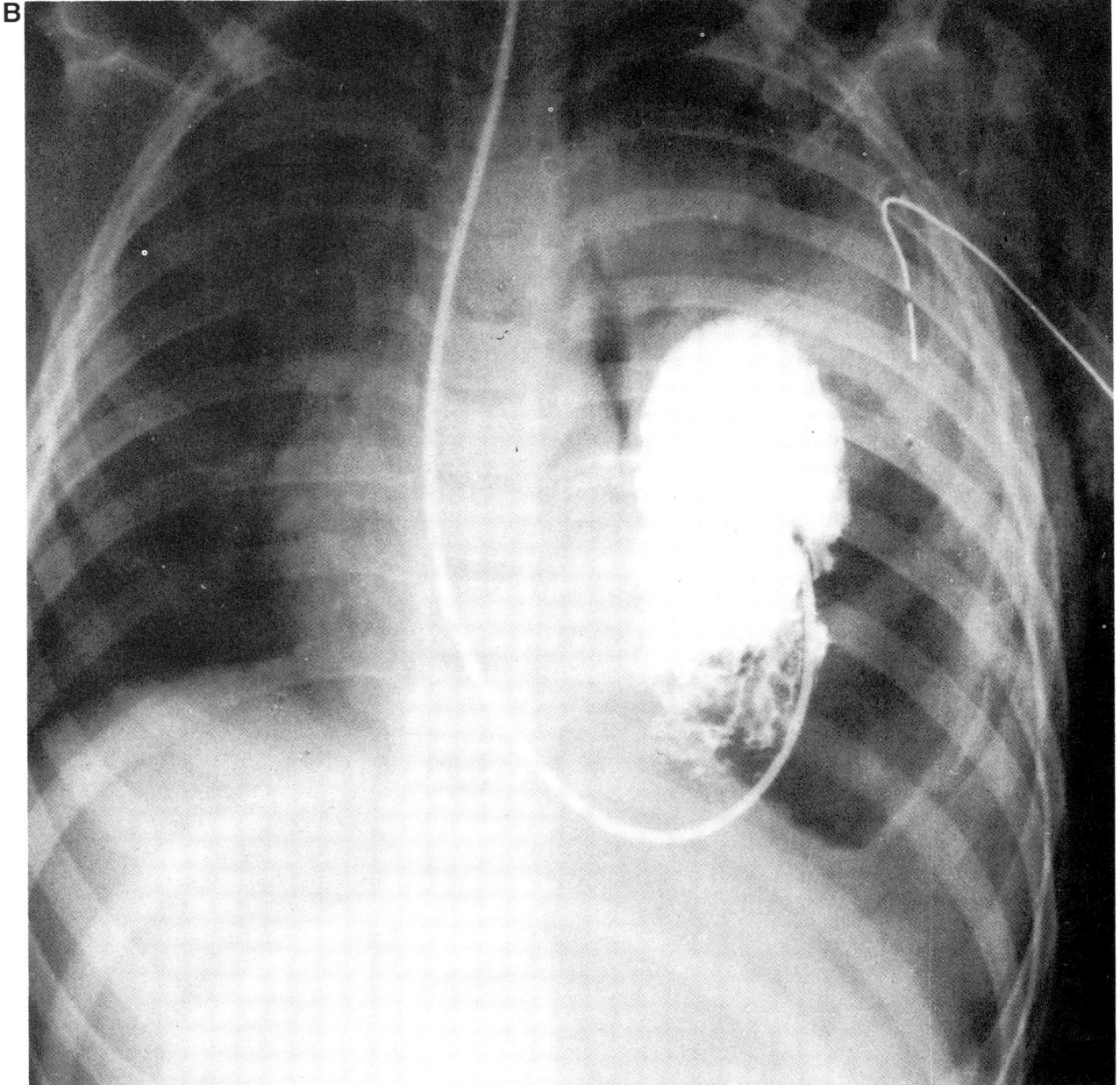

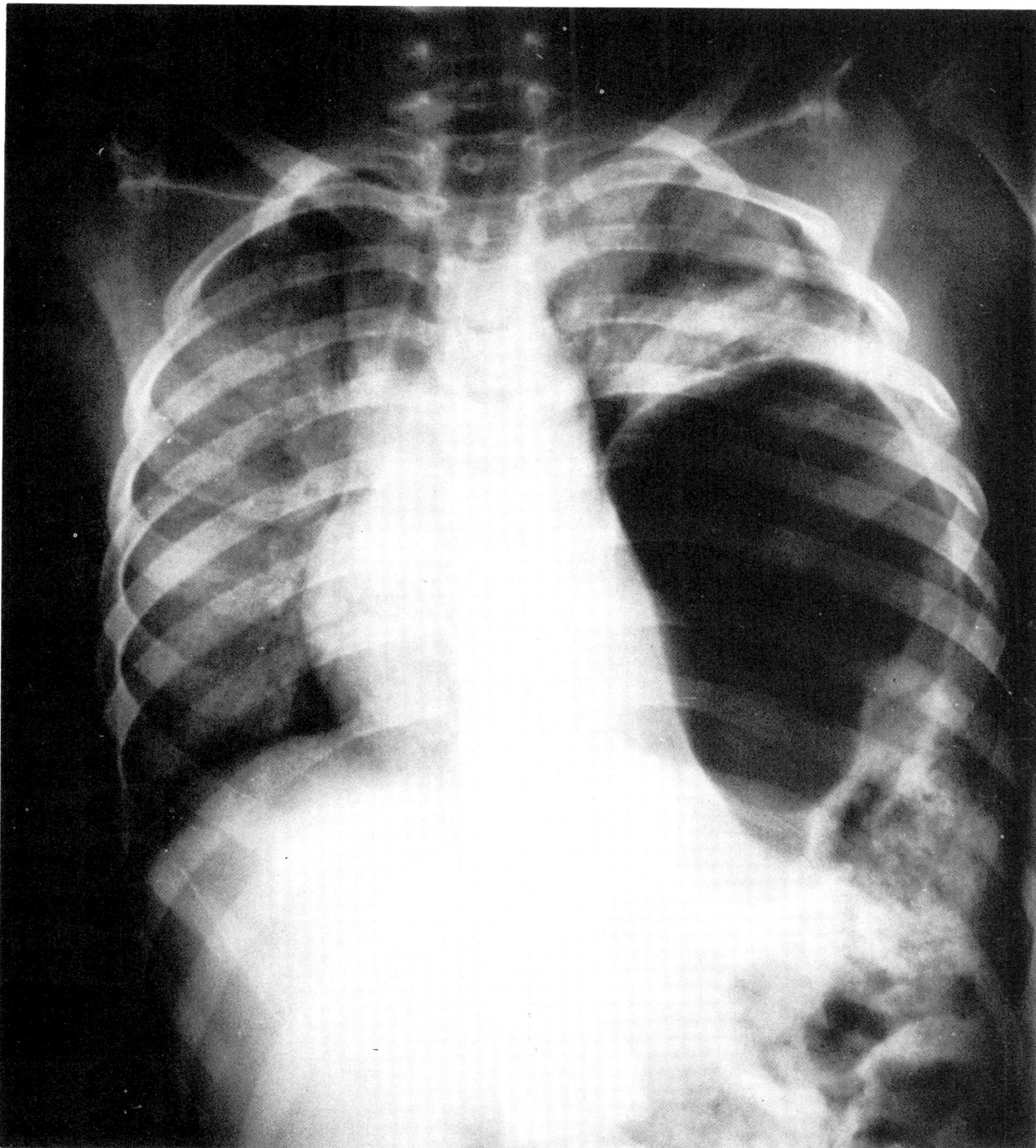

This child presented following a serious road traffic accident.

- Describe the chest X-ray.
- What is your emergency management?

A17

The child's chest and abdomen had been run over by a truck wheel. The chest X-ray shows the result of traumatic rupture of the left diaphragm, with the stomach herniating into the left chest. The trachea and mediastinum have been displaced to the right.

Application of positive pressure ventilation and decompression of the stomach by a nasogastric tube resulted in marked improvement and Film B was taken at this stage, 15 minutes after X-ray A. Opacification of the right lung is due to lung contusion. At surgery a lateral tear in the diaphragm was found.

Traumatic diaphragmatic hernias occur in children following falls and crushing injuries. Any segment of the diaphragm may be lacerated, but about 90% of such hernias are on the left side and extend radially from the central tendon to the periphery. Early repair is advisable because initially small tears gradually enlarge.

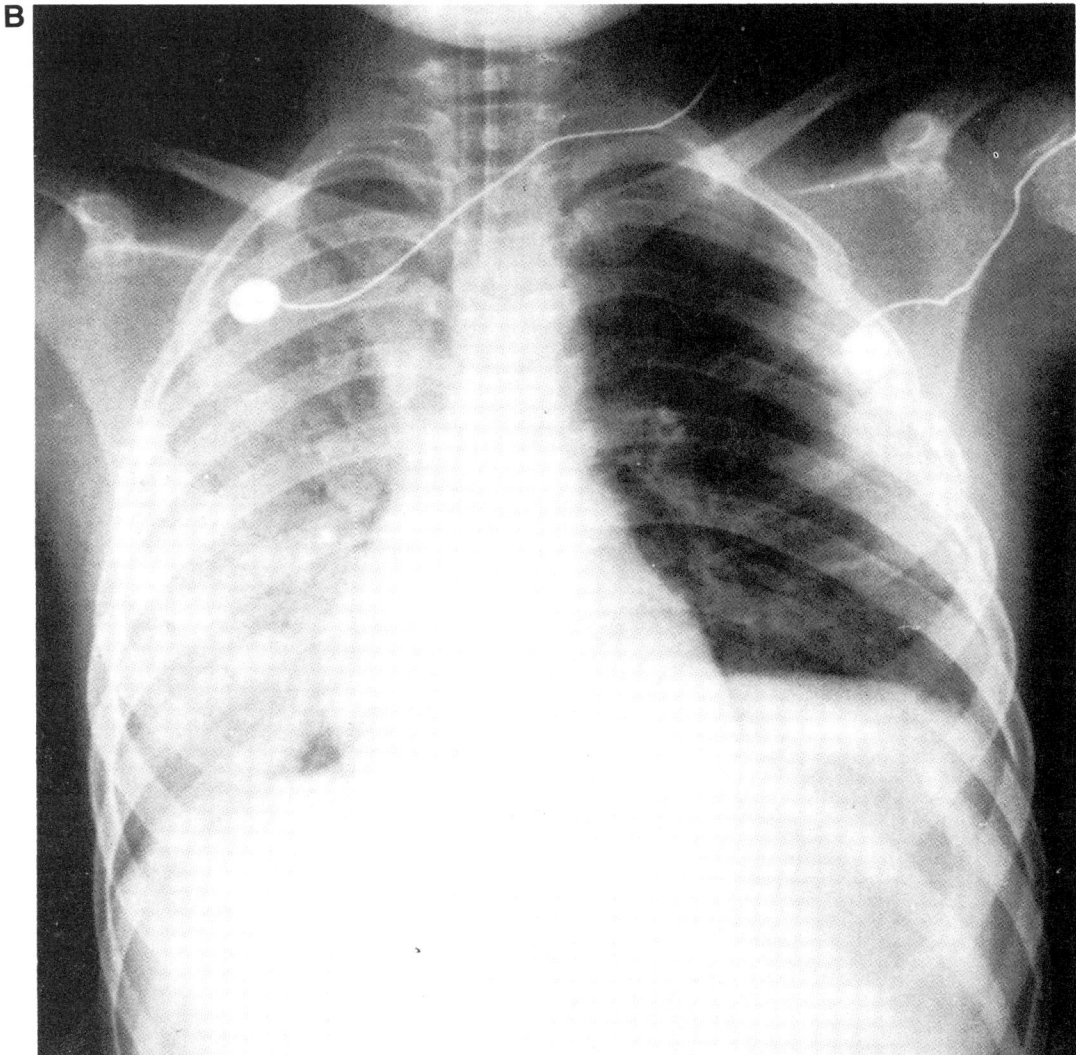

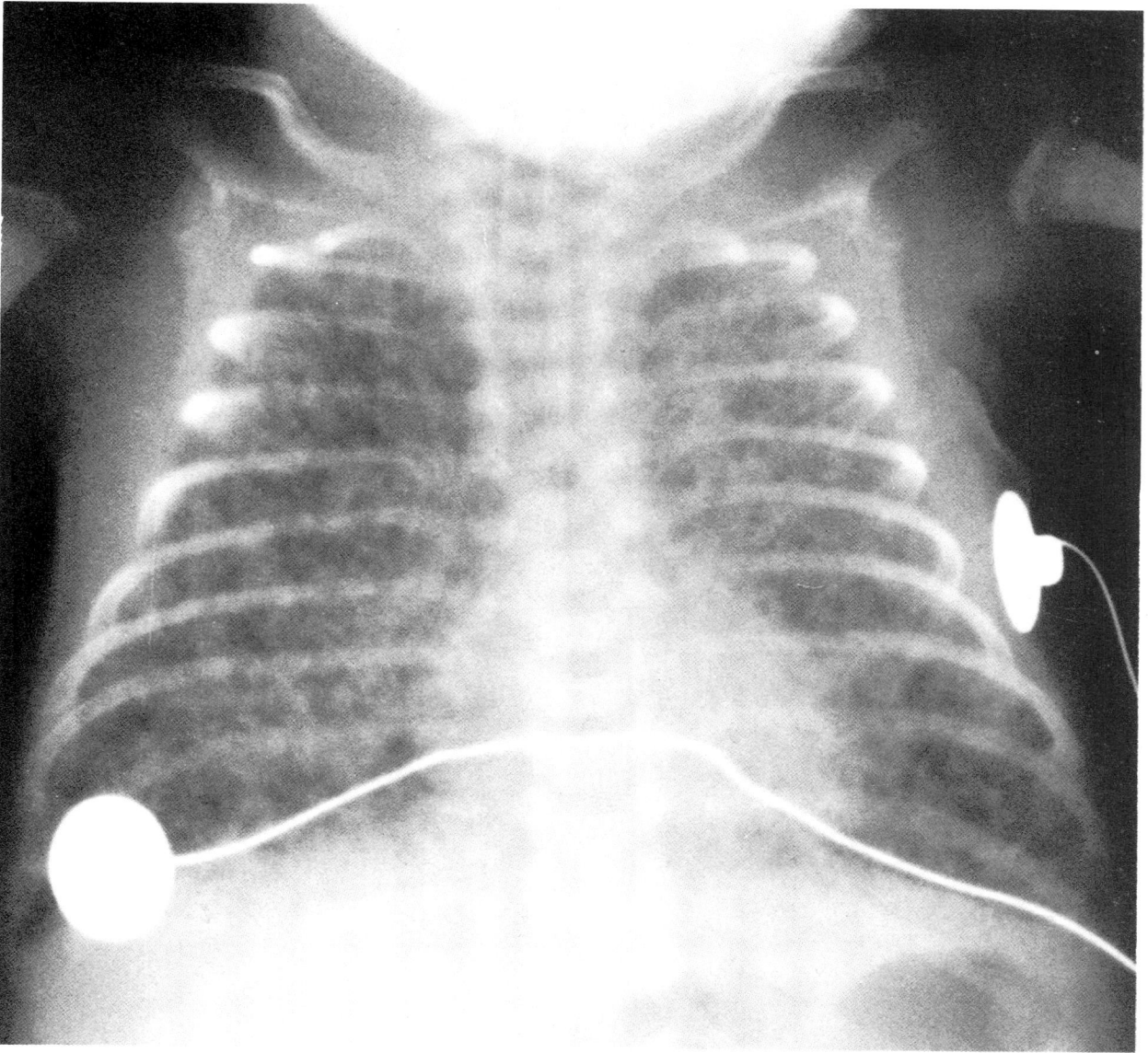

This is the chest X-ray of a 26 week gestation neonatal patient taken at 6 weeks of age.

- What is the diagnosis?

- This infant died at the age of 3 months. What findings would you expect on post-mortem examination of the lungs?

A18

The patient is being ventilated. He had developed broncho-pulmonary dysplasia (BPD), which is a form of chronic lung disease seen in early infancy and usually follows intensive therapy for respiratory difficulties in the neonatal period. The chest X-ray in such patients shows increased hyperexpansion and focal hyperlucency alternating with strands of opacification. This final stage is preceded by three other gradually progressive stages. Initially the films are consistent with respiratory distress syndrome. From 4-10 days the lungs become more consolidated. From 10-20 days numerous cystic areas of various sizes appear and the lung fields may look hyperinflated.

Post-mortem examination revealed fibrous adhesions in both pleural cavities and, macroscopically, the lungs had a cobblestone appearance. Histology demonstrated marked distortion of the alveolar pattern with focal areas of over-distension alternating with collapse. There was marked hypertrophy and fibrosis of smooth muscle. The pulmonary artery showed considerable thickening of the muscular coats indicating hypertension.

Q19

A

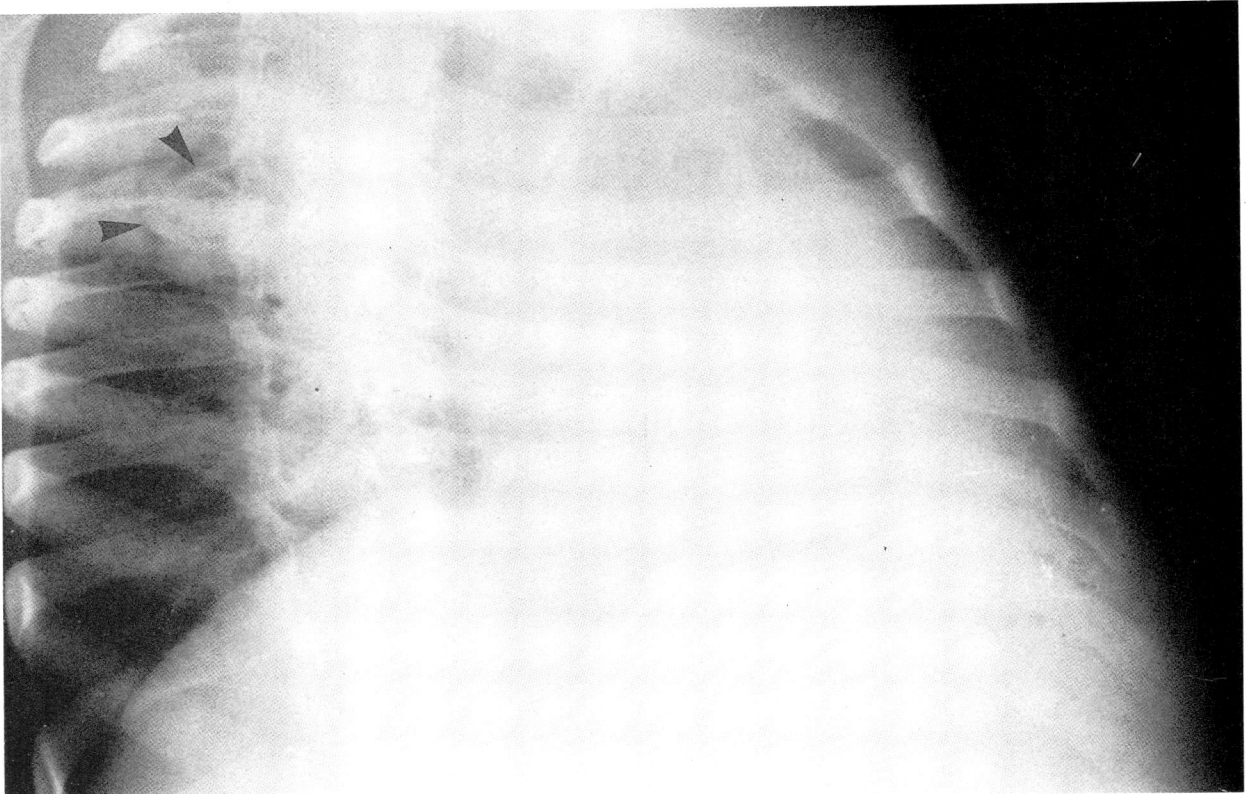

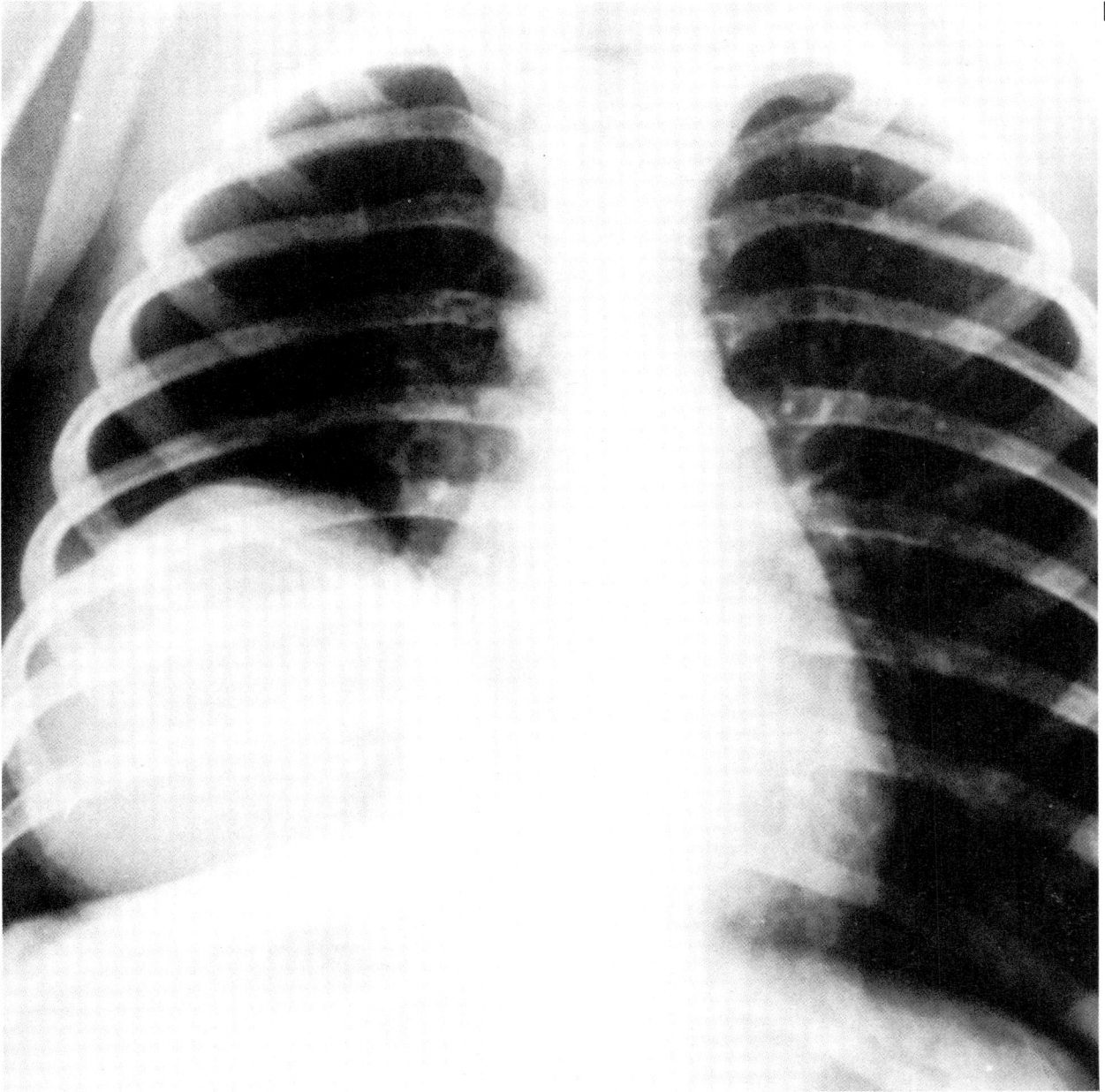

Patients A and B have a similar disease. Patient A was a young girl who presented to casualty coughing up blood and watery fluid. A blood film revealed an eosinophilia.

- What is the diagnosis?

- What radiological features are seen in this condition?

- What other investigations would support your diagnosis?

A19

Patient A has a ruptured hydatid cyst. The cyst had ruptured into her bronchus causing haemoptysis. She was also coughing up the watery content of the cyst. Following rupture in patient A the cyst appears as a rounded air-filled cavity with a fluid level. The collapsed endocyst appears as a wrinkled shadow on the surface of the fluid level – the 'water lily' sign (arrowed). The exocyst and pericyst have come apart forming a translucent line (arrowed). This is known as the meniscus sign.

A chest X-ray may show a cyst as a round uniformly opaque mass (patient B).

Eosinophilia is present in over 70% of patients. The Casoni test may be performed by giving a 0.2ml intradermal injection of sterile hydatid cyst fluid. A positive test is shown by a wheal of not less than 2cm with a surrounding flare of more than 1cm. This usually develops within 30 minutes of injection, and is positive in approximately two thirds of patients with hydatid cysts. False positive results may occur. The hydatid complement fixation test is more reliable than the Casoni test and is positive in over 50% of patients with hydatid disease.

Q20

A

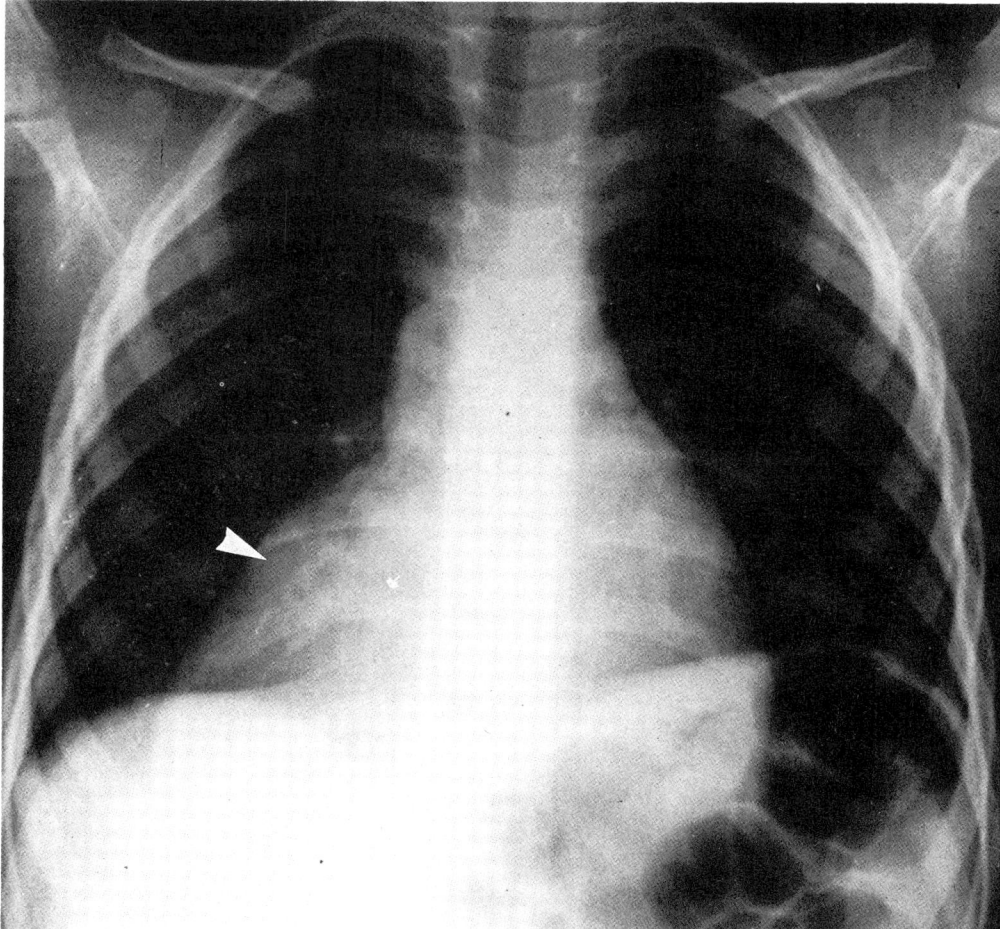

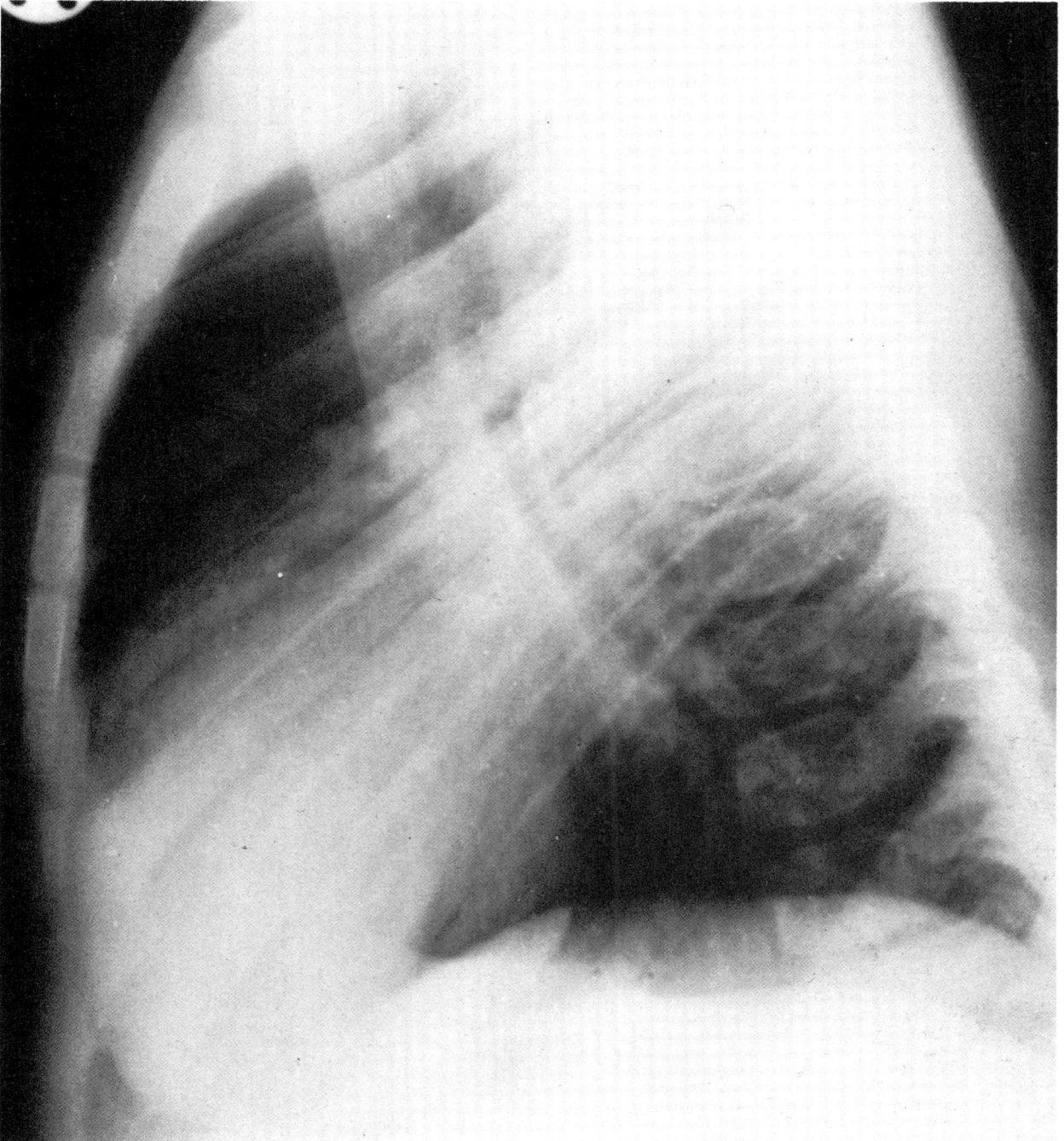

This child had a chest X-ray taken because of a recent cough which improved without treatment. Describe the anomaly seen in the right lung (arrowed).

- What is the differential diagnosis of a mediastinal mass in this position?

- The mass was found to be inseparable from the cardiac image in all projections. What diagnoses should be considered?

A20

The child has a mass present in his right peri-cardiophrenic angle. The differential diagnosis of a lower anterior mediastinal mass includes a pericardial cyst, a fat pad and a Morgagni hernia with herniation of the left lobe of the liver. A CT scan showed it to contain water and a diagnosis of pericardial cyst was made.

Failure of a pericardial lacuna to coalesce with the main pericardiac coelom results in later dilation and formation of a thin-walled sac lined by flat epithelium. It is a benign condition.

Q21

A

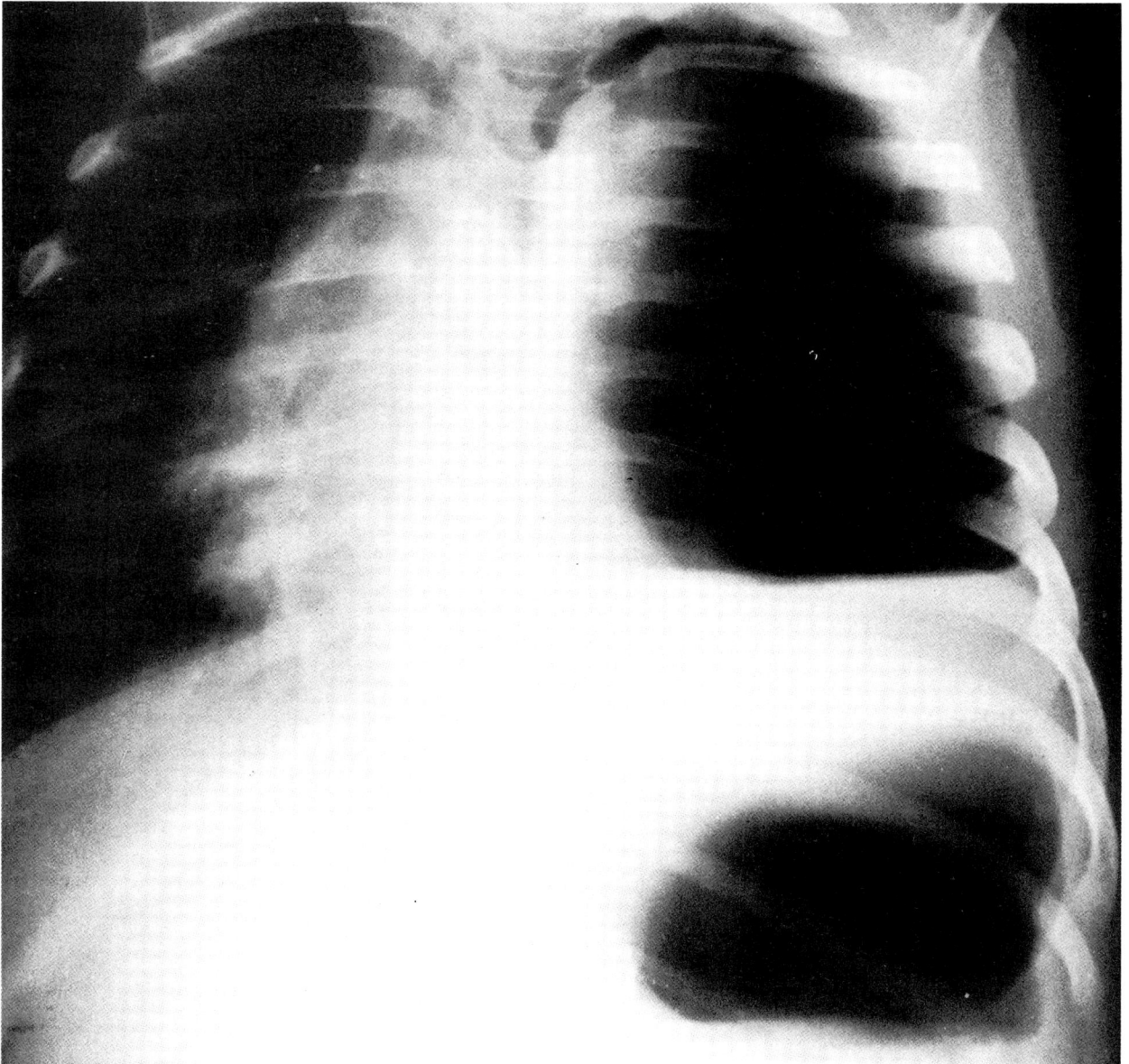

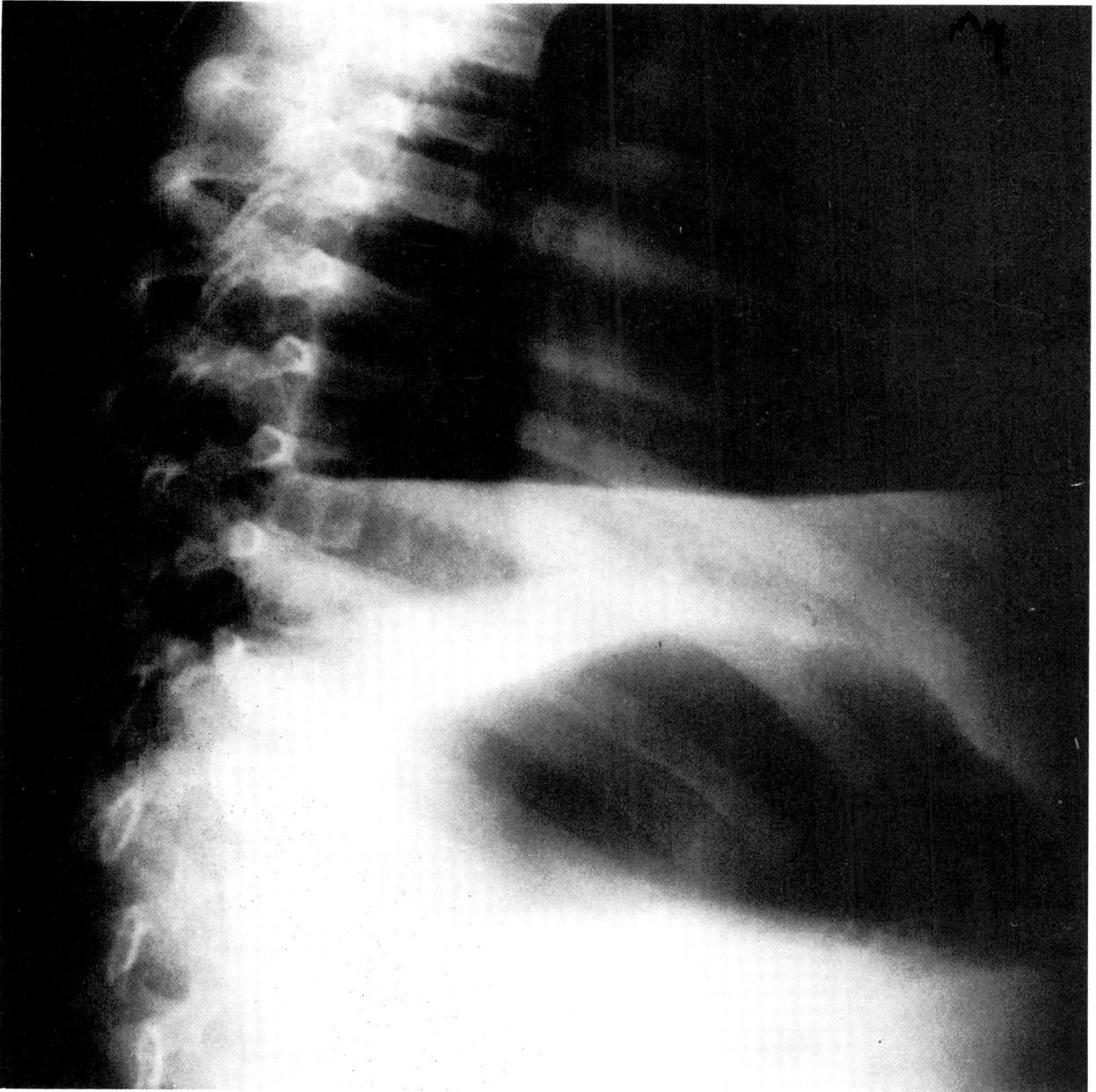

This young child was an inpatient receiving antibiotics for pneumonia. She became breathless.

- What has caused the deterioration in her condition?
- How would you manage this patient?

A21

This child has developed a pyopneumothorax. The increased intra-pleural tension is shown by displacement of the heart and mediastinum to the opposite side. The long horizontal air fluid levels are visible in both projections.

Pyopneumothorax may be generalised or loculated. This patient was treated by insertion of an intercostal drain, relieving the tension pneumothorax and draining the purulent fluid.

Management of para-pneumonic effusions and empyema includes effective antibiotic therapy and general supportive care. In childhood approximately 70% of cases of pleural empyema occur in the first 2 years of life. *Staphylococcus aureus* is the major pathogen in the first 6 months of life. *Haemophilus* and *Streptococcus pneumoniae* cause more than half the cases in infants from 7-24 months. In the exudative phase, when fluid is thin (containing few cells) as much fluid as possible should be aspirated. In the fibrinopurulent stage the fluid is thicker and fibrin is deposited in the pleura and loculation sometimes occurs. These cases require an intercostal catheter to be inserted with underwater drainage. Ultrasonography can be useful to identify areas of loculation or abscesses and may help in repositioning the catheter to drain these. The third stage in the pleural reaction to infection is that of organization when fibroblasts form layers in the pleural space.

If there is a large amount of pus under pressure, rupture into the lung or through the chest may occur. In some centres early thoracotomy is performed to break down adhesions and to remove pus and fibrinous material. The prognosis for full recovery of lung function is good.

Film C shows a loculated empyema containing only pus. Note the slight rib crowding and the spinal curve towards the side of the empyema.

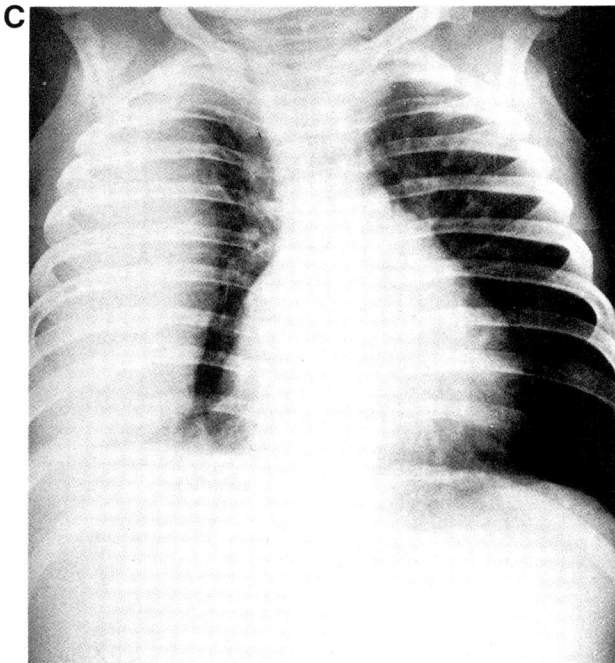

C

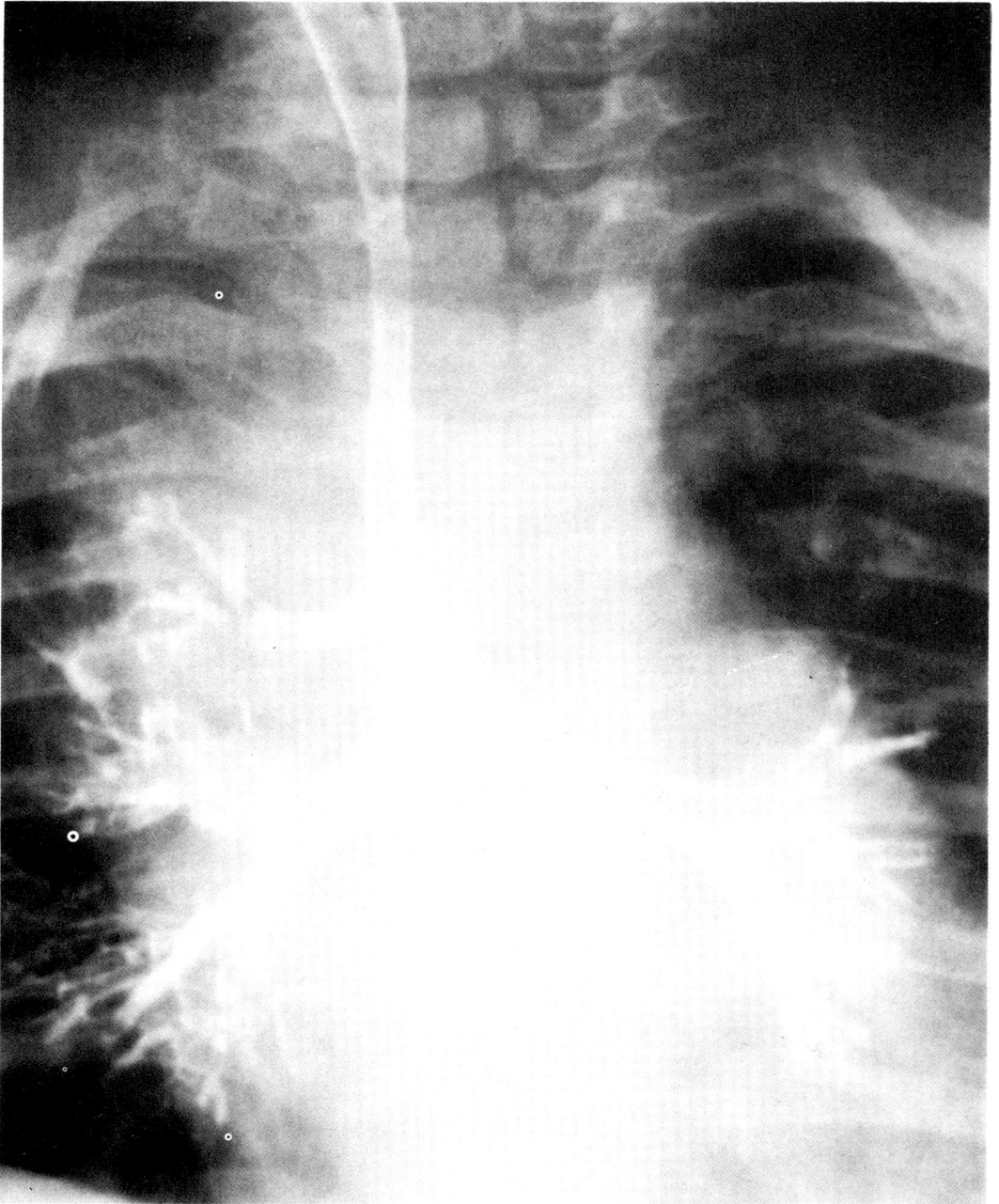

This child presented with stridor, and at bronchoscopy complete cartilaginous rings were noted in the upper thoracic trachea, which was stenosed and would not admit the instrument. The carina could not be accurately visualised and this was the indication for this study.

- What study has been performed?
- What other abnormality has been detected?

A22

A bronchogram has been performed. This shows the tracheal stenosis. The aberrant right upper lobe bronchus arises from the trachea. Tracheal bronchi are right sided and usually of no clinical significance. A tracheal bronchus is normal in most clovenhoofed animals and is often referred to as a 'pig' bronchus.

Q23

A

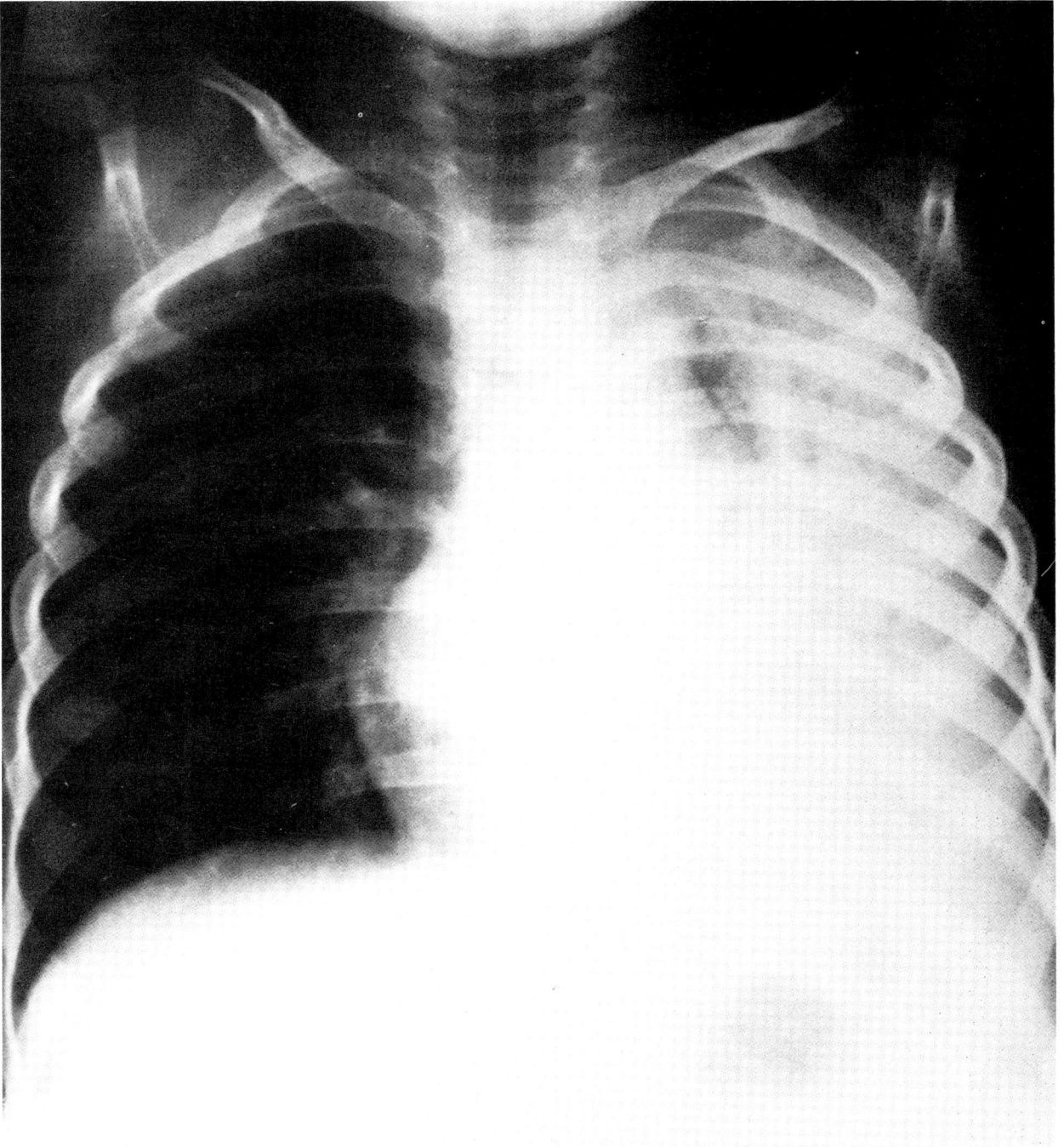

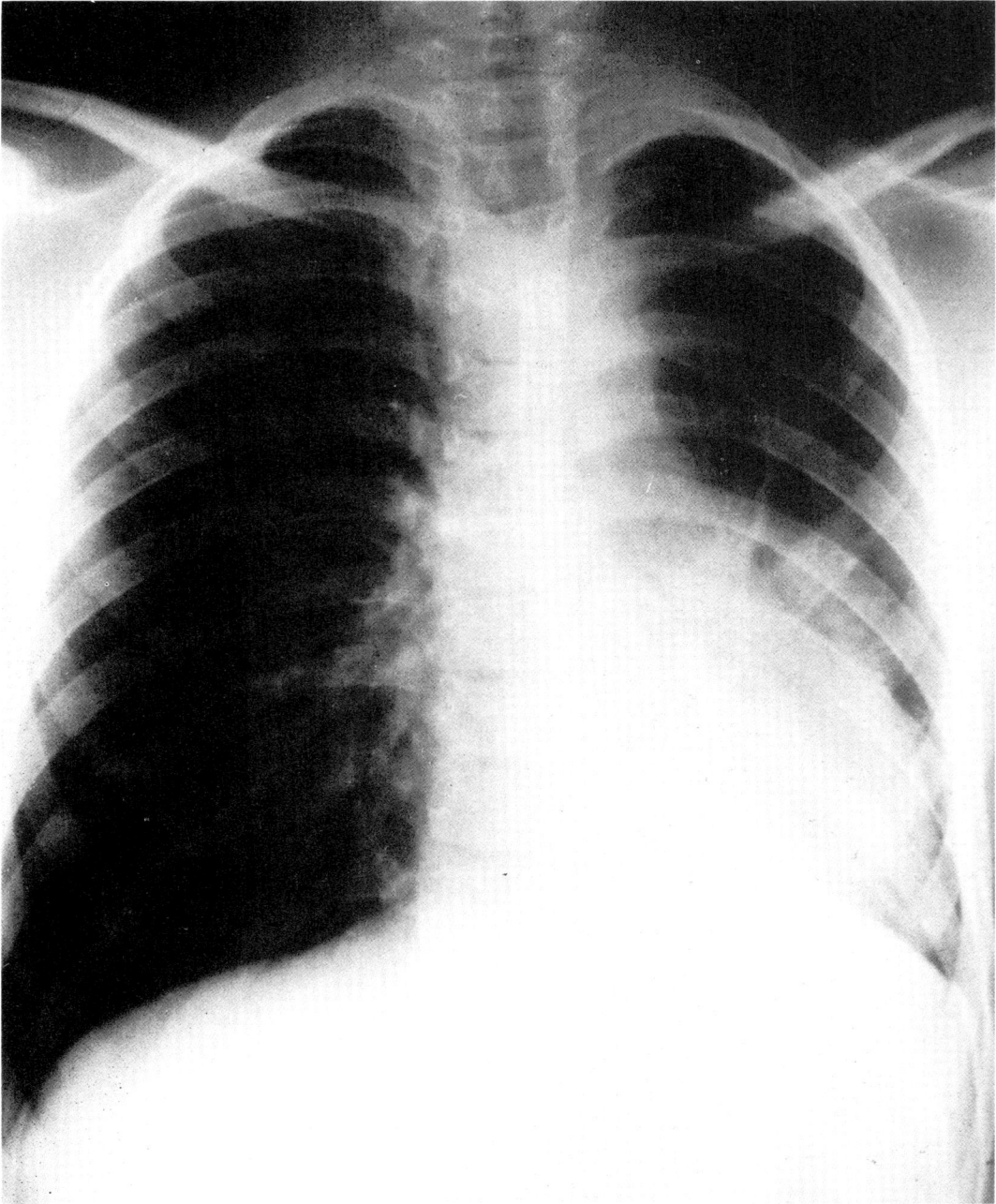

At 2 years of age this boy developed a severe left sided pneumonia (Film A). When seen at 10 years of age he was suffering from recurrent chest infections and a productive cough.

- Describe the X-ray changes of film B.

- What is the diagnosis?

A23

The child has dense and persistent collapse of his left lower lobe with uniform dilation of the bronchi. Taken with the clinical findings a diagnosis of bronchiectasis can be made. Only when medical treatment for bronchiectasis has failed and surgery is being considered should a bronchogram be done.

Primary infection does not usually cause extensive destruction of the bronchial wall. Collapsed lobes re-expand as the infection resolves and bronchial dilation disappears. If the condition remains untreated for more than 6-12 months, permanent bronchiectasis may develop. Therefore, early diagnosis, appropriate antibiotic treatment and physiotherapy to help to re-expand the lung are essential. The ability of the airways to return to normal size is known as 'reversible bronchiectasis'.

Q24

A

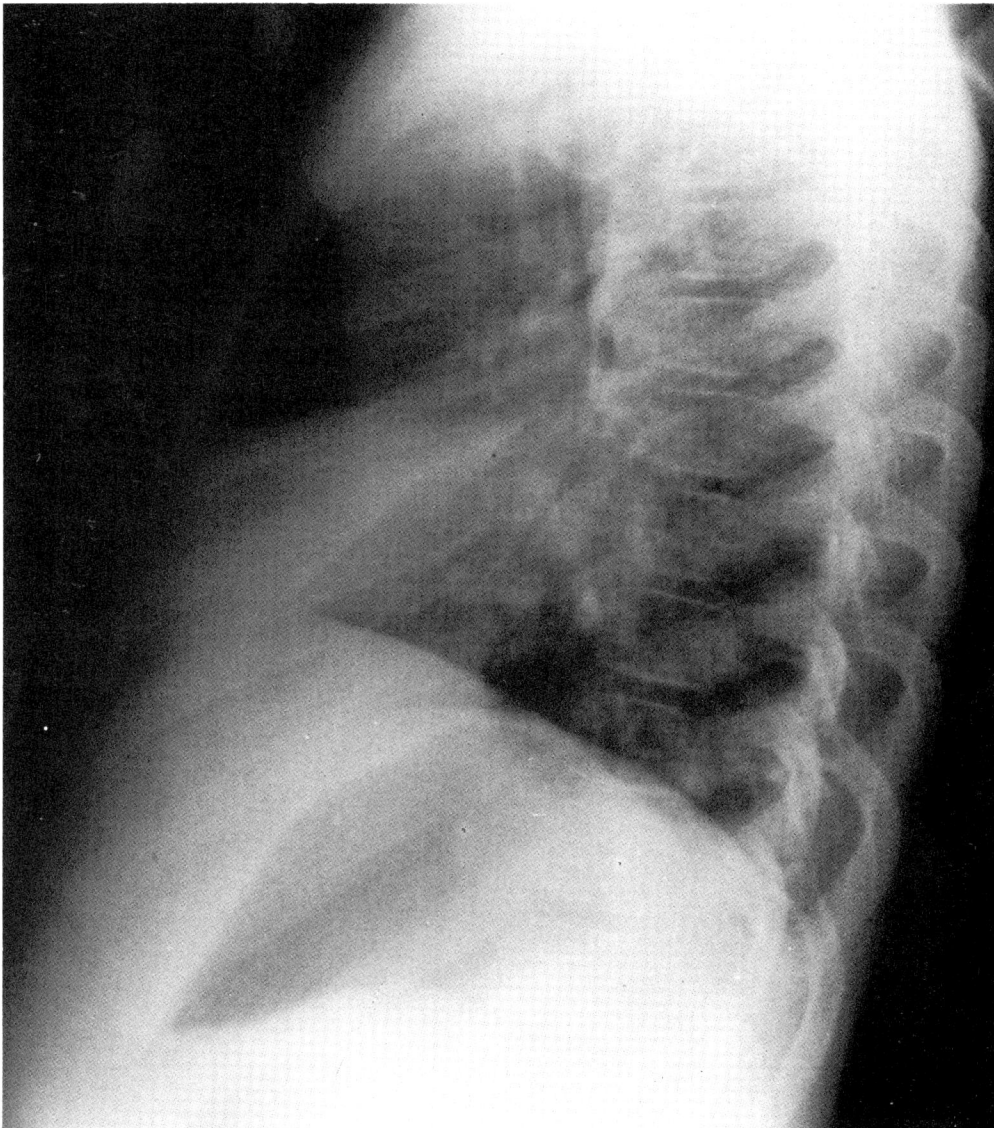

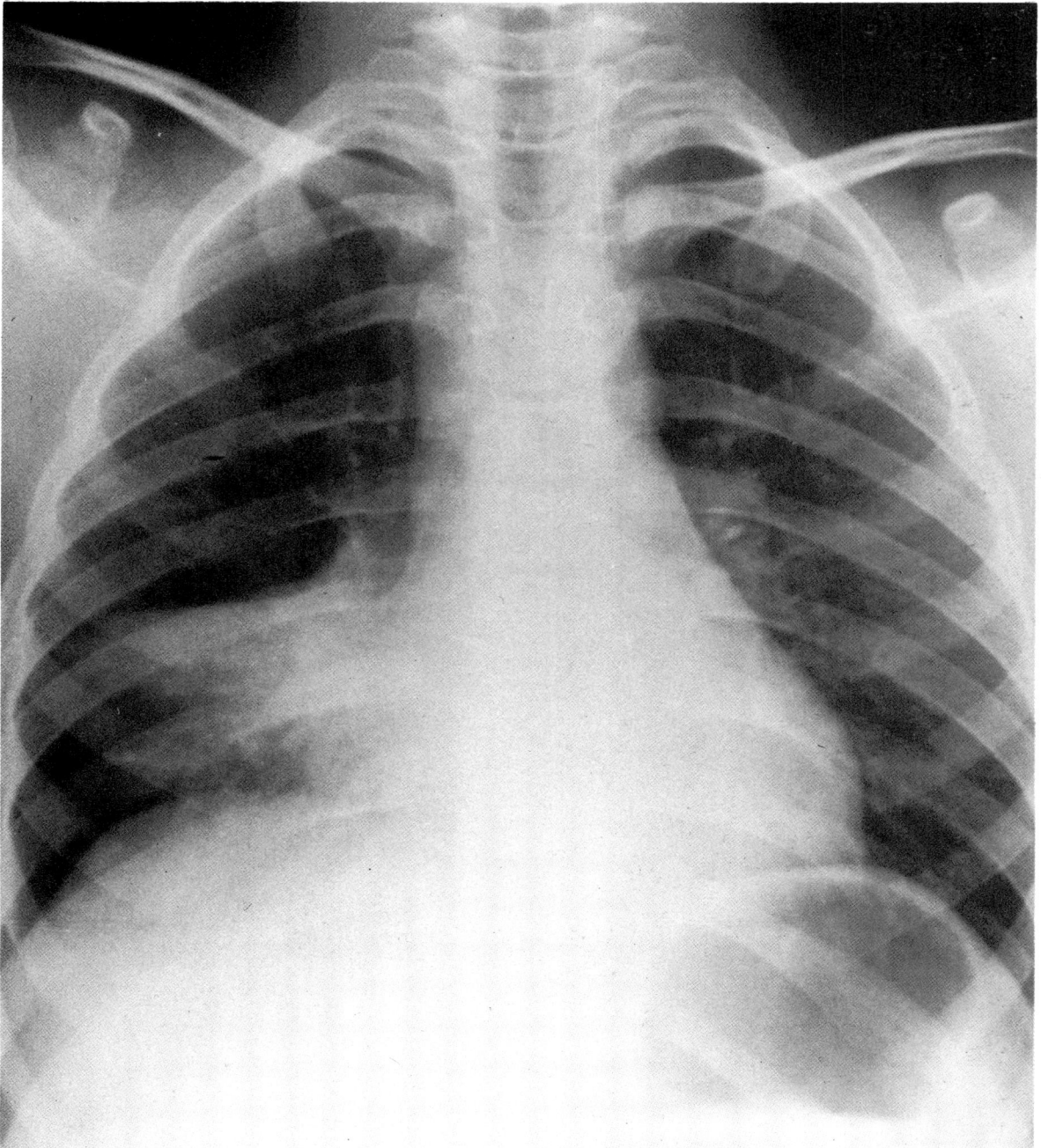

This child presented with cough and fever.

- What abnormality is seen on the chest X-rays?

- In some patients this may become a recurrent problem. What pathophysiological features predispose to this?

A24

This child has collapse and consolidation of her right middle lobe. This is seen as loss of her lower right heart border on AP chest X-ray where the heart is in contact with the right middle lobe (Film B).

Middle lobe syndrome is a vicious circle of recurrent collapses and subsequent infections. It may lead to damage of the bronchi, fibrosis or bronchiectasis. The bronchus of the right middle lobe is small in diameter, short, and takes off from the intermediate bronchus at an acute angle. The right middle lobe bronchus is surrounded by lymph nodes that drain it, as well as the lower and upper lobes. When these lymph nodes enlarge compression of the right middle lobe bronchus results. The lobe is also isolated by fissures from the right upper and lower lobes and thus from the aerating effects of collateral ventilation (air drift).

Q25

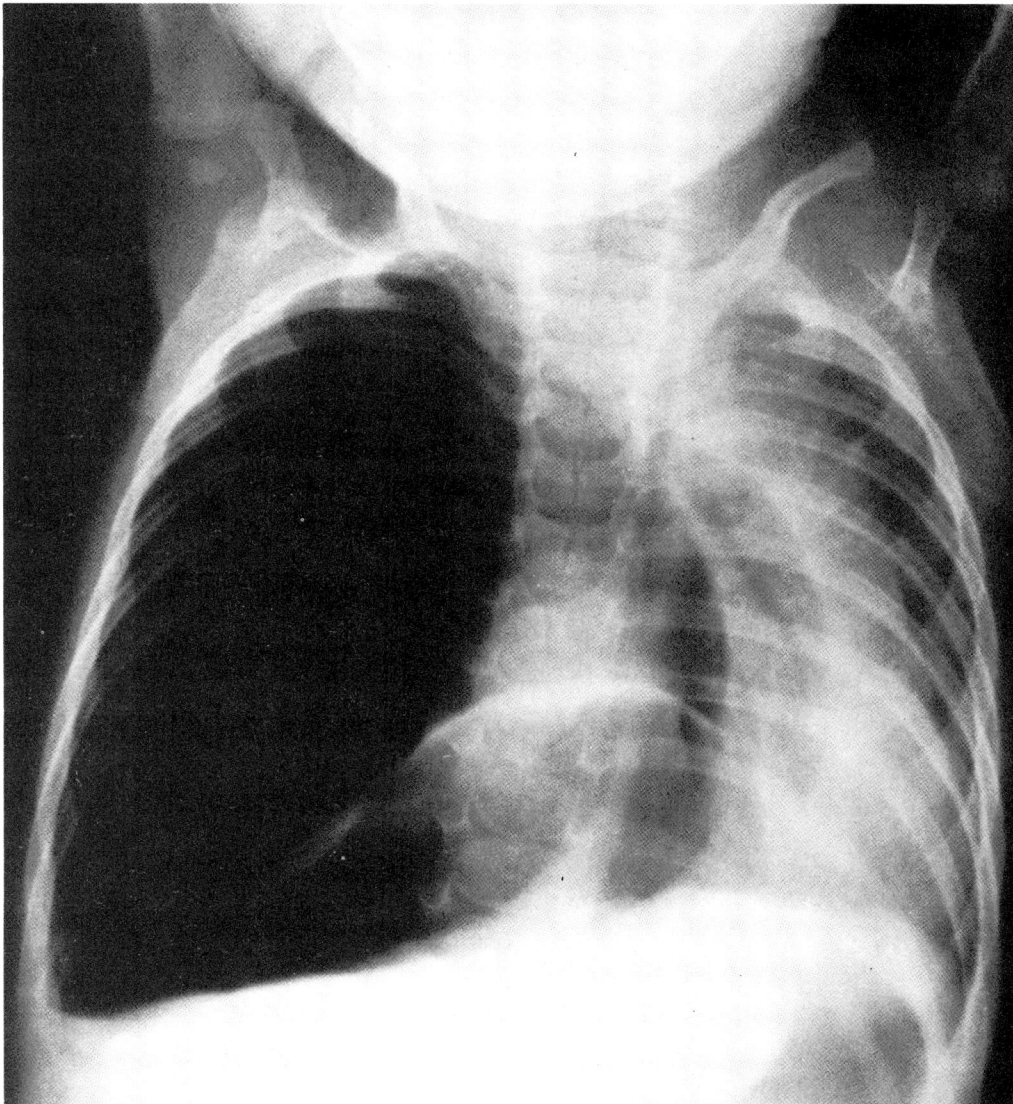

Patient A

Patient A: This 5 month old child presented to casualty with increasing respiratory distress. There was a 2 week history of difficulty with feeds, occasional vomiting and loss of weight.

- What is causing his respiratory distress?

Patient B: This 8 year old child had suffered from a similar problem on 3 previous occasions.

- What is responsible for his respiratory distress?

- What is the common underlying cause of these patients' problems?

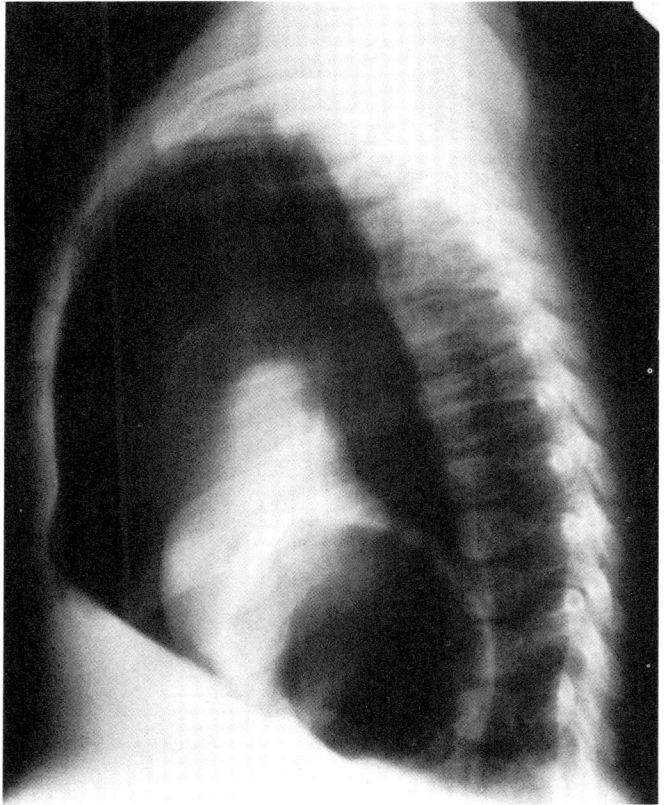

Patient A

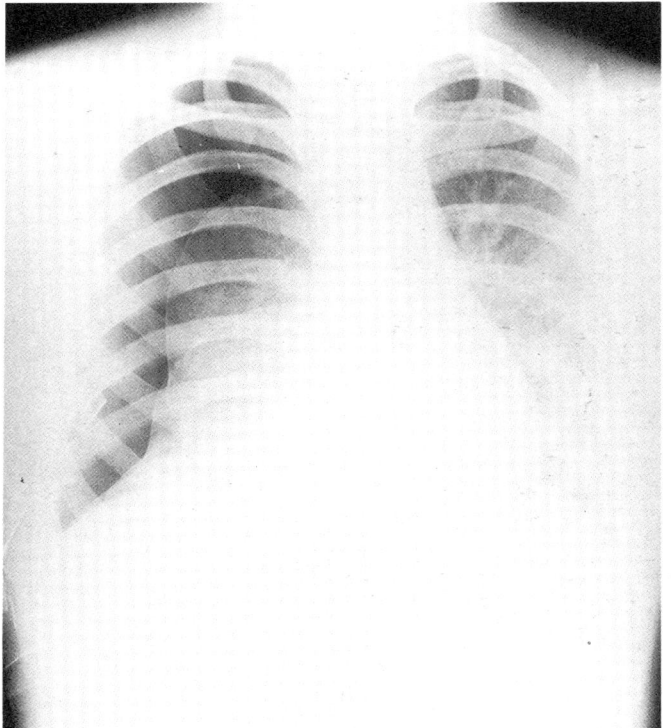

Patient B

A25

The X-ray of patient A reveals a huge right tension pneumothorax. The trachea, heart and mediastinum have been pushed into the left thorax compressing the left lung with resultant respiratory distress, which was relieved by insertion of a chest drain.

A thin-walled cystic shape is seen in the right hemithorax. The differential diagnosis is between a lung cyst and a diaphragmatic hernia. Spontaneous pneumothoraces are very rare in childhood. A cause for pneumothorax must always be sought. The possibility of a congenital cystic lesion must always be considered. This is especially true if pneumothoraces are recurrent and if underlying problems such as intra-bronchial foreign body, cystic fibrosis, histio-cytosis with honeycomb lung and asthma are excluded.

In this patient surgical excision of a foregut duplication cyst was carried out.

Patient B also has a right sided pneumothorax. This recurred and was due to a lung cyst which can be seen sitting on top of the collapsed right lung.

Q26

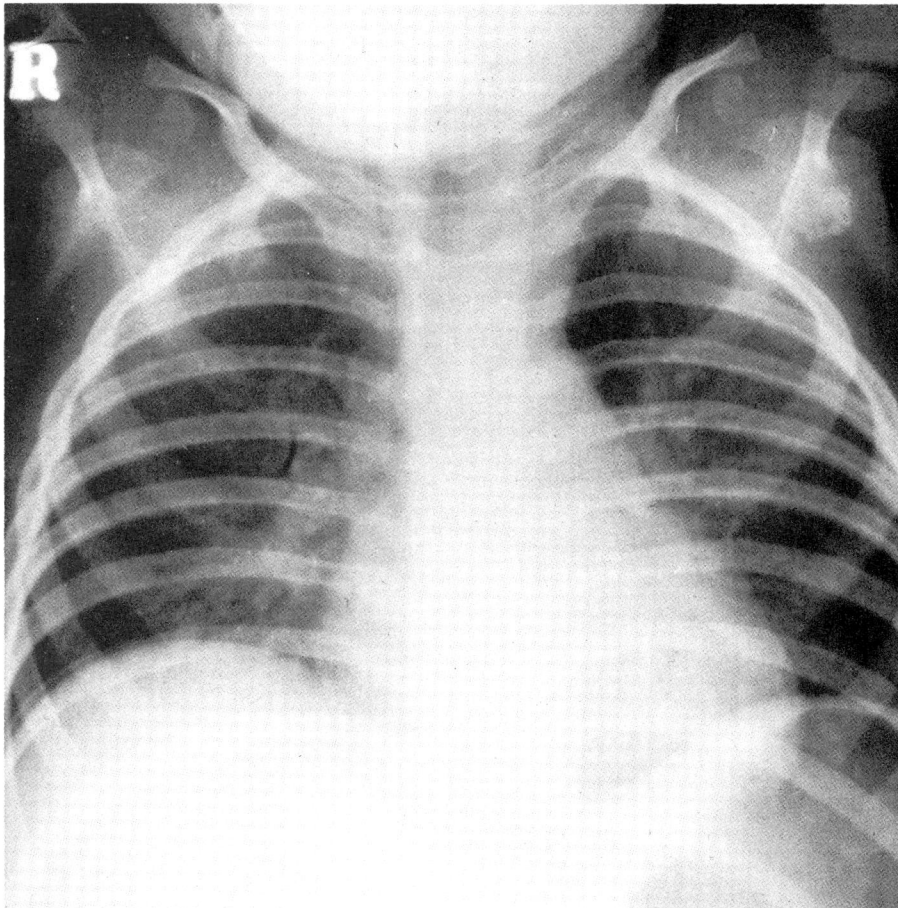

This infant, born in England, was found to have bronchiolitis caused by respiratory syncitial virus infection.

- What is the family background of this infant?

- If the chest X-ray was taken in 10 years' time would it be possible to guess his racial origin?

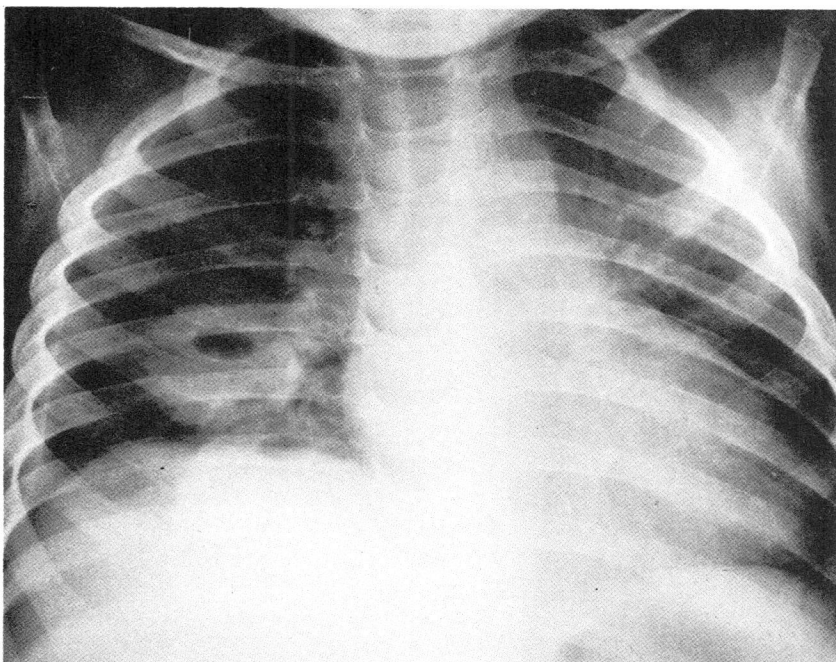

Q27

This child presented with sudden onset of fever, malaise, cough and dyspnoea.

- What does the chest X-ray show?

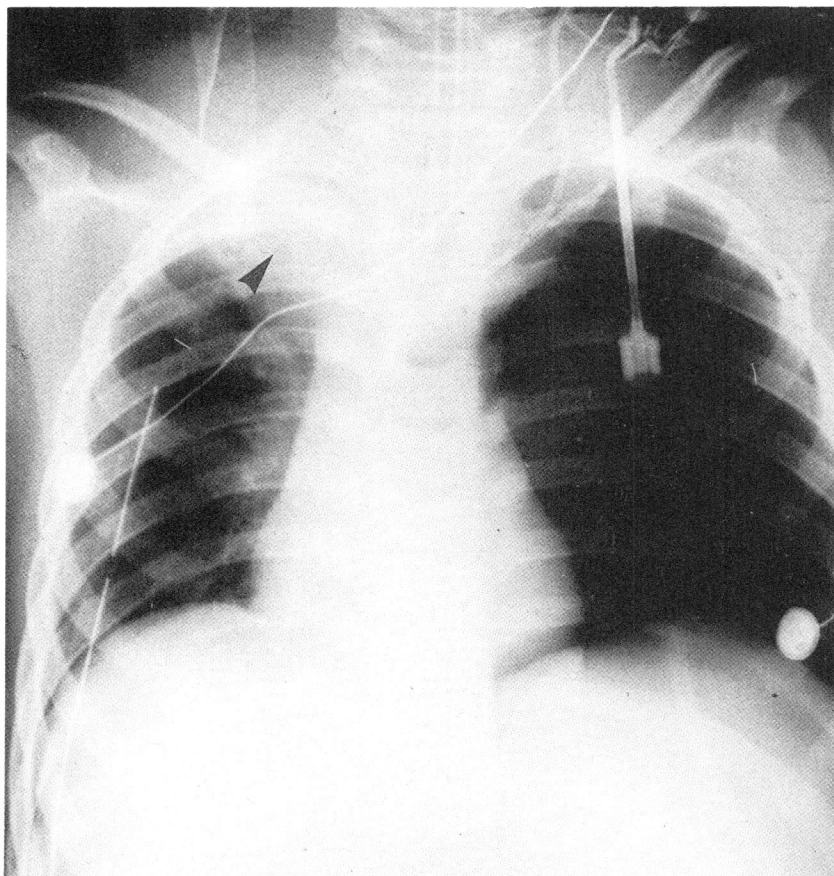

Q28

This child required a central venous line. It was successfully placed following attempts on both sides of the neck.

- What iatrogenic complications have occurred?

A26

The infant has a calcified lymph node in his left axilla. Calcification can be found in nodes regional to inoculations with BCG vaccine. This patient was inoculated with BCG into the skin of the left forearm on the 10th day of life. Calcifications residual to BCG tend to disappear more quickly than those associated with natural infections in the lungs. It is unlikely that an X-ray at 10 years of age would reveal calcification. In the United Kingdom the majority of BCG inoculations are given shortly after birth to children of Asian parents, and to any other child at particular risk of TB infection from within the family.

A27

Chest X-ray reveals an abscess in the right lung with an air fluid level. There is loss of volume of the right lung. The most common cause of lung abscesses is *Staphylococcus aureus*.

A primary abscess is usually solitary and occurs in an otherwise healthy child. Secondary abscesses may be solitary or multiple and occur in a compromised child, for example, due to immunosuppression or prematurity.

Radiologically the abscesses appear as thick-walled cavities in the lung and may vary in size from 1-20cm or more in diameter. Solitary abscesses occur more often in the right lung than the left, and an air fluid level is often present. Compressive atelectasis is often seen around the abscess.

Children with primary lung abscesses usually do well with antibiotics alone and there is no evidence that drainage is necessary for complete resolution.

A28

Three catastrophes occurred:
1   A right sided pneumothorax which required underwater drainage via an intercostal tube.
2   An apical haematoma on the right side (arrowed).
3   A left sided pneumothorax that required drainage.

The child made a full recovery.

Q29

This premature baby developed severe respiratory distress within the first 4 hours of life.

- What is the diagnosis?
- What does the X-ray show?

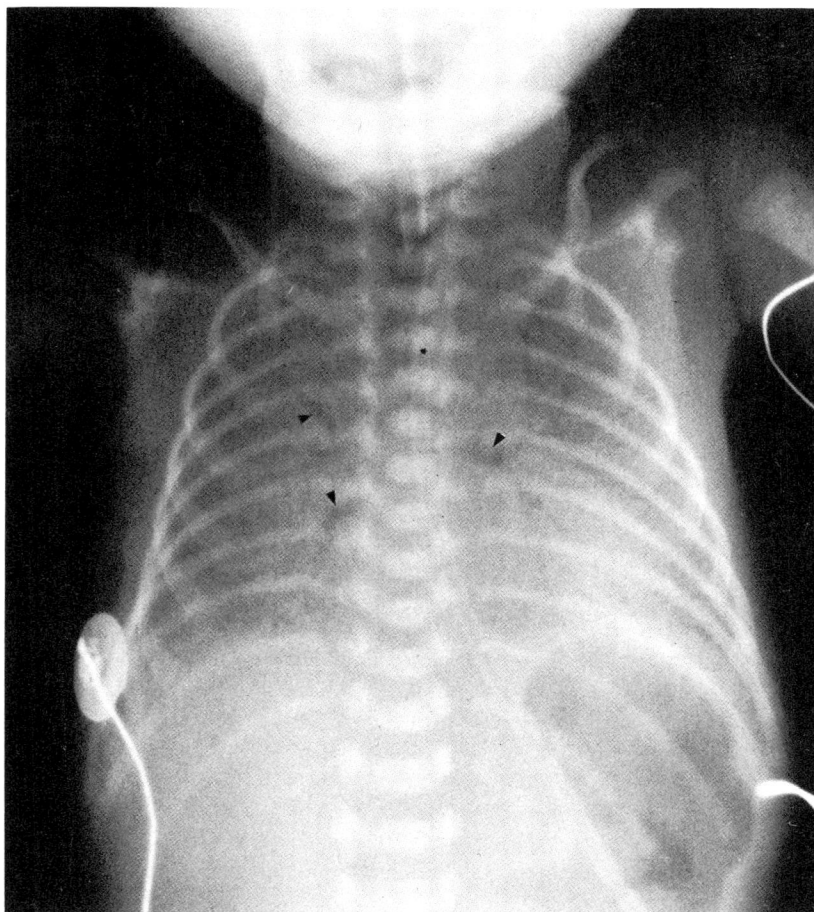

Q30

This child presented with a short history of increasing stridor.

- What is the diagnosis?
- What features help in the diagnosis?
- How would you manage this patient?

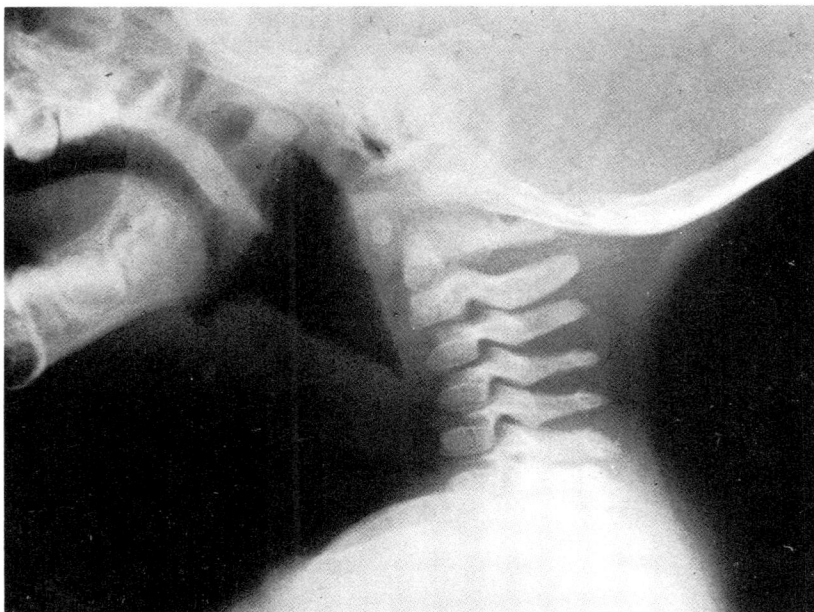

A29

This X-ray and clinical history are characteristic of the respiratory distress syndrome (RDS).

There is a diffuse, fine reticular granular (ground glass) appearance involving both lung fields with air bronchograms (arrowed). The main purpose of the chest X-ray in a baby with respiratory distress syndrome is to confirm the diagnosis and also to exclude other causes of respiratory distress such as a pneumothorax or diaphragmatic hernia which requires surgical intervention.

Neonatal pneumonia may give a similar appearance irrespective of birth weight. In practice therefore most of these babies are treated with antibiotics.

A30

The lateral X-ray shows that the epiglottis is swollen confirming the diagnosis of epiglottitis.

The onset of epiglottitis is usually rapid over a few hours. The patient is pyrexial (usually over 38.5°C) and lethargic, refusing to drink because of a sore throat. Upper airway obstruction becomes obvious with a soft inspiratory stridor and an expiratory element resembling a snore. The child prefers to sit upright and is often drooling saliva. The voice is weak and there is no harsh cough such as that heard in patients with croup. The epiglottis is swollen and cherry coloured. Staff and facilities capable of relieving the obstruction must be at hand before inspection as this may precipitate complete airway obstruction.

Unlike epiglottitis, the child with croup will have upper respiratory tract infection for 1-2 days before developing a harsh barking cough and hoarse voice. With more severe airway obstruction chest wall recession occurs and stridor may be inspiratory and expiratory. The child is restless and drooling occurs. Symptoms usually develop at night and fever is usually below 39°C. Hypoxia may cause tachypnoea, tachycardia, restlessness and eventually cyanosis.

Many hospitals intubate all patients with epiglottitis. This decision is made on clinical grounds. Lateral X-rays are not usually performed to aid diagnosis. Intubation is required for 6-18 hours. Tracheostomy is also a satisfactory (and sometimes essential) method of relieving the obstruction. Intravenous chloramphenicol is given to treat the causative *Haemophilus influenzae* type B infection.

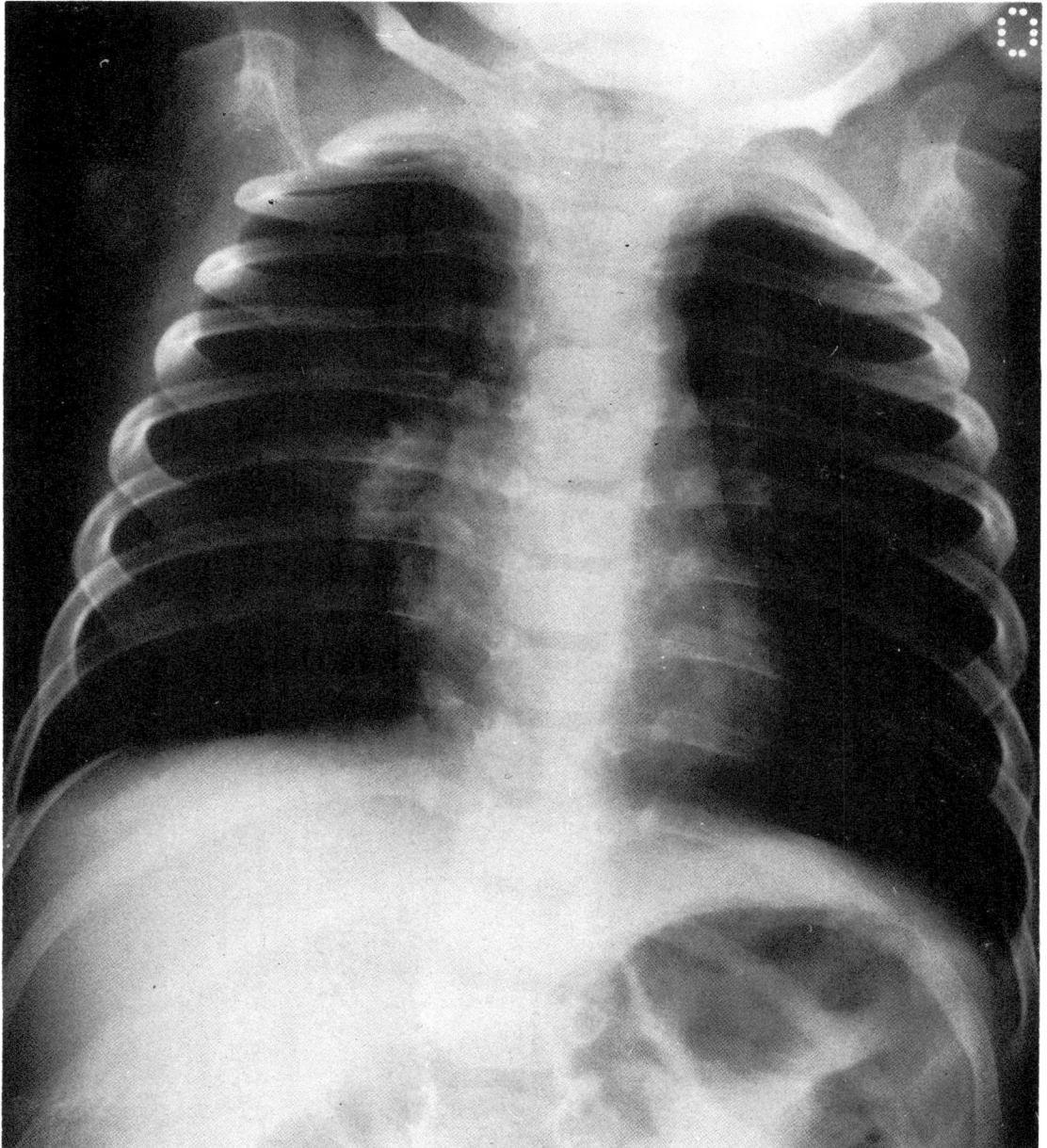

This 3 month old infant had respiratory distress following an upper respiratory tract infection. She was tachypnoeic (130/minute), had difficulty with feeds and fine crepitations were heard all over the chest.

- What is the diagnosis?
- How does the chest X-ray help in diagnosis?

A31

This patient has acute bronchiolitis which is the commonest severe lower respiratory tract infection in infancy. The large majority of infections are due to respiratory syncitial virus and occur in epidemics each year which last 3-4 months. The peak incidence coincides with the coldest month of the year.

The virus invades the entire respiratory tract with the main assault on the bronchioles. These develop oedema, necrosis and shedding of epithelial cells. Mucous secretions block the bronchiolar lumen. This leads to gross hyperinflation but also to areas of local collapse.

Diagnosis is based on the clinical findings including some fever, tachypnoea, hyperinflation and fine crepitations. Heart failure and pneumonia need to be excluded. This child's X-ray shows a depressed diaphragm, horizontal ribs and some hilar shadowing. Over 60% of infants with bronchiolitis show marked hyperinflation of the lungs with depression of the diaphragm and a pad of air in front of the heart on the lateral film. Peribronchial thickening is seen on 50% of films with areas of consolidation in 25% and an area of segmental or lobar collapse in 10%.

Many of these infants are seriously ill needing supportive treatment with head box oxygen and nasogastric or intravenous fluids when feeding is difficult. Few require ventilation and mortality is usually confined to infants with underlying respiratory and cardiac defects. Up to 80% of these infants will have recurrent attacks of cough and wheeze over the next 2-3 years.

Q32

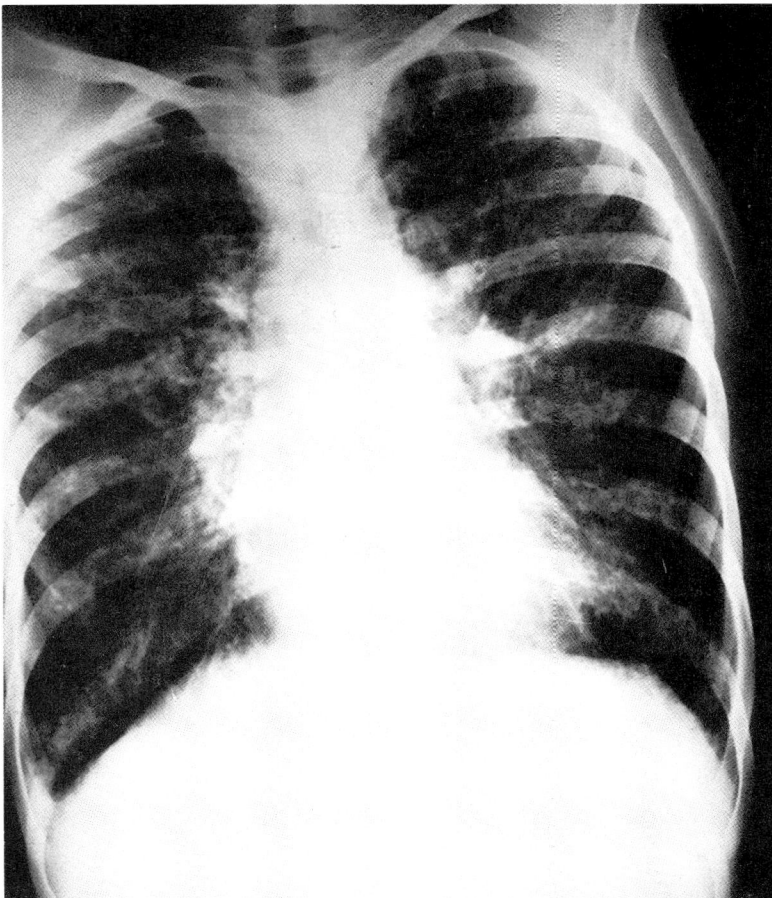

This patient had a productive cough for many years. Sputum contained *Pseudomonas aeruginosa*.

- What is the diagnosis?

Film A is the chest X-ray of an Asian child who had emigrated to England. She had malaise and weight loss.

- What radiological features help you to make a diagnosis?

- What simple test will help to confirm the diagnosis?

Contact tracing was carried out and film B was the chest X-ray of one of her cousins.

- What does it suggest?

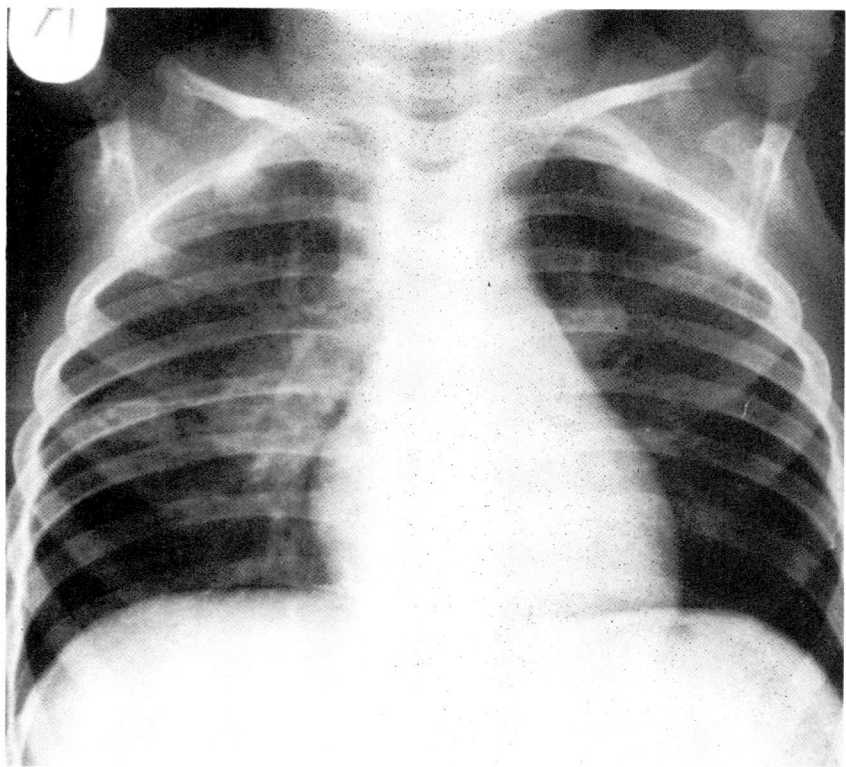

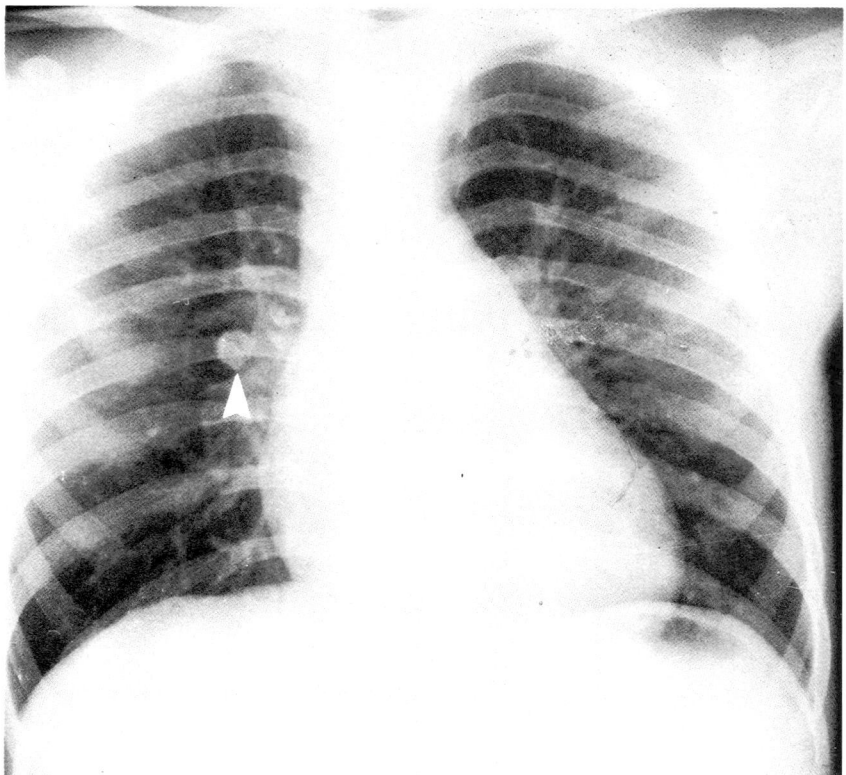

A

B

A32

This patient has cystic fibrosis. The heart is relatively small due to hyperinflation of the lungs. The hilar glands are enlarged due to infection. Peribronchial thickening extends from the hilar region towards the periphery. Multiple small opacities extend throughout both lung fields during episodes of acute infection.

In the periphery of the lung many ring shadows are visible.

A33

The patient had tuberculosis. The chest X-ray shows right hilar and paratracheal lymph node enlargement and a primary focus in the right mid-zone following tuberculosis infection. This was confirmed by a strongly positive reaction to a Mantoux test.

In approximately 60% of children the primary lesions of TB in the lungs are detected, not as a result of symptoms but on routine survey of schoolchildren or contacts.

Her cousin has a small calcified gland in the right hilum (arrowed, Film B) and a strongly positive Mantoux test.

The recognition of primary lesions may not be easy. The radiological appearance may resemble other types of inflammatory disease.

Q34

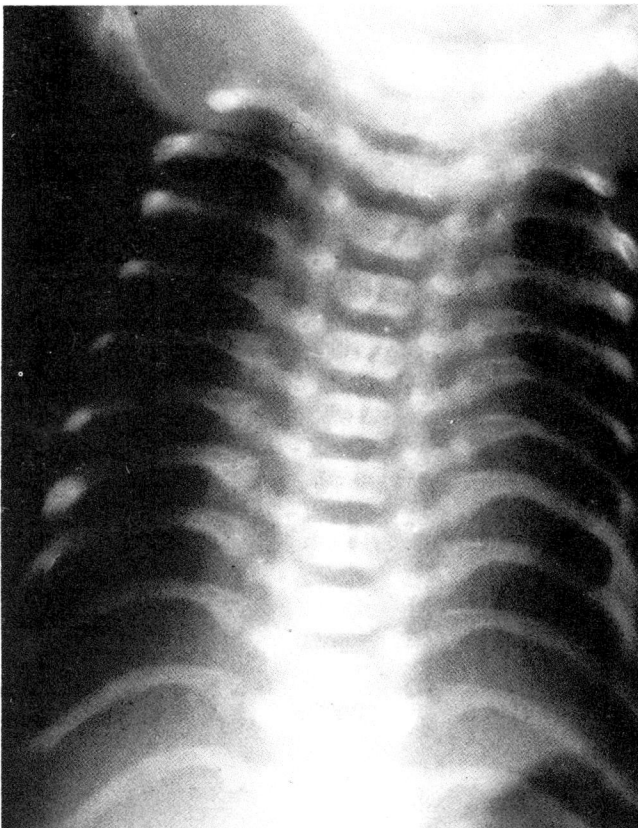

This is the chest X-ray of a child who was in extreme respiratory distress with severe tachypnoea.

- Describe the X-ray.
- What is your differential diagnosis?

Chest X-ray showed this child to have a persistent hyperlucent left lung. A diagnosis of McLeod's syndrome was made.

- What is the differential diagnosis in this case?

- What is the commonest cause of McLeod's syndrome?

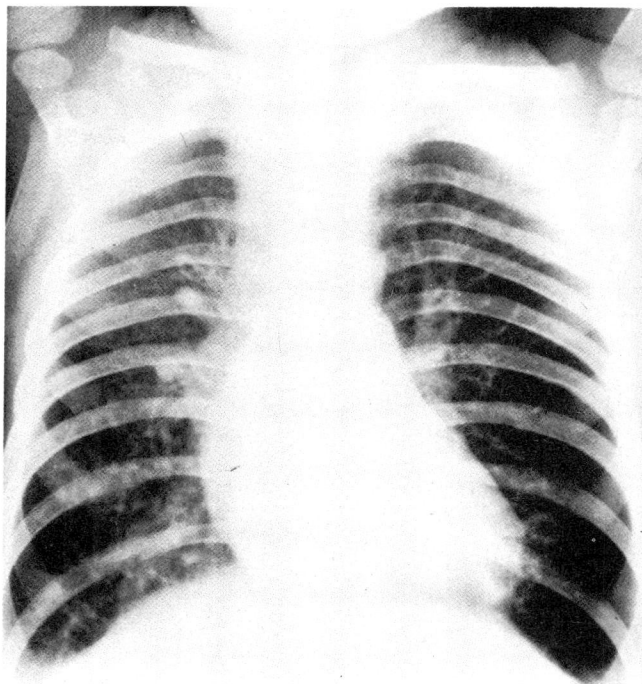

Q36

This child presented at 6 weeks of age with a paroxysmal cough, tachypnoea, diffuse rales and conjunctivitis. The patient was afebrile. Investigations revealed a peripheral blood eosinophilia and elevation of immuno-globulins IgG and IgM. The conjunctivitis did not respond to neomycin eyedrops.

- What is the likely diagnosis?

- What is the probable cause of the conjunctivitis and how would you treat it?

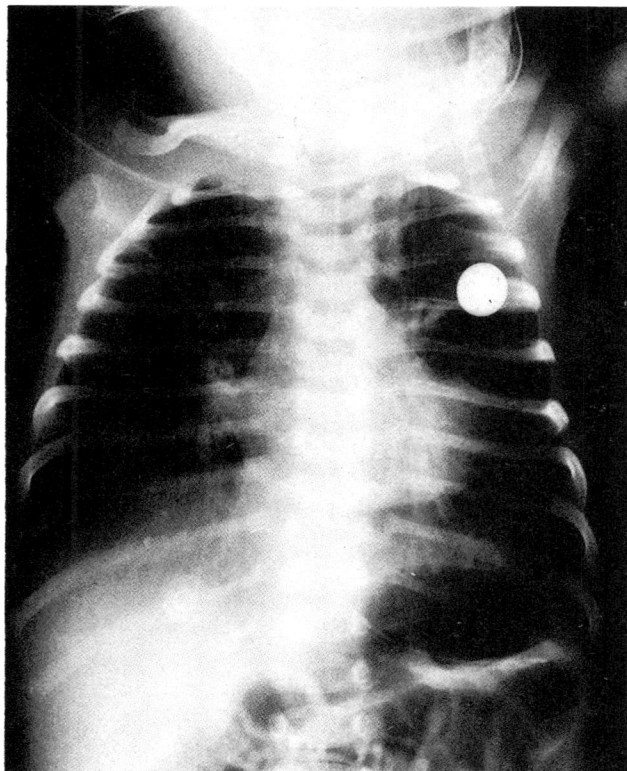

A34

This child has a short-ribbed asphyxiating thoracic dystrophy. The ribs are short but the spine is normal. In 1954 Jeune described a generalised chondrodystrophy with a small thorax. These children may die in infancy from respiratory failure. However, after the first year of life the respiratory problems decrease due to the improved growth of the thorax and lungs, and a normal life span may be possible.

The patients are short with some shortening of the limbs. Renal cystic dysplasia may be present and lead to renal failure and hypertension. The condition is thought to be autosomal recessive.

The differential diagnosis includes other bone dysplasias with a small thorax, namely:
— Ellis van Creveld syndrome
— thanatophoric dwarfism
— metatropic dwarfism
— diastrophic dwarfism
— Achondrogenesis II.

A35

In McLeod's syndrome one lung is small and hyperlucent, the other is radiologically normal.

It is most important to remember that not all children with one hyperlucent lung have this condition. The most common cause of this appearance is a patient rotated at the time of filming. Full investigation of these children is needed to exclude a treatable cause. Endoscopy may show bronchial stenosis, segmental bronchomalacia and an inhaled foreign body. A bronchogenic cyst compressing a bronchus may be responsible for air trapping. In these conditions the hyperlucent lung is usually the larger as in this case. This patient had a bronchogenic cyst not seen on the AP chest X-ray but revealed by barium swallow.
Rarely, congenital lobar emphysema or a large lung cyst may appear as a hyperlucent lung.

In McLeod's syndrome there is overdistension of the alveoli in the affected lung and decreased pulmonary blood flow with a relatively small pulmonary vascular tree. It is due to an obliterative bronchiolitis complicating viral infection in infancy. The most common cause is adenovirus infection followed by *Mycoplasma pneumoniae* infection.

A36

Towards the end of the 1970s *Chlamydia trachomatis* was recognised as a cause of pneumonia in infants less than 6 months of age.

It is acquired from the mother's genital tract. Infants usually present between 4 and 16 weeks of age with an 'afebrile pneumonia'. A chlamydial conjunctivitis is present in up to half of the infants with pneumonia. The other typical features are as in the question. Most chest X-rays show, as in this case, bilateral hyperexpansion. Also diffuse infiltrates show a variety of radiographic patterns including reticular nodular, atelectasis and bronchopneumonia. Pleural effusions or lobar consolidations are not found. The radiological features often suggest a more serious illness than observed clinically.

In infants aged 1-3 months and hospitalised with pneumonitis the clinical presentation and course, laboratory investigations and X-ray changes seen in infants with pneumonitis due to *Chlamydia trachomatis* also occur in those with *Pneumocystis carinii*, cytomegalovirus and possibly *Ureaplasma urealyticum* infections.

In this patient conjunctivitis was caused by *Chlamydia* which is not sensitive to neomycin. Oral erythromycin, and chloramphenicol eye drops, were curative. Erythromycin eliminates the organism from the respiratory tract secretions and may significantly shorten the course of chlamydial pneumonia.

Mother and partner also require treatment.

This neonatal patient was found to be acidotic.

- What is the cause of her acidosis?

- What treatment is required?

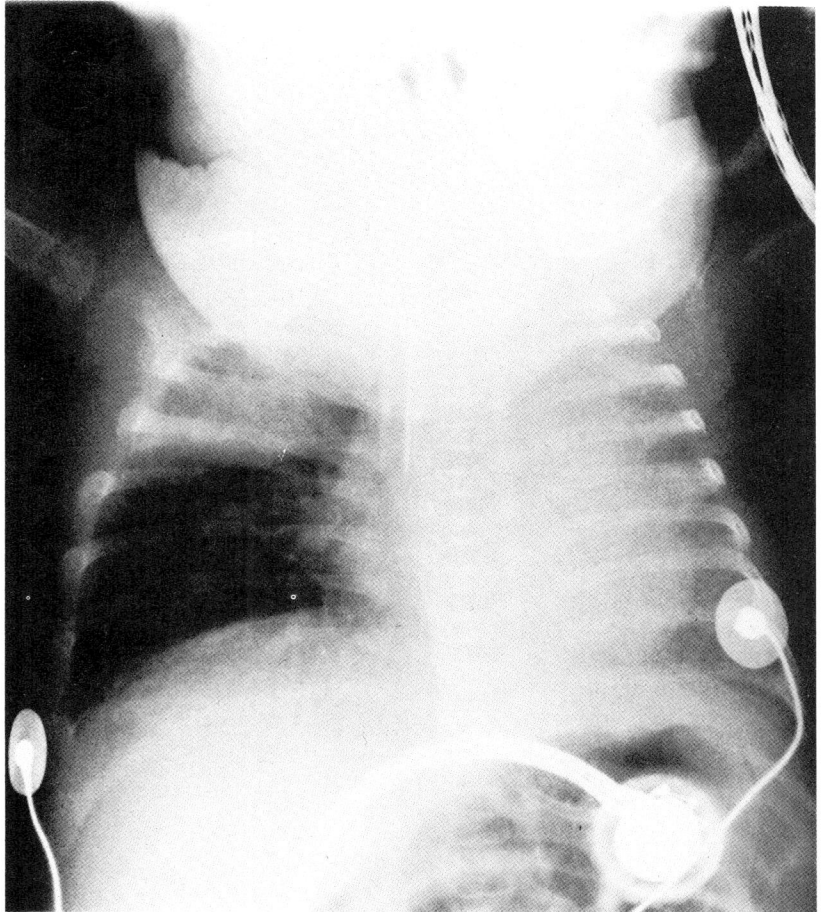

Q38

The mediastinum has a distinctive shape.

- What is the cause of this?

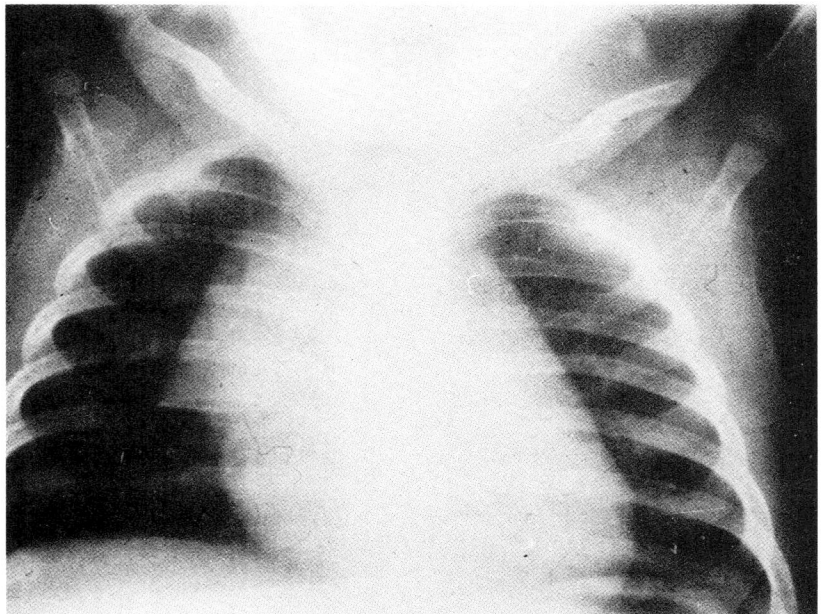

A37

The endotracheal tube has been pushed into the right main bronchus. There is collapse of the left lung and the right upper lobe. The acidosis is due to a high CO_2 level because of poor ventilation. Pulling the endotracheal tube back 2cm re-expanded the left lung and right upper lobe. The improved ventilation reduced the CO_2 level and corrected the respiratory acidosis.

A38

The thymus is seen as a triangular opacity in the upper mediastinum, with its basal angle projecting laterally over the lung field to give the well recognised 'sail' shape. On the lateral film the thymic shadow lies anteriorly behind the manubrium sternum. Thymic shadows in the mediastinum in infancy may cause difficulty in interpretation of the chest film. The thymus may present as a lateral convexity with no angle at all, or may just cause a general widening of the mediastinum. The thymus may be indented by the costochondral junctions resulting in a scalloped outline which confirms the opacity lies in the anterior mediastinum. The thymus is visible radiologically in over 50% of neonatal patients of normal birth weight.

The thymus is very sensitive to protracted stress and may atrophy following infection and starvation. The thymus often hypertrophies with recovery of the patient and may occasionally appear pathologically enlarged.

The differential diagnosis of such a shadow includes cysts and tumours of the anterior mediastinum, segmental consolidation of the upper lobes and aberrant thyroid tissue. Distension of the superior vena cava in some cases of total anomalous pulmonary venous drainage widens the upper mediastinum.

This child presented with tachypnoea.

- What is your differential diagnosis of a mass in this part of the mediastinum?

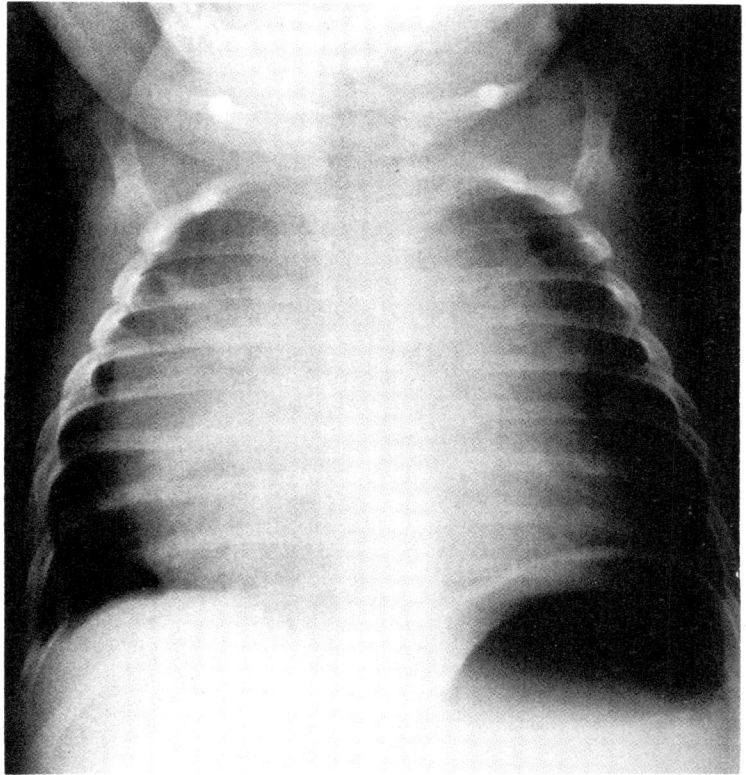

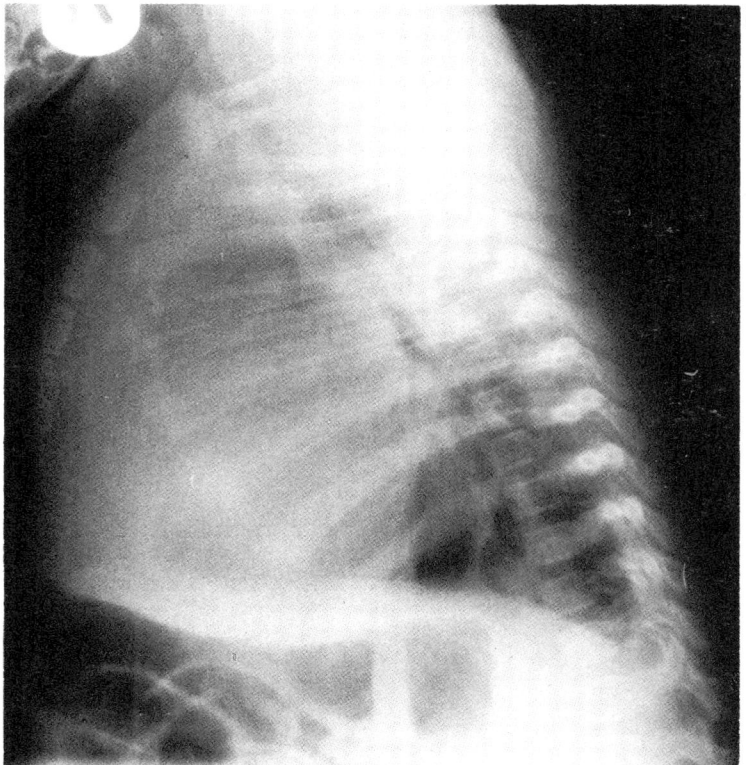

A39

The chest X-ray shows a massively enlarged mediastinal shadow. The lung fields are normal. The lateral X-ray confirms that the mass occupies the anterior mediastinum.

The differential diagnosis of masses in the anterior mediastinum in children include:
— teratoma
— thymoma
— thyroid
— lymph node enlargement either by infection or malignancy
— cystic hygroma extending down from the neck.

If the mass is lower in the mediastinum the following should be considered:
— pericardial cyst
— fat pad
— Morgagni hernia.

In this case a CT scan revealed a mass which appeared separate from the heart and lying in the right side of the chest. At operation a very large bilobed smooth teratoma was removed. Histology showed it to have many cysts and a wide range of tissues. Malignancy is uncommon in such teratomas. They may be asymptomatic and even discovered on routine X-ray. Compression of adjacent structures causes dyspnoea, cough, stridor, wheeze, cyanosis, and engorgement of head and neck veins. Symptoms are more often seen when large tumours occur in small infants, as in this case.

A

B

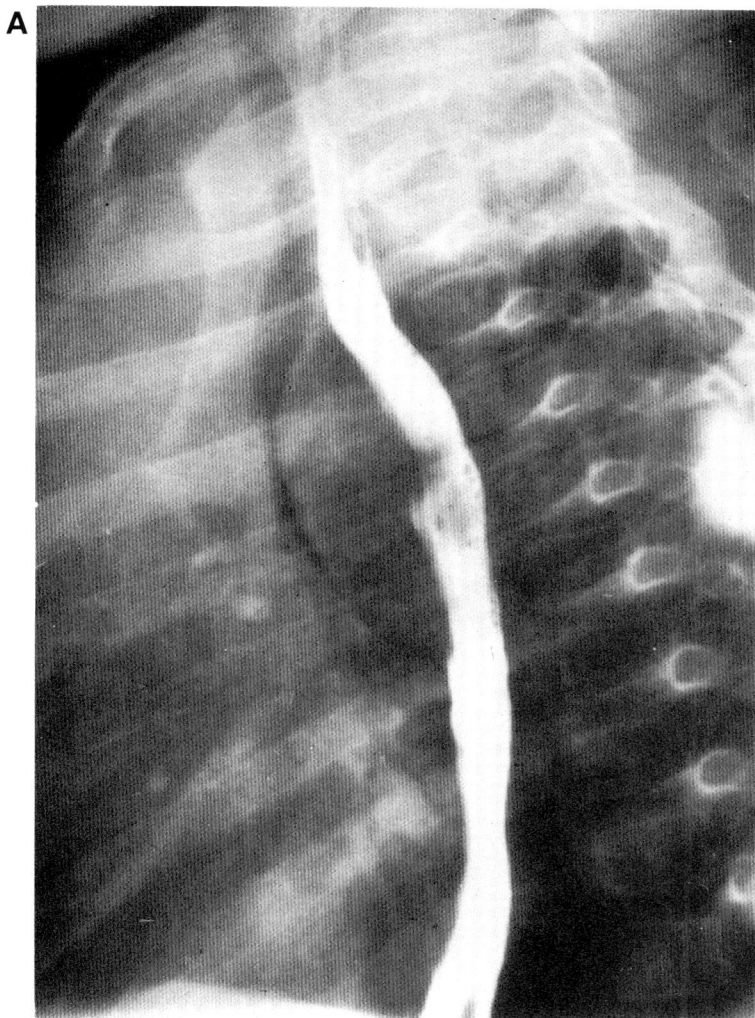

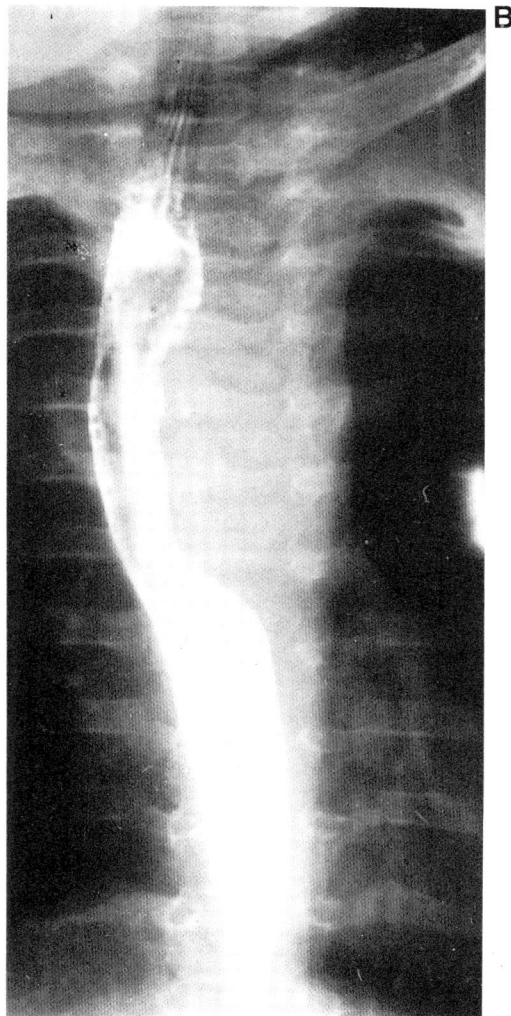

This child had cough and 'wheeze'. She failed to respond to anti-asthma therapy and was investigated further.

- What investigation has been performed and what does it show?

- What is the differential diagnosis of a mass in this part of the mediastinum?

A40

The barium swallow shows that the oesophagus from the level of the aortic arch to just below the carina is bowed to the right. The lateral film shows the oesophagus to be bowed backwards and the trachea bowed forward and narrowed. There is a mass between the oesophagus and trachea. At thoracotomy a bronchogenic cyst was found to be compressing the trachea from behind causing stridor. In many patients with a bronchogenic cyst the typical plain chest X-ray shows hyperinflation of one lung. This may be intermittent. The cyst itself may be seen on a plain chest radiograph. Barium swallow shows most foregut 'duplication cysts' particularly on lateral projection, as here. Treatment is surgical.

The differential diagnosis of masses in the middle mediastinum include:
— oesophagus – duplication cysts
— great vessels – aneurysmal dilatation
— hila – enlarged lymph nodes, leukaemia, lymphoma, tuberculosis etc
— trachea – bronchogenic cysts.

Q41

A

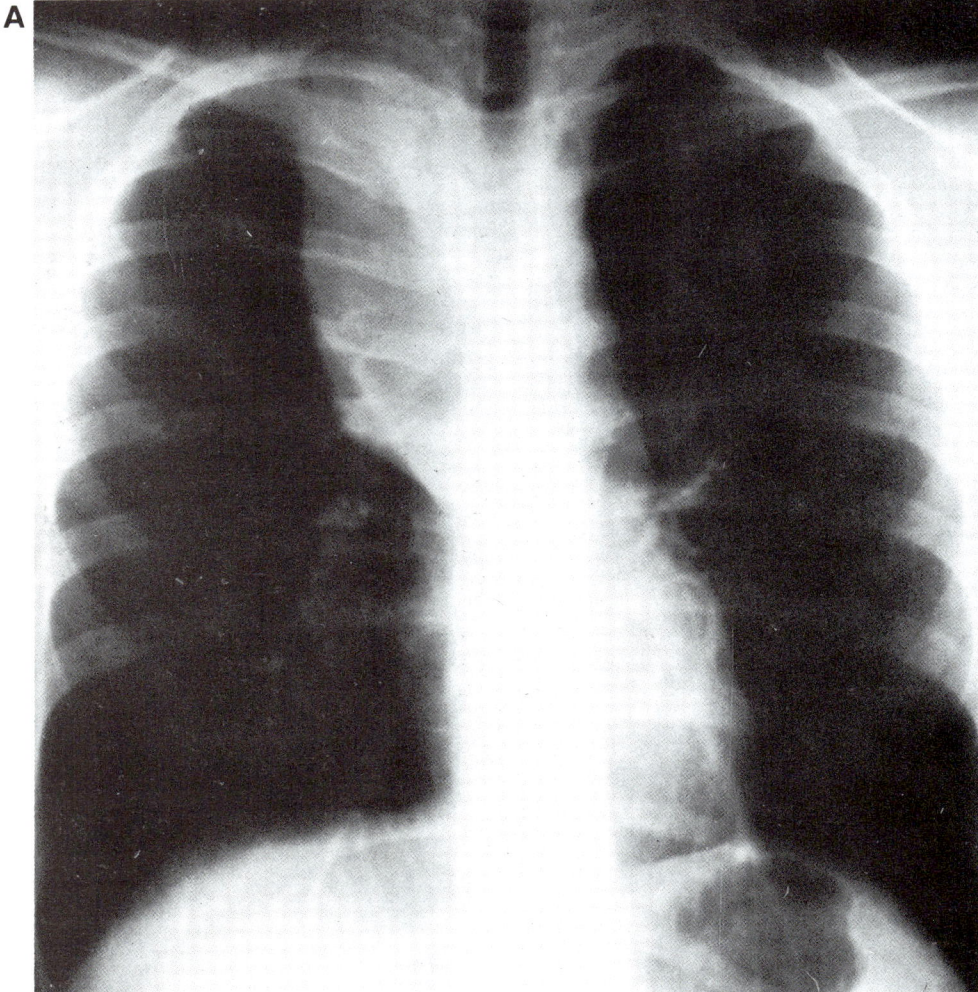

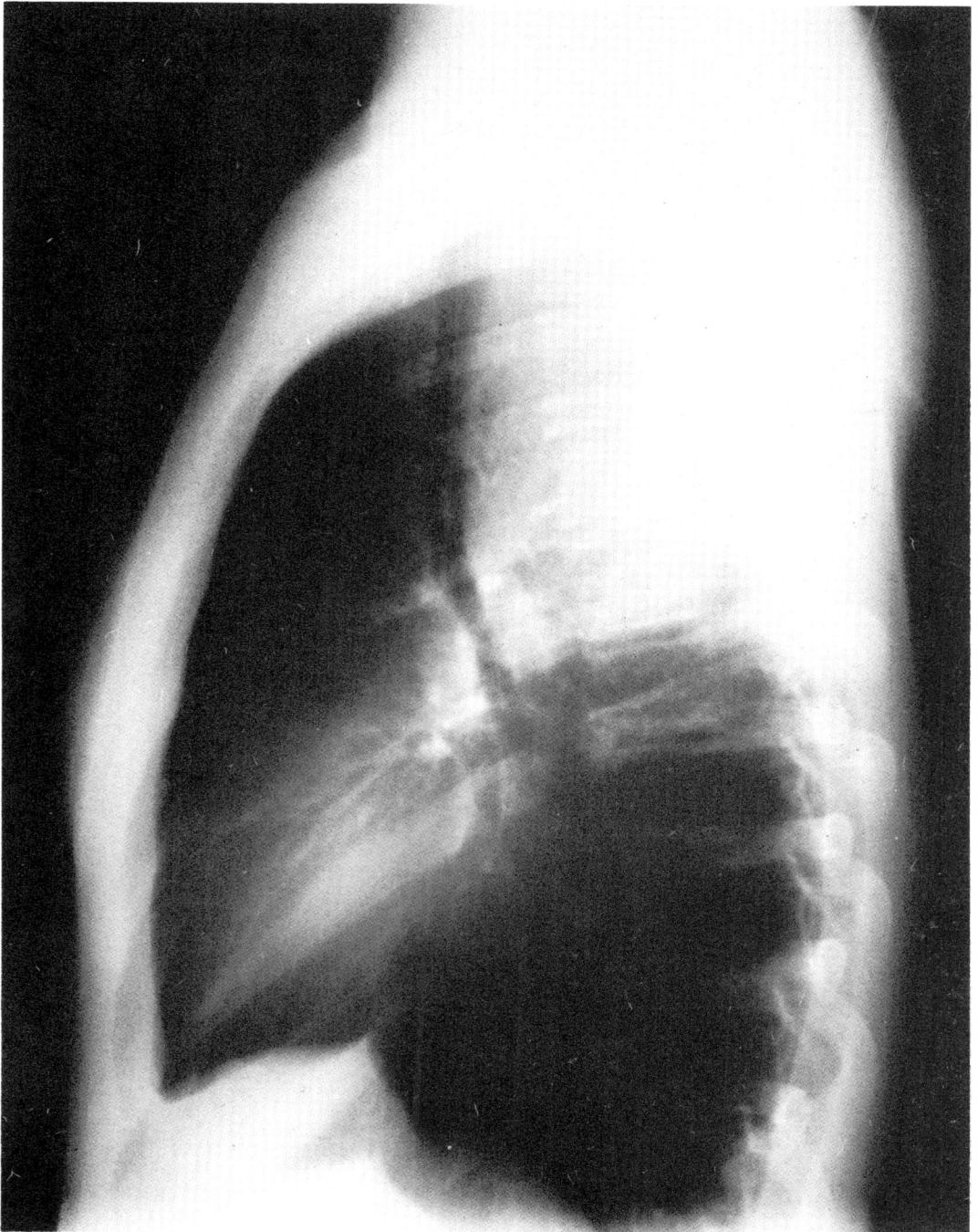

This 12 year old child had suffered from a cold hand since birth and this chest X-ray was taken to exclude a cervical rib.

- Describe the X-ray findings.

- What is your differential diagnosis?

A41

A right sided superior mediastinal mass is present. It lies posteriorly. There is widening of the intercostal space between the third and fourth ribs. There is no forward displacement of the trachea. The patient had no neurological signs.

The differential diagnosis of such a mass in the mediastinum includes:
— ganglioneuroma
— neuroblastoma
— neurofibroma
— spinal infectious disease, e.g. tuberculosis, which may produce a bilateral paravertebral mass.

A ganglioneuroma was excised. A ganglioneuroma is a benign tumour which typically arises in the paravertebral gutter and may also expand through a vertebral foramen into the spinal canal. This may result in two solid elements connected by a narrow isthmus in the intervertebral foramen, a so-called 'dumb-bell' tumour.

This 2 week old boy had tachypnoea shortly after birth which became worse, with recession and an asymmetrical chest. He was afebrile throughout the postnatal period. There was an expiratory wheeze over the right side of his chest.

- What is the diagnosis?
- Are further investigations required?
- What treatment do you recommend?

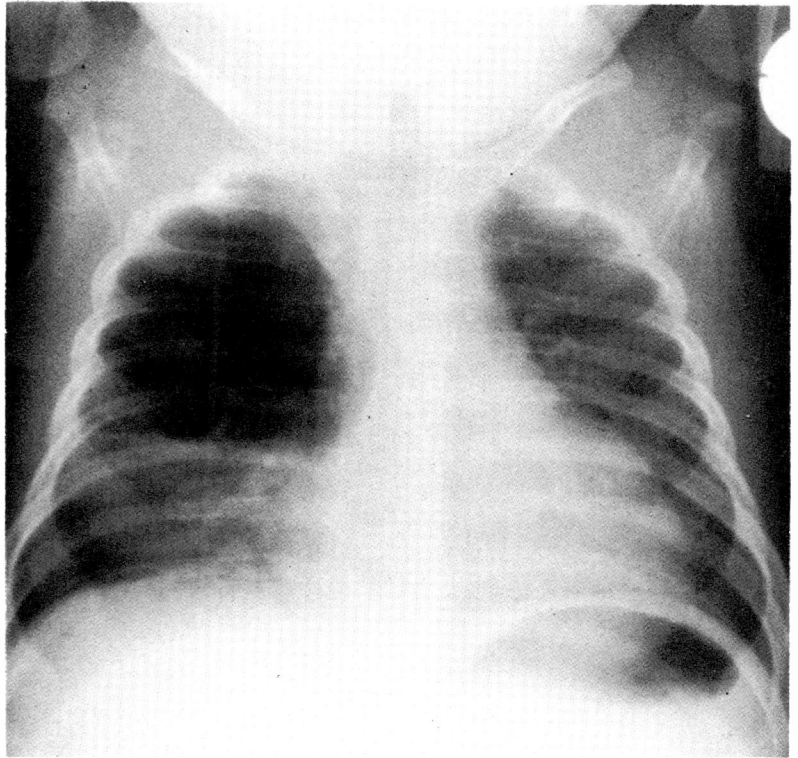

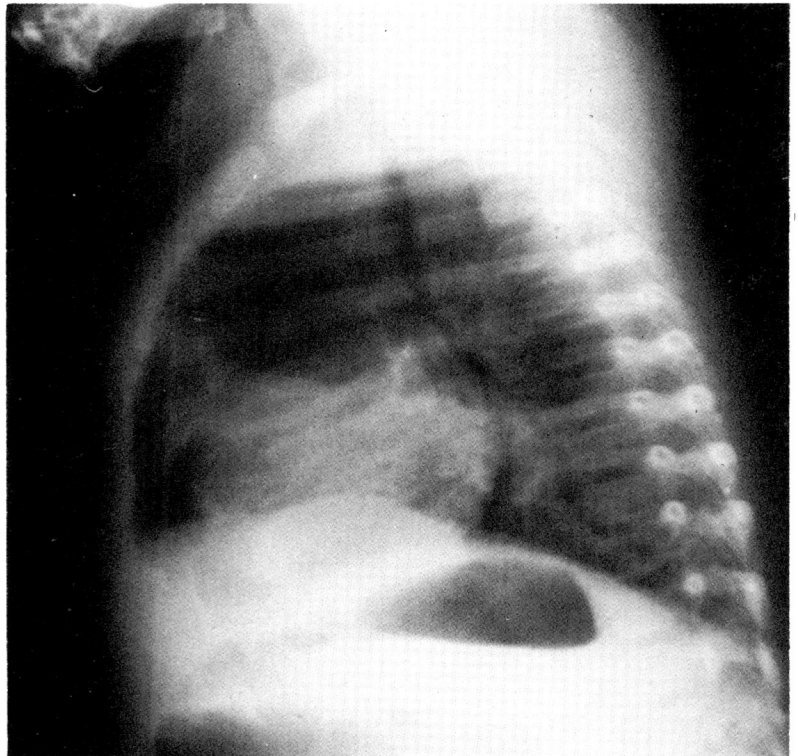

A

B

A42

The infant has congenital lobar emphysema. Chest X-ray shows a hyperinflated area in the right upper zone. It may be difficult to determine the lobar nature of the lesion. Adjacent lobes are compressed and the mediastinum displaced. The hyperinflated lobe often extends across the anterior mediastinum. In congenital lobar emphysema the involved lobe is massively and uniformly dilated. The most constant pathological finding is cartilage deficiency. About 14% have an associated cardiac anomaly which appears to be unrelated to the hyperinflated lobe.

This clinical picture associated with typical radiological findings and absence of respiratory infection allows the diagnosis to be made. Bronchography and bronchoscopy are hazardous in small infants and are contraindicated. Further air trapping in the affected lobe during anaesthesia may cause increasing respiratory distress. Fluoroscopy reveals air trapping at the site of hyperinflation with little change in volume during the respiratory cycle. A ventilation/perfusion scan may help in assessment when the need for surgery is in doubt.

Lobectomy is indicated in symptomatic infants. Percutaneous drainage prior to surgery is usually contraindicated.

Q43

A

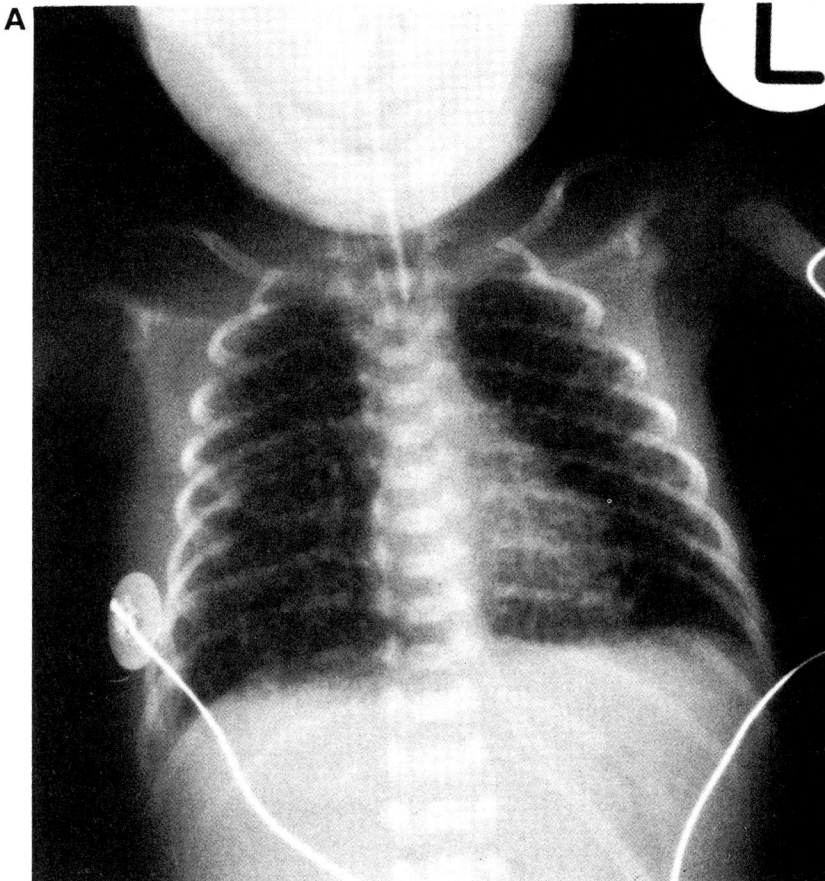

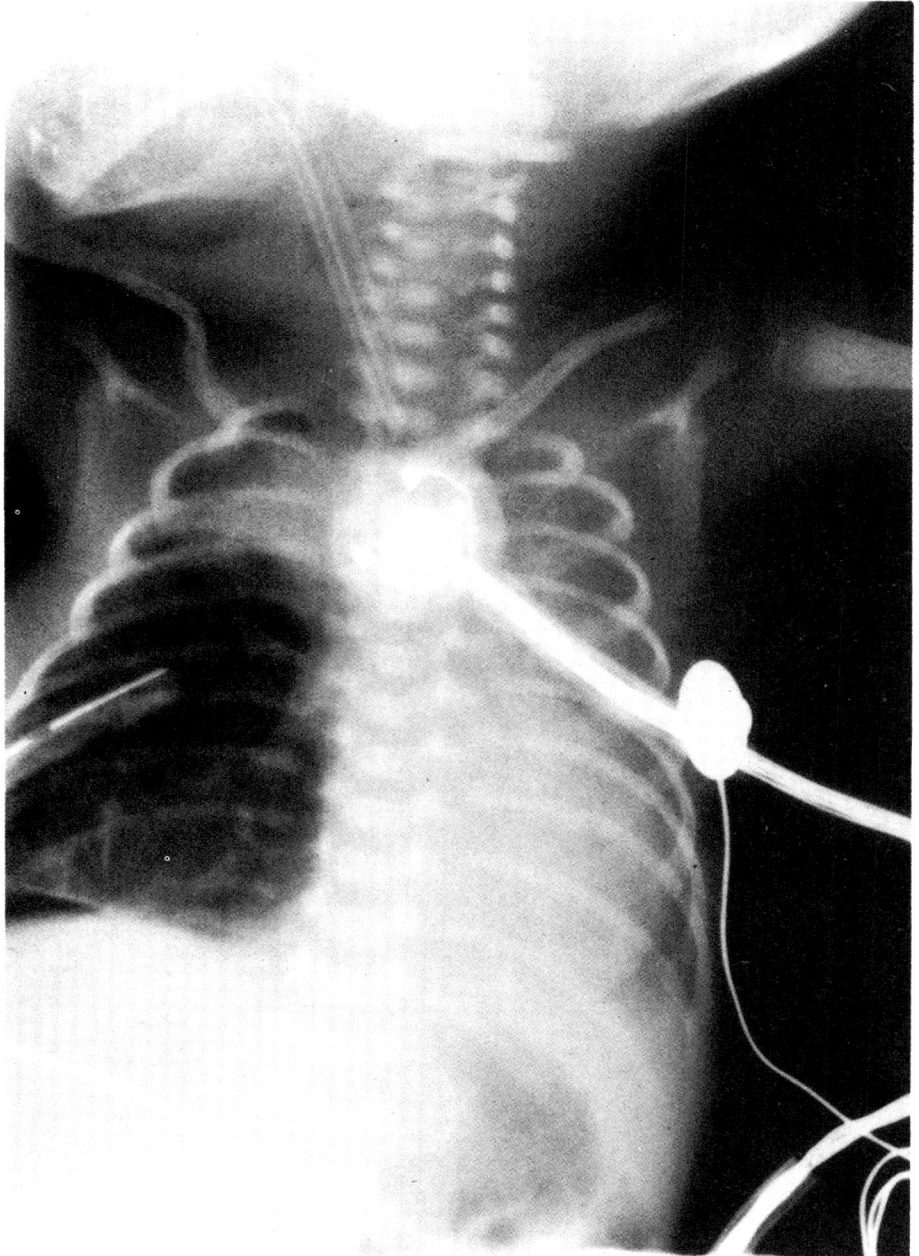

Film A is of a 10 day old premature baby. Ventilation was necessary from birth.

- What is the diagnosis?

- What are the possible outcomes of patient A's chest problem?

- Film B is of a premature baby on the same unit. A similar X-ray appearance to that seen in film A was noted 2 days before. What has happened?

A43

Film A: This premature baby developed respiratory distress syndrome (RDS) which required ventilation. Pulmonary interstitial emphysema (PIE) developed. PIE is commonly found in ventilated premature babies. When gas leaks out of an alveolus, in a neonate, it tracks along the lymphatics and bronchovascular bundle, only rarely rupturing subpleurally. If air is trapped within a bronchovascular bundle because of damage by IPPV or because there is more interstitial connective tissue in very premature lungs, PIE develops.

Radiologically PIE is recognised by two patterns. First, a linear pattern consisting of streaky radiolucent lines lacking the classic branching pattern of air bronchograms. Second, and much more common is a cystic pattern consisting of small rounded or oval lucencies.

There are three possible outcomes of PIE:
1 Resolution.
2 Pneumomediastinum, pneumopericardium and pneumothorax.
3 Progression in severity with emphysema.

X-ray B shows the patient has developed two complications of PIE, (1) a pneumothorax that has been drained and (2) an acquired lobar emphysema.

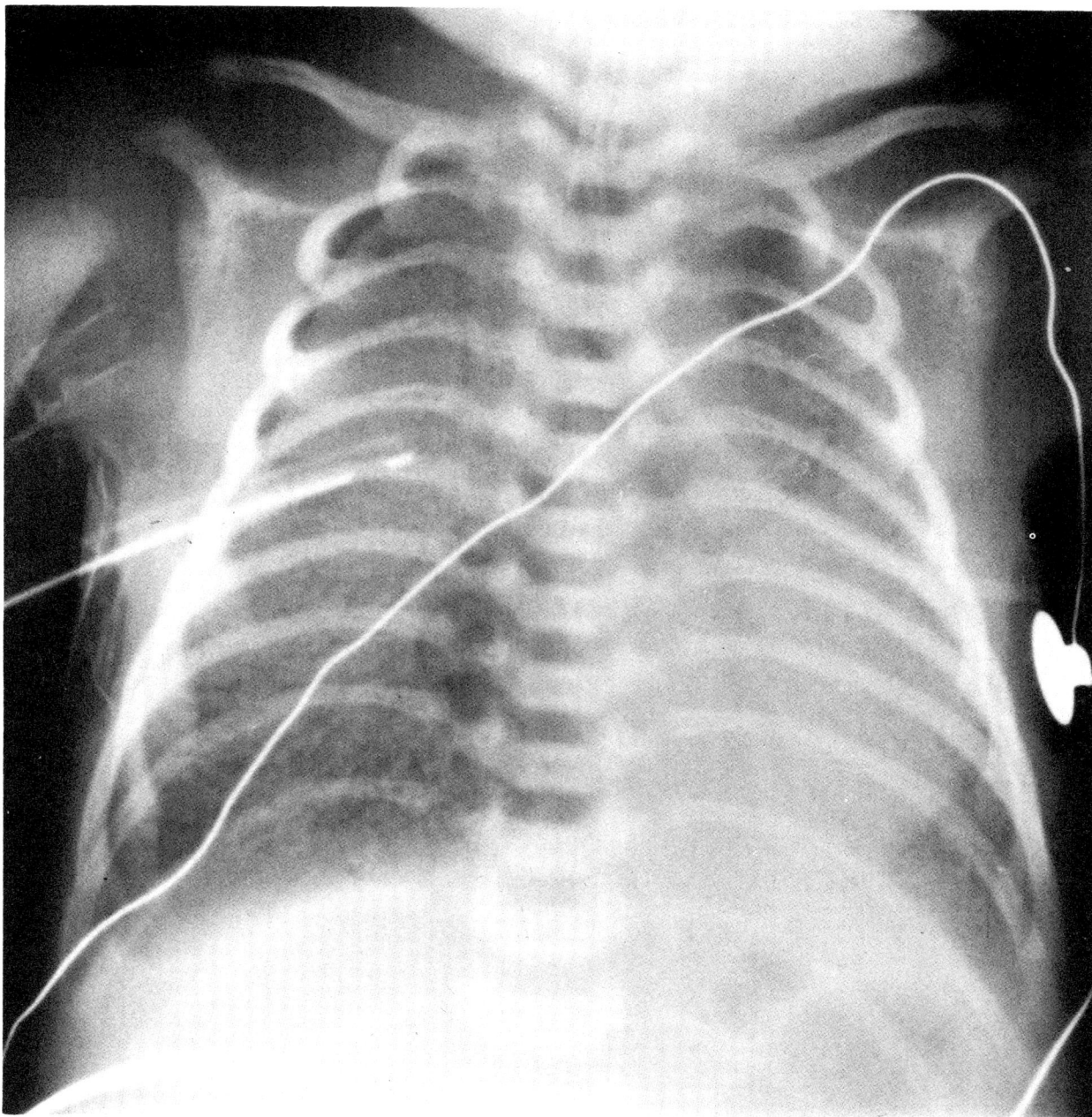

This neonatal patient was still difficult to ventilate following insertion of a chest drain for a tension pneumothorax.

- Describe the chest X-ray.

- What other investigation may help?

A44

This child is suffering from the respiratory distress syndrome (note the air bronchogram seen through the heart) and pulmonary interstitial emphysema. He is intubated and has an intercostal drain inserted. However the right pneumothorax has not been completely drained and the right diaphragm is depressed, indicating that tension may still persist on this side.

A lateral chest X-ray shows that the pneumothorax had not been fully drained (see free air anteriorly in Film B). Insertion of a further chest drain controls the pneumothorax.

In a lateral radiograph of a supine baby the air accumulates above the lung which is partially collapsed and lies at the back of the chest. The consequence is that in film A the large amount of air free in the pleural space and above the lung is not shown.

B

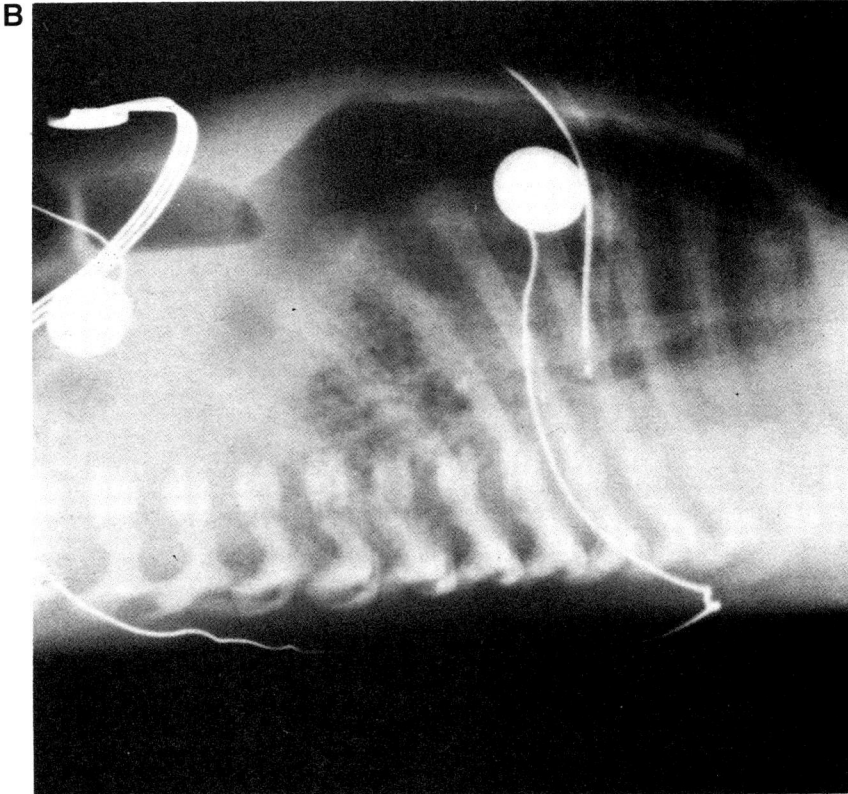

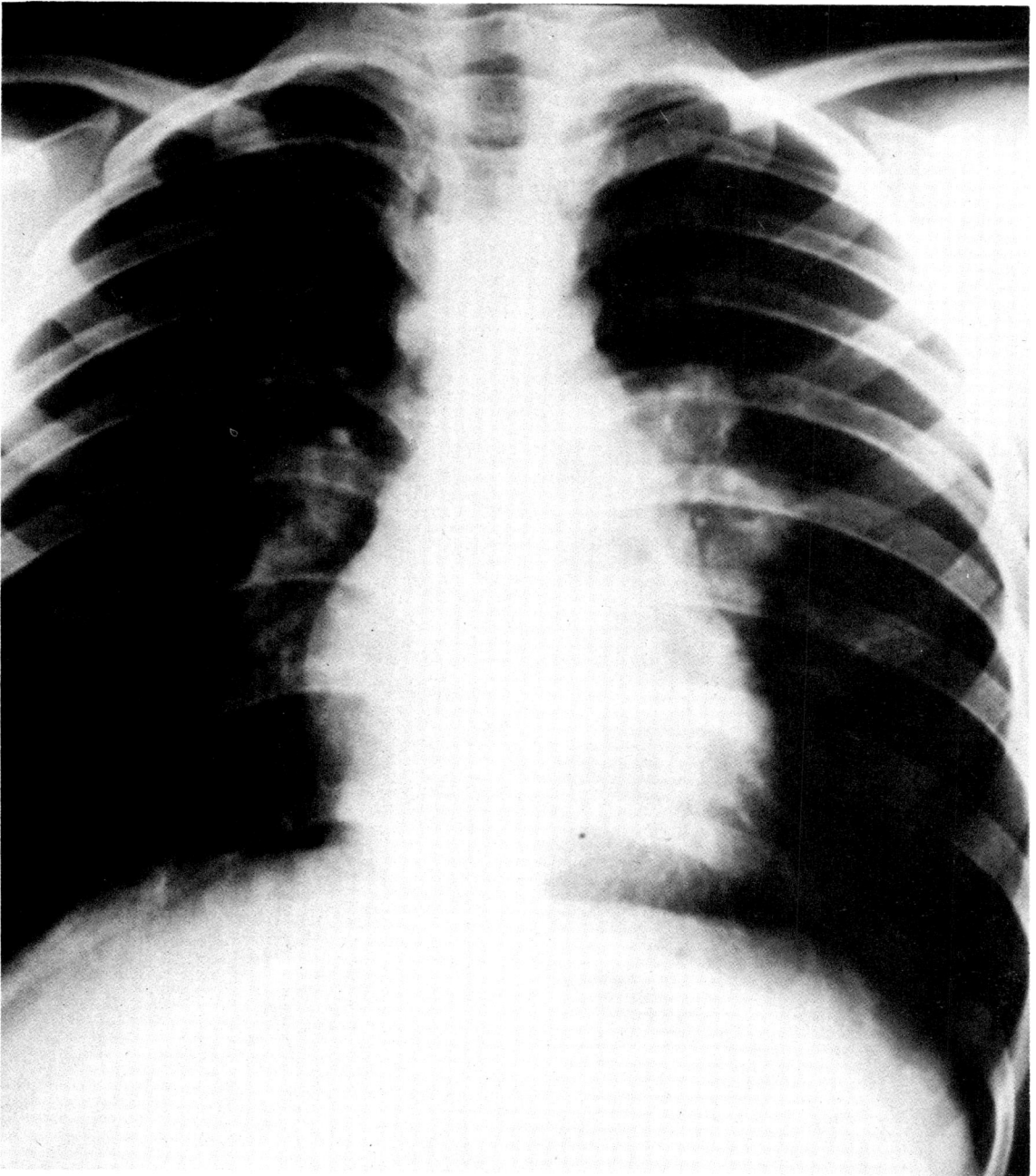

This is the chest X-ray of a young person suffering from uveitis. A Mantoux test was negative.

- What is the diagnosis?
- What treatment is required?
- What other symptoms may be present?

A45

This child had sarcoidosis and erythema nodosum. Large hilar nodes are seen on her chest X-ray. Sarcoidosis is a chronic non-caseating granulomatous disease with a predilection for intrathoracic organs, associated with depressed cell mediated immunity.

Uveitis and keratitis are the commonest eye signs and may lead to blindness, therefore systemic corticosteroids are indicated.

The radiological changes in sarcoidosis may be classified as:
Stage 1, hilar and mediastinal lymphadenopathy.
Stage 2, diffuse mottling and strand-like opacities also present.
Stage 3, diffuse pulmonary disease without lymphadenopathy.
Stage 4, bullae, fibrosis and emphysema.

Sarcoidosis may occur at any age but is more common in older children, adolescents and young adults. Fatigue, malaise, lethargy, weight loss, cough, fever, abdominal pain and peripheral lymphadenopathy are the commonest presenting symptoms. Hepatomegaly may be found and dyspnoea and chest pain may occur. Sarcoid is generally a benign disease in childhood and adolescence but some develop progressive lung disease.

Q46

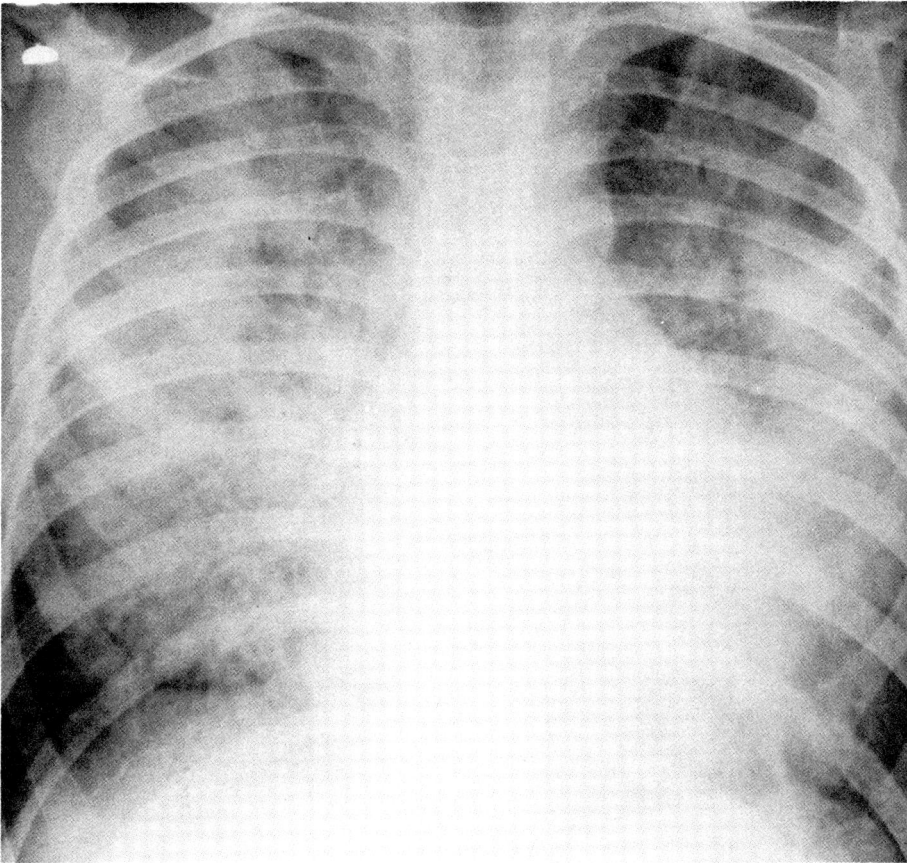

This child presented with haematuria and oliguria. A diagnosis of acute glomerulonephritis was made. His condition deteriorated and he became hypertensive.

- What does the chest X-ray show?
- What is the cause of this appearance?

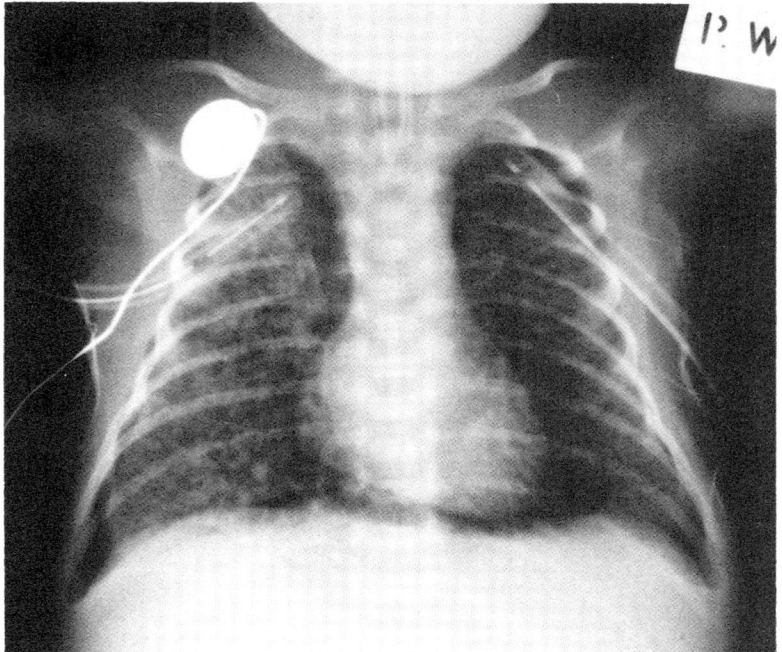

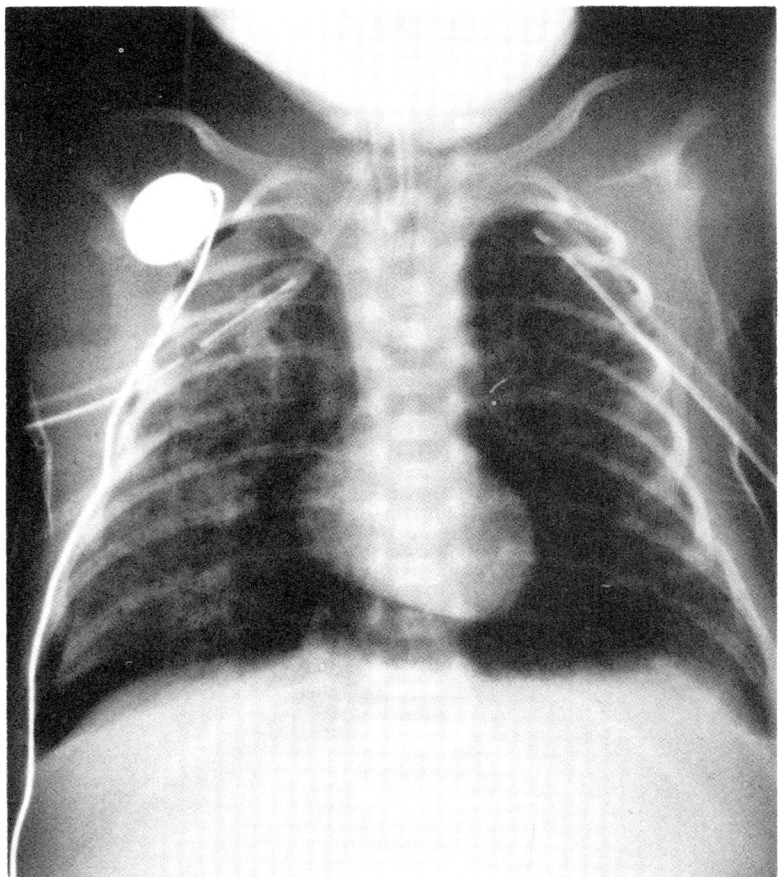

This premature baby had pulmonary interstitial emphysema.

Two hours after film A was taken she suddenly deteriorated.

- What has caused the deterioration? (Film B)

- How would you manage this child?

A46

The child is in acute heart failure. Severe bilateral pulmonary oedema is seen. When the excessive fluid in the lung is confined to the interstitial tissues, the radiographic appearance is a diffuse ground glass increase in density, initially perihilar. Hypervolaemia and oedema in acute glomerulonephritis is due to salt and water retention in the oliguric state before sodium and water have been restricted.

The child was also found to have a raised ASO titre consistent with the diagnosis of a post-streptococcal glomerulonephritis.

A47

Chest X-ray A shows the patient to be ventilated and have bilateral chest drains in situ. A pneumomediastinum can be clearly seen as a dark area around the heart. Collapse was due to cardiac tamponade produced by gross pneumomediastinum (film B).

Pneumomediastinum appears occasionally after the onset of pulmonary interstitial emphysema or other air leak and tends to be limited to infants who are being ventilated for severe respiratory disease. The diagnosis should be suspected whenever a severely ill ventilated neonatal patient shows rapid deterioration. Blood pressure drops rapidly due to cardiac tamponade as does Pao_2. Death may then occur quickly. Urgent needle aspiration of the air is required. If air reaccumulates a suction tube and drain may be required.

Other causes of a sudden deterioration include tension pneumothorax, blocked airway, intraventricular haemorrhage, cardiac arrhythmias, hypovolaemia, and cardiac failure.

- What abnormality is seen on this lateral chest X-ray?
- What may cause this condition?

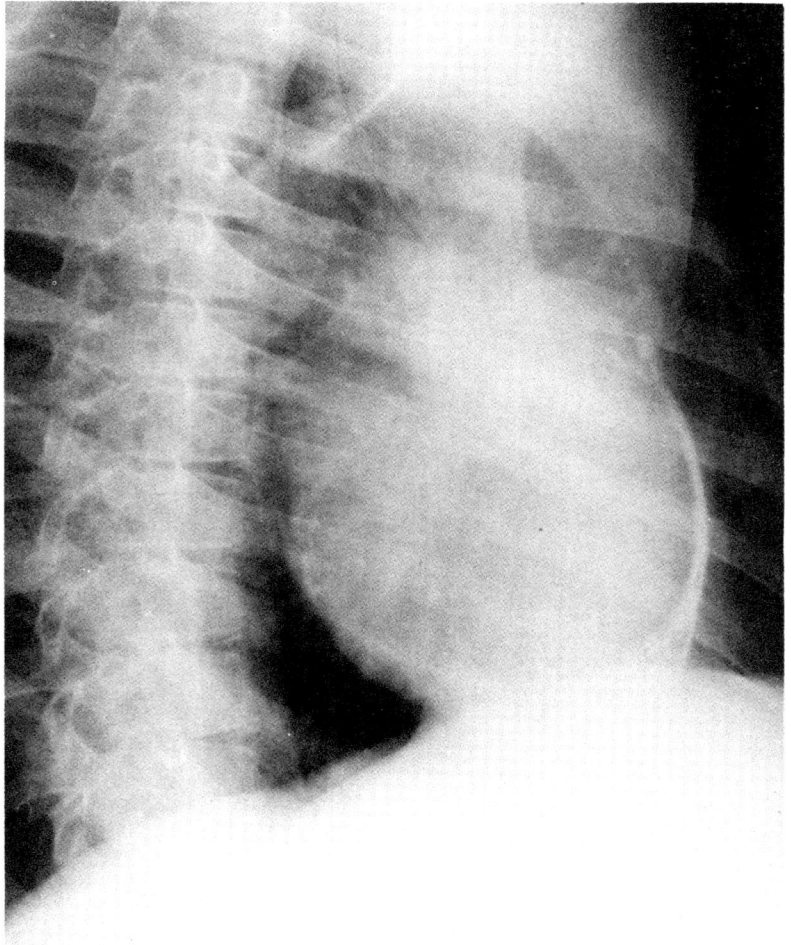

Q49

This is the chest X-ray of a child presenting to casualty following a road traffic accident.

- What is the likely diagnosis?
- What further investigation is indicated?

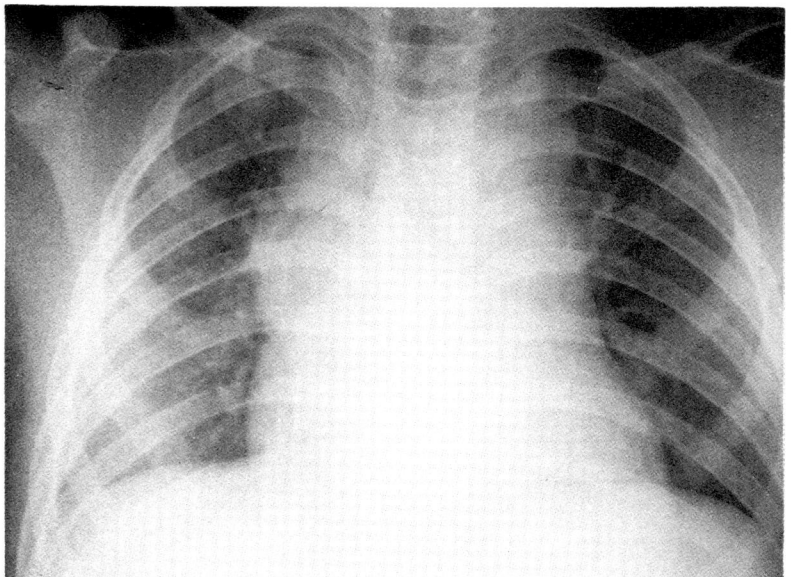

A

A48

The lateral chest X-ray shows pericardial calcification that is maximal along the anterior and inferior pericardial borders. It is often impossible to see the calcification on an anterior/posterior chest film but commonly it is well seen at fluoroscopy. Calcification usually occurs in a patchy nature even though the pericardium is often thickened and rigid all over the heart.

Calcification of the pericardium is usually post-infective in origin, with TB and Coxsackie infections being the commonest causes.

Calcific pericarditis is a feature of constrictive pericarditis which presents quite frequently with ascites. The detection of a raised JVP should alert the clinician to the diagnosis.

A49

The child has mediastinal widening following trauma. Aortography is indicated and has established the diagnosis of aortic rupture. Venous bleeding which does not require emergency surgery can cause similar radiological features.

Rupture of the aorta can occur with remarkably mild trauma. Fractures of the sternum or ribs may not be present. Occasionally, aortic rupture is diagnosed months or years after the injury when the development of an aneurysm is noted.

The thoracic aortogram demonstrates the aortic leak and almost complete transection just distal to the origin of the subclavian artery (film B).

Digital vascular imaging in a child may give similar information to that shown by this aortogram.

B

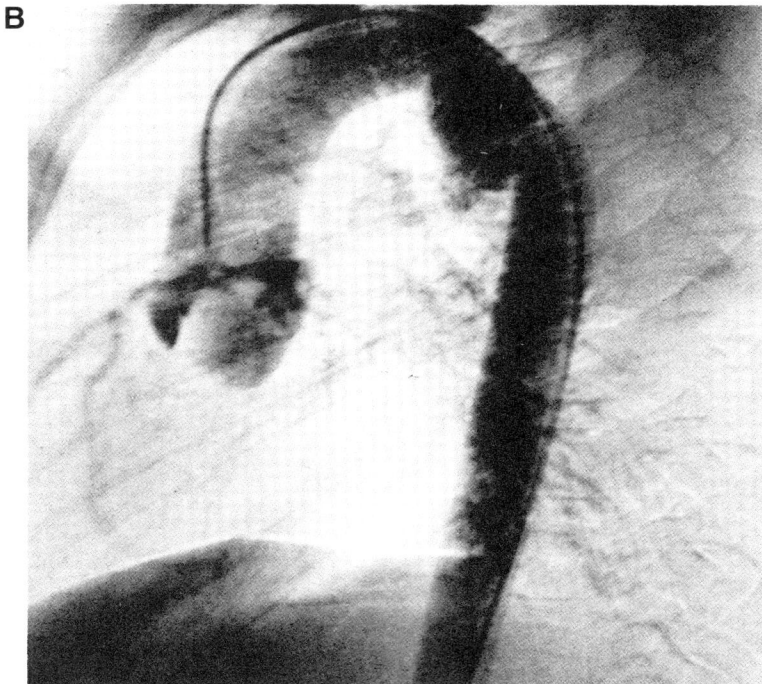

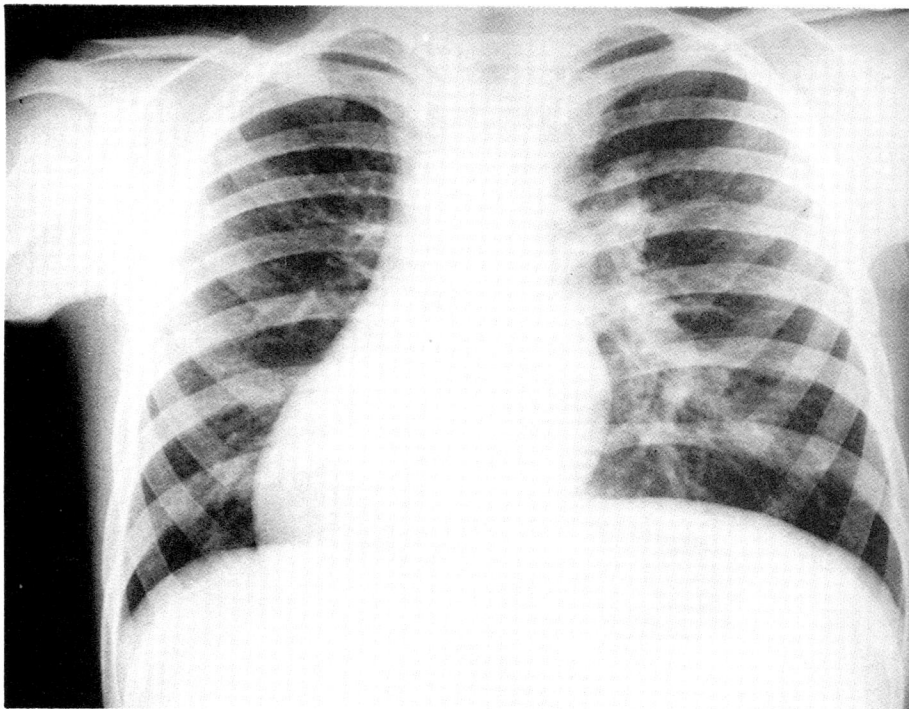

Q50

- Describe this child's chest X-ray.
- The heart was found to be a mirror image. Do you think the heart will be normal?

Q51

Film A is the chest X-ray of a 2 year old child with a history of marked snoring. A recent ECG demonstrated right atrial and right ventricular hypertrophy. Echocardiography revealed a structurally normal heart. She presented to casualty with increasing respiratory distress and cyanosis.

- Why is the child unwell?
- What is the underlying diagnosis?

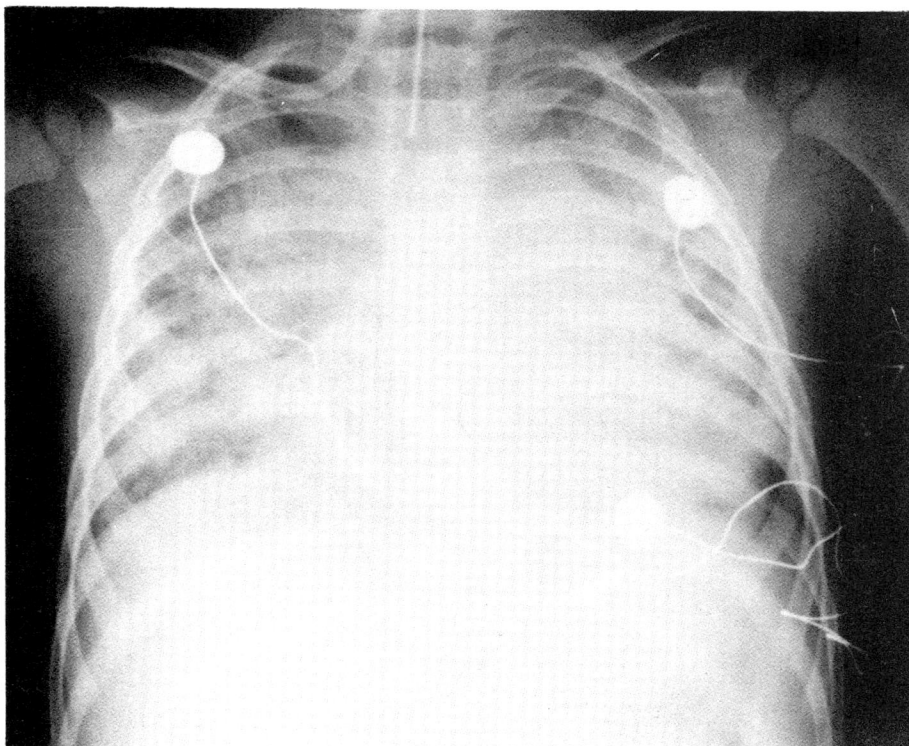

A

A50

This child has 'isolated dextrocardia' without transposition of the abdominal organs. In such circumstances the heart may be normal. If a cardiac lesion is present it is likely to be complex with transposition variants being among the lesions frequently seen. Such children may occasionally have asplenia or polysplenia, which may be indicated by the presence of Howell-Jolly bodies in the red blood cells.

It is of interest that the right diaphragm is lower than the left. The diaphragm is usually higher on the right because the heart pushes the left diaphragm down. In this case the right diaphragm is lower.

A51

The child has acute pulmonary oedema secondary to an obstructive sleep apnoea. The child has been intubated (Film A). Following ventilation with high positive and expiratory pressures and antifailure treatment her condition improved dramatically (Film B).

This child had an adenoidectomy for snoring 5 months previously when signs of pulmonary hypertension were noted. This resulted in some improvement. On this admission she was distressed and cyanosed with marked stridor.

Examination revealed the cause of her problems to be large tonsils meeting in the midline. After removal of her tonsils there were no further problems.

Many centres now routinely remove both tonsils and adenoids initially because of the possibility of subsequent tonsillar hypertrophy.

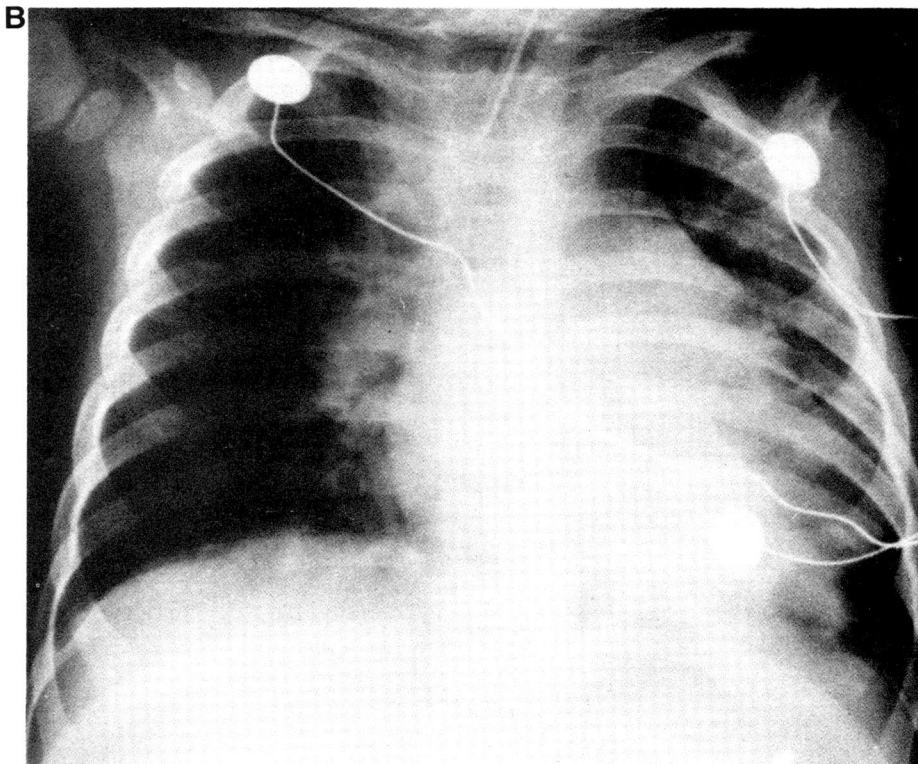

A

B

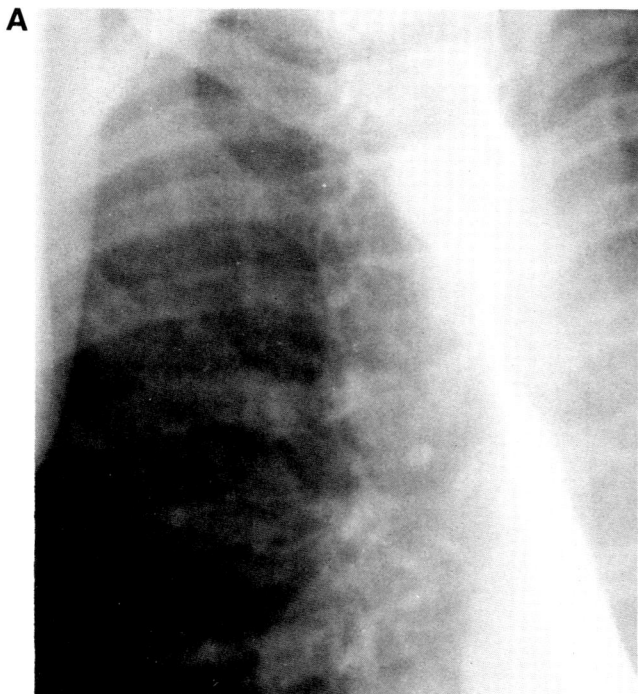

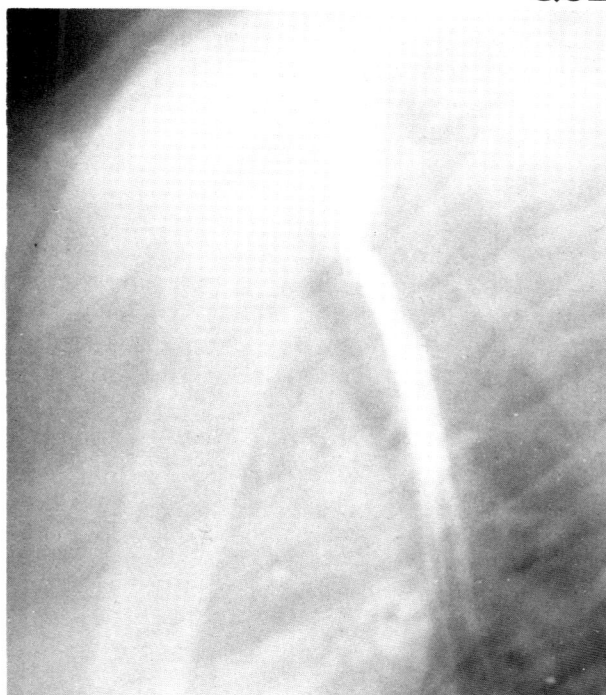

This child suffered from stridor since birth and recurrent lower respiratory tract infections.

- What investigation has been performed?
- What is the diagnosis?

Q53

A

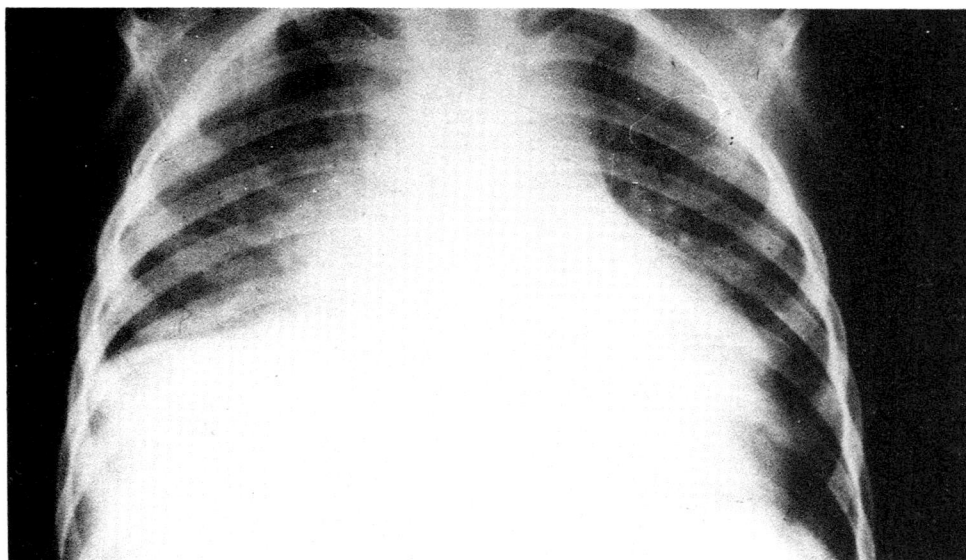

This chest X-ray was taken 5 days after successful repair of a ventricular septal defect.

- What abnormality is seen?
- How would a lateral decubitus film help with the diagnosis?

A52

A barium swallow has been performed and shows the child has a vascular ring. There is a posterior indentation of the oesophagus seen on the lateral film. There is an indentation to the right of the oesophagus at the level of the aortic arch seen on the PA film (right aortic arch). The diagnosis is either a double aortic arch or a right sided aorta with an aberrant left subclavian artery.

A53

The chest X-ray shows the presence of a large right subpulmonary effusion. A subpulmonary effusion is said to be present when there is free pleural fluid but little or no fluid is seen to run up the chest wall. The upper border of fluid is much the same shape as the normal diaphragm, and since the true diaphragmatic shadow is obscured by the fluid it may be difficult or impossible to tell from the standard erect film if any fluid is present at all (Film A). The diagnosis is confirmed by a lateral decubitus film where the pleural fluid moves to lie between the lateral chest wall and the lung edge (Film B).

Subpulmonary effusions occur after major heart surgery in up to 10% of children. The effusions are usually left sided. On the left side a clue to their presence is an increased distance between the lung and stomach bubble on an erect chest X-ray. They are also commonly seen in children with nephrotic syndrome.

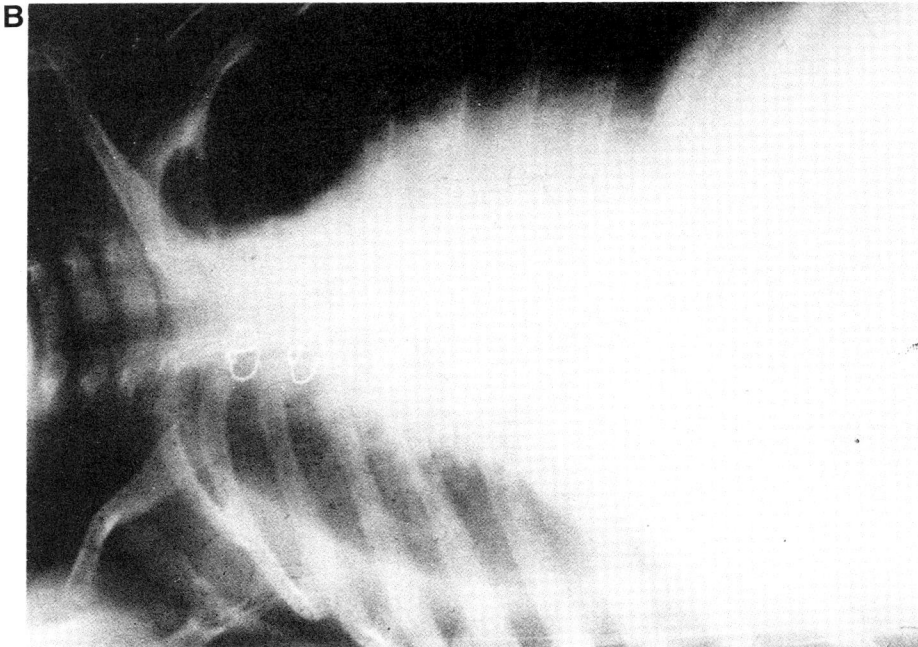

B

This child had a systolic ejection murmur in the pulmonary region, fixed splitting of the second heart sound, and a parasternal heave of right ventricular hypertrophy.

- What is a likely diagnosis?
- Describe the radiological findings and comment on the pulmonary vessel size.
- What ECG findings would you expect?

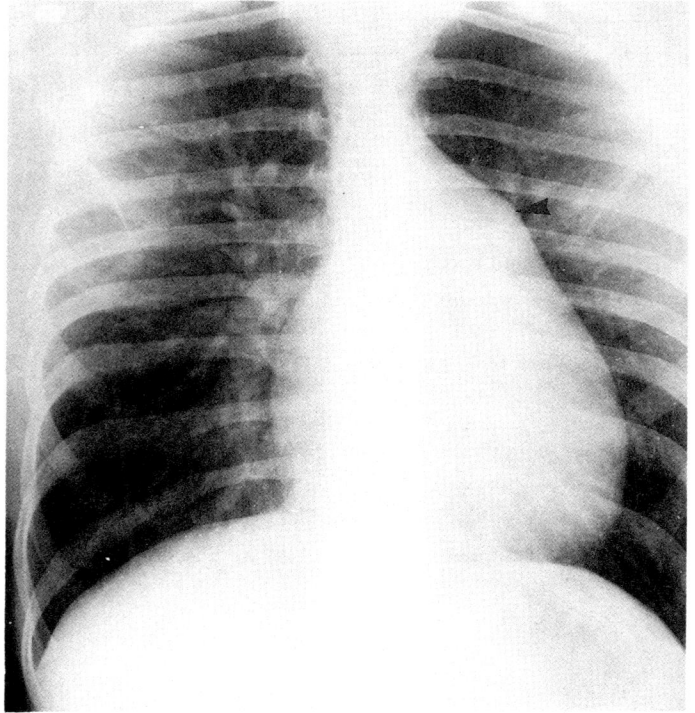

A

Q55

This child presented with cough and pyrexia. There was a past history of recurrent chest infections and sinusitis.

- Describe the radiological findings.
- What is the most likely diagnosis?
- What additional investigation will confirm the diagnosis?

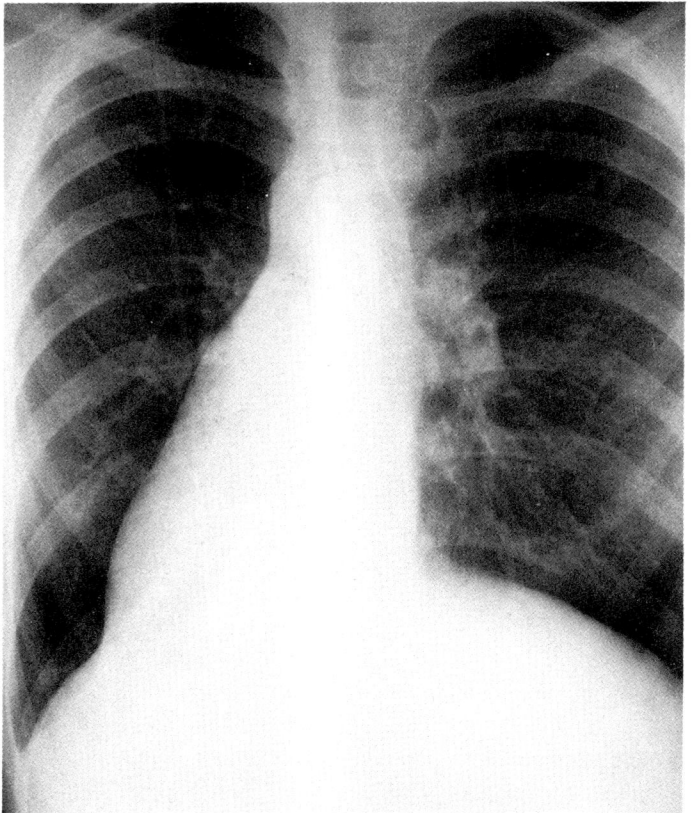

A54

This young girl has an atrial septal defect. The plain film of the chest shows a heart with a slightly increased transverse diameter. Both lateral borders of the heart are convex due to enlargement of the right atrium, right ventricle and right ventricular outflow tract. This has dilated causing a bulge obliterating the normal concavity of the left atrial appendage (arrowed).

The ECG findings are; right axis deviation, right atrial and right ventricular hypertrophy, first degree atrioventricular block, and incomplete right bundle branch block. The latter ECG finding is almost always present in cases of atrial septal defects. At cardiac catheterisation the pulmonary systemic blood flow ratio was greater than 2:1 and the defect was subsequently closed by direct suture.

A55

The child has dextrocardia associated with transposition of all the thoracic organs. He also had abdominal situs inversus but this cannot be seen on this film. There is collapse of the lower lobe of the right lung, which has only an upper and lower lobe due to transposition of the thoracic organs. These findings are suggestive of Kartagener's syndrome which was first described in 1933 as the combination of situs inversus, bronchiectasis and sinusitis. Inheritance is autosomal recessive and there may be considerable phenotypic variation. The basic defect appears to be due to a primary ciliary abnormality, such as a deficiency of the dynein arms of the microtubule doublets of the cilia.

A nasal biopsy of ciliated cells studied under the electron microscope will reveal ultrastructural abnormalities. In some centres facilities are available for assessing the beat frequency of the cilia and can be used to screen for samples needing study by electron microscopy. The abnormal cilia have a lower beat frequency.

Associated cardiac abnormalities are uncommon.

Film B is a bronchogram of another patient with Kartagener's syndrome showing bronchiectasis in the right lower lobe.

B

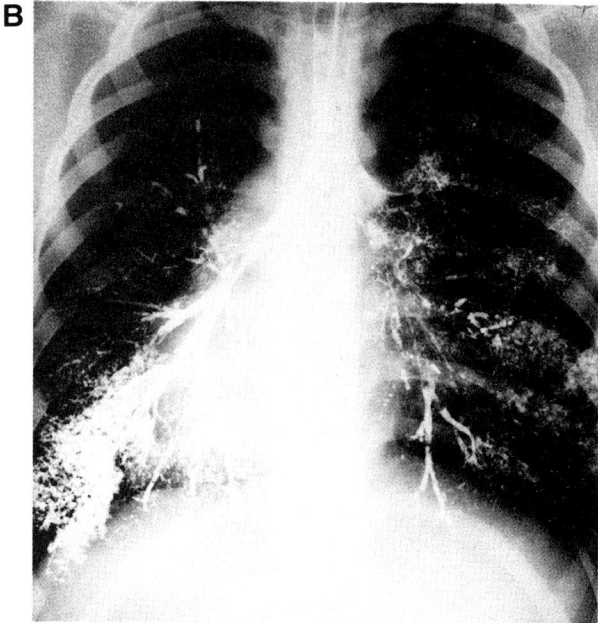

A

Patient A presented shortly after birth with cyanosis and dyspnoea. A very loud pulmonary component of the second heart sound was heard. Patient B was older than patient A, had mild cyanosis and was not ill. He had physical signs similar to an ASD. A nitrogen wash-out test confirmed arterial desaturation with a Pa_{O_2} < 150 mm Hg in 100% oxygen.

- Describe the X-ray findings of the two patients.

- What abnormality do they have in common?

- Why is their presentation different?

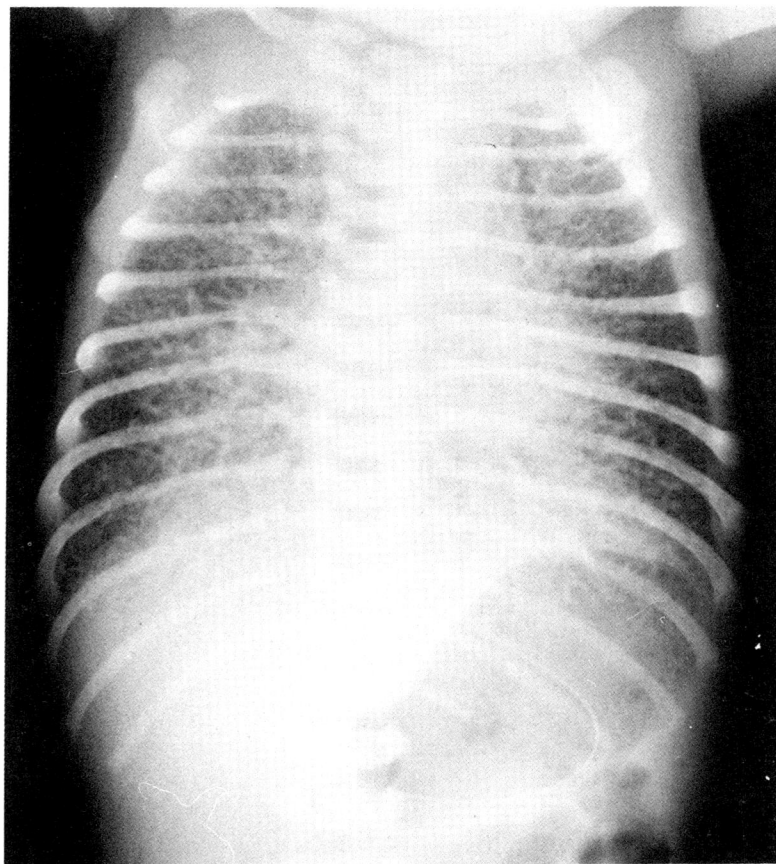

B

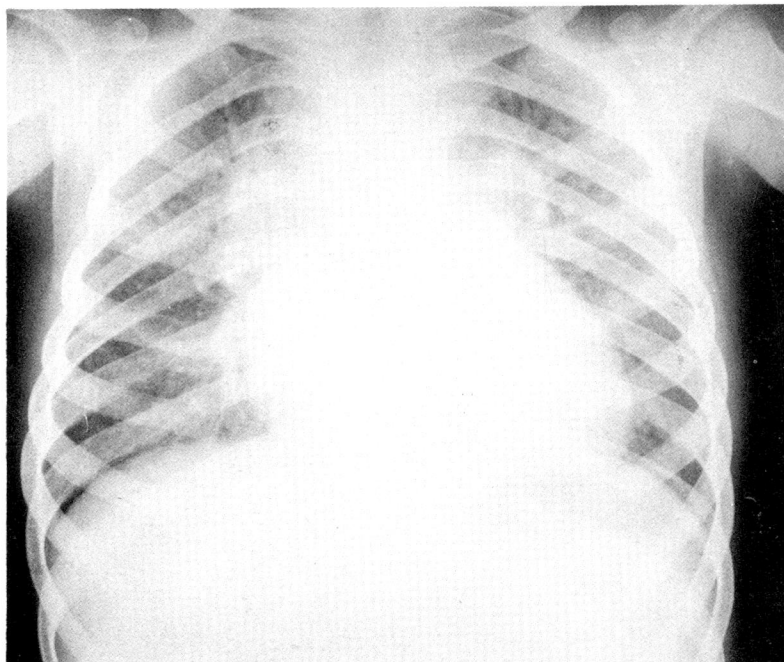

A56

These patients both have total anomalous pulmonary venous drainage.

Patient A has obstructed infra-diaphragmatic total anomalous pulmonary venous drainage. The chest X-ray shows pulmonary oedema with a normal sized heart. It is important to differentiate this condition from hyaline membrane disease. In pulmonary oedema the periphery of the infant lung is relatively clear. A nitrogen wash-out test will help to confirm the diagnosis.

In total anomalous pulmonary venous drainage the oxygenated blood returning from the pulmonary veins enters the right atrium instead of the left. In isolated total anomalous pulmonary venous drainage an atrial septal defect has to be present for blood to reach the left side of the heart. The defect is divided into supra-diaphragmatic and infra-diaphragmatic forms. In supra-diaphragmatic drainage the pulmonary venous blood drains into a common pool. This channel may drain into the superior vena cava, azygous, or innominate veins. The rarer form is infra-diaphragmatic, where blood drains from the common pool via a descending vein, through the diaphragm and enters the inferior vena cava, having passed through the liver circulation or the ductus venosus. When the ductus venosus closes post-natally (day 2-3) all pulmonary blood must flow through the liver with resulting obstruction.

Patient B has an anomalous vein ascending into his left innominate vein and the superior vena cava carries the total pulmonary venous return. These vessels are large and produce the so-called 'cottage-loaf' appearance (broad upper mediastinum). Despite the plethora seen in such cases the heart may be of normal size and the 'cottage-loaf' appearance is often obscured by thymic shadow.

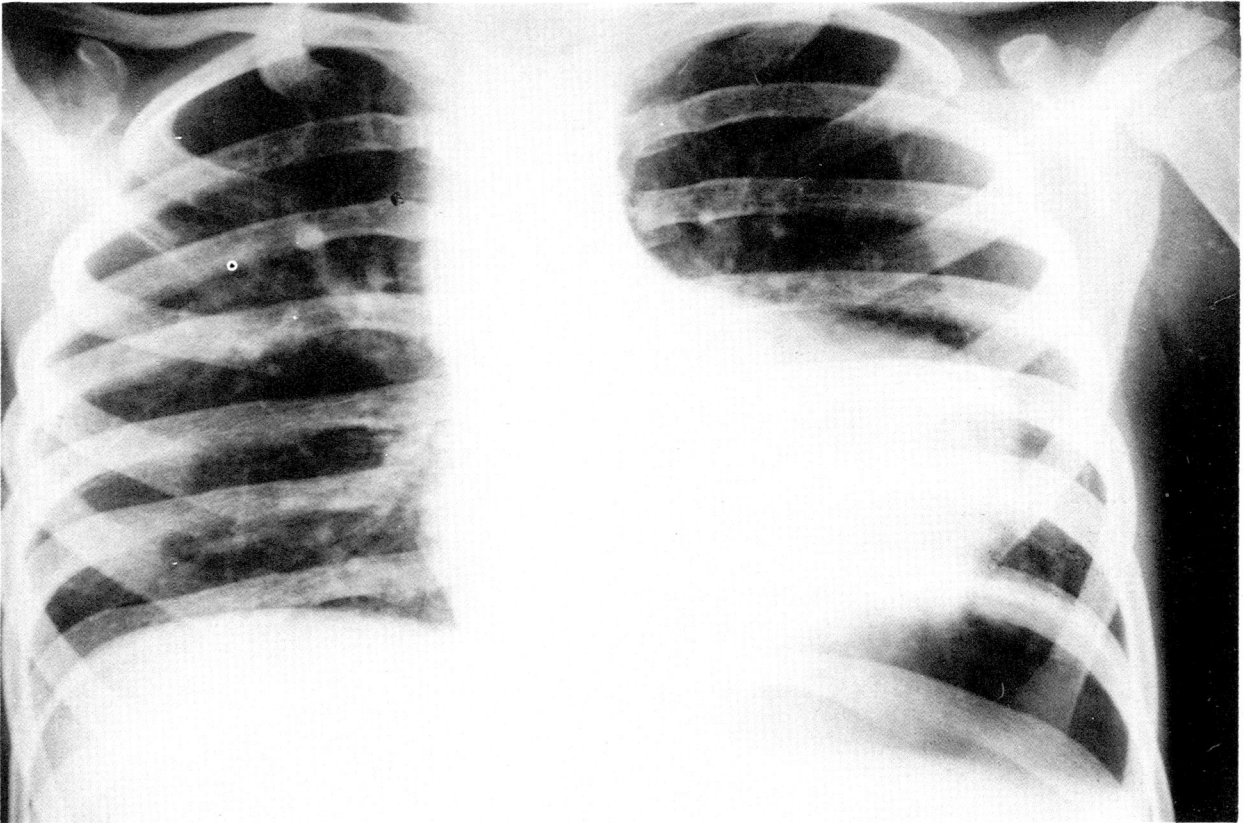

This patient was cyanosed. The cyanosis had developed in the previous 4½ years.

- What does the X-ray show?
- What is the likely diagnosis?

A57

This patient has a tetralogy of Fallot, which comprises:

1 Ventricular septal defect.
2 Pulmonary valve or infundibular stenosis ensures the right ventricular pressure is high.
3 An aorta that overrides the ventricular septum.
4 Right ventricular hypertrophy is the consequence causing the apex of the heart to be high and lateral.

Pulmonary vessels are narrow and pulmonary blood flow is low. Small bronchopulmonary collateral arteries have developed, giving an appearance of multiple small nodular opacities. Heart size in patients with tetralogy of Fallot is normal in almost all cases.

Film B is the lateral angiogram of a patient with tetralogy of Fallot. The catheter has entered the right ventricle which has a rugged contour because of right ventricular hypertrophy. The contrast medium injected passes upwards through the infundibular stenosis of the right ventricular outflow; then through the thick pulmonary valve (arrowed).

The contrast medium passes from the right ventricle through the VSD (small arrow) then into the outflow tract of the left ventricle to opacify the rest of the aorta. Note that the anterior aspect of the root of the aorta lies anterior across the VSD and overrides the right ventricle.

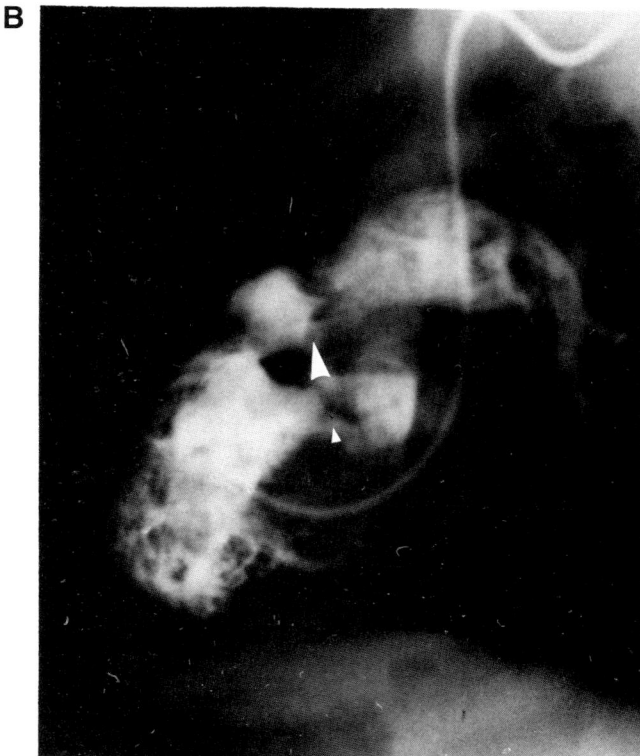

B

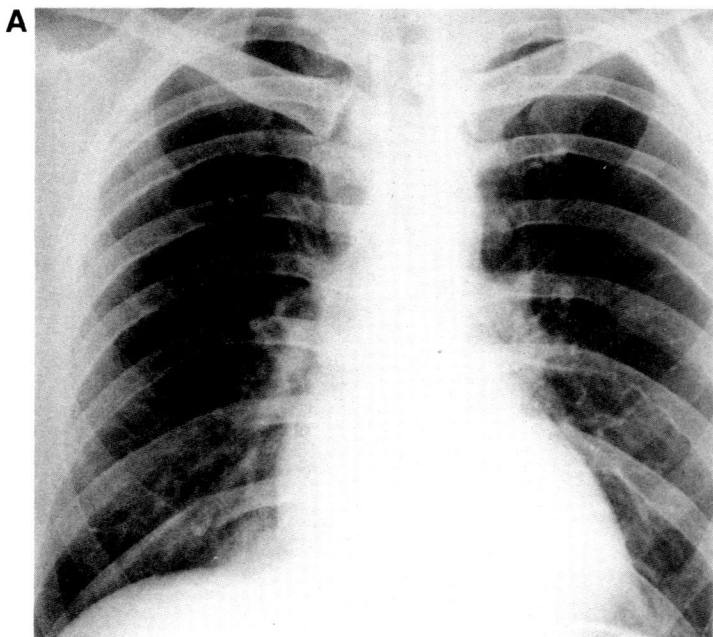

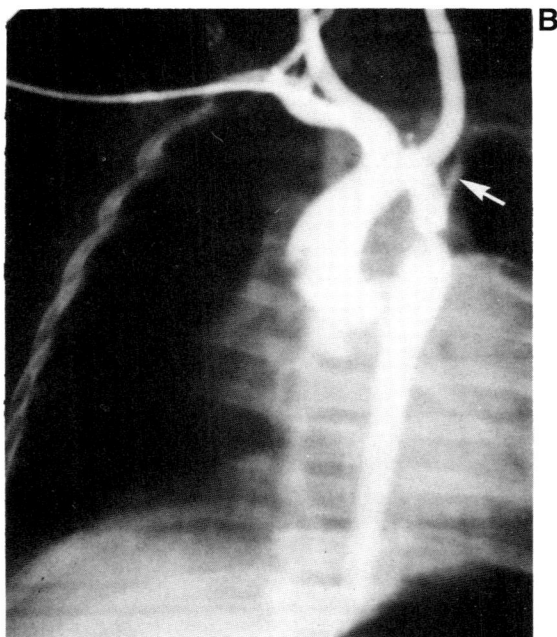

These 3 X-rays are from different patients with the same diagnosis.

- What is the diagnosis?
- What radiological features suggest the diagnosis in each case?

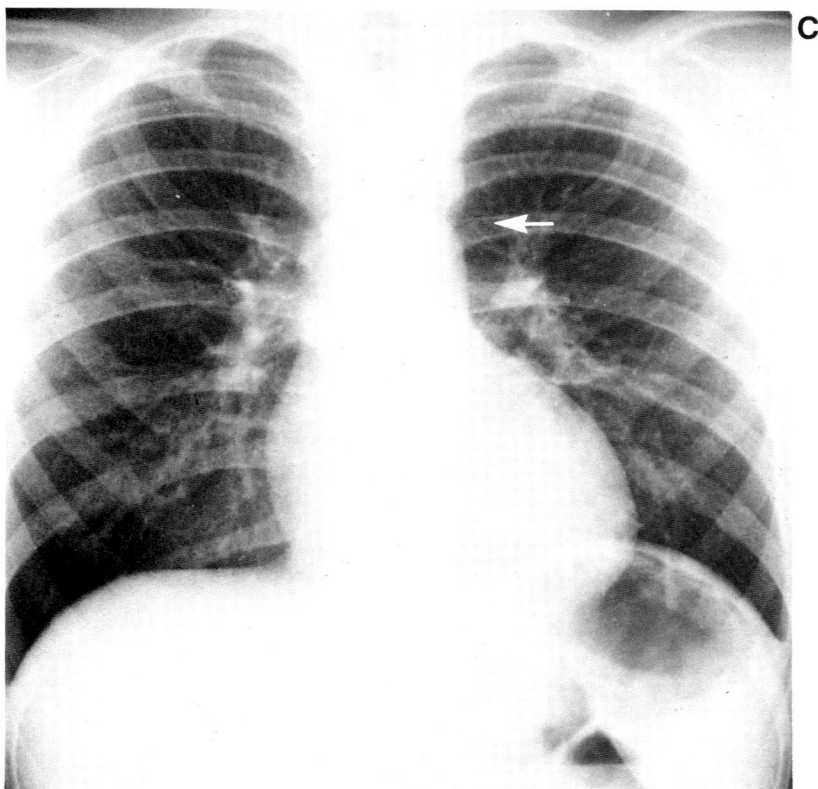

A58

These patients all have coarctation of the aorta.

Patient A has marked rib notching seen on ribs 4-8. Due to the coarctation a collateral circulation develops with retrograde blood flow in the intercostal arteries supplying the descending aorta. These arteries become tortuous and erode the inferior surface of the ribs producing notching in their middle and posterior parts. Notching of the ribs is usually found on the medial 4cm of the inferior rib margin. Rib notch is uncommon under the age of 8, and its absence in older patients does not exclude the diagnosis. The apex of the heart is low and rather lateral due to left ventricular hypertrophy in this 10 year old child. There is no pulmonary oedema.

Patient B, an infant, presented with breathlessness, mild central cyanosis and signs of pulmonary oedema and cardiac failure. The femoral pulses were diminished and delayed. The systolic blood pressures of the right and left arms were 100 and 85 mm Hg respectively. The systolic blood pressures of the lower limbs were 60 mm Hg. Cardiomegaly with a right ventricular pulsation and a diffuse apical impulse was found. The second heart sound was accentuated in the pulmonary region and a quiet precordial murmur was heard. This is the presentation of a pre-ductal coarctation. It is important to realise that the lower limb blood pressures may be higher than expected due to blood flow into the aorta distal to the coarctation via the ductus.

The angiogram shows the site of the coarctation well. The very narrow left subclavian artery is arising from the region of the duct (arrowed).

In patient C the chest X-ray shows a double shadow at the aortic knuckle (arrowed) representing a dilated left subclavian artery origin and a dilated descending aorta. This is an exceptional finding on a plain chest X-ray since most patients will be operated on earlier in life.

This neonatal patient developed a fever and was given antibiotics. Blood cultures grew methicillin resistant *Staphylococcus aureus* (MRSA). Several days after discontinuing antibiotics the patient again became septicaemic and a pustule on her arm grew MRSA. She had microscopic haematuria. No heart murmur was heard, however an echocardiogram was performed.

- What is the echo-bright round lesion (arrowed)?
- What is the diagnosis?

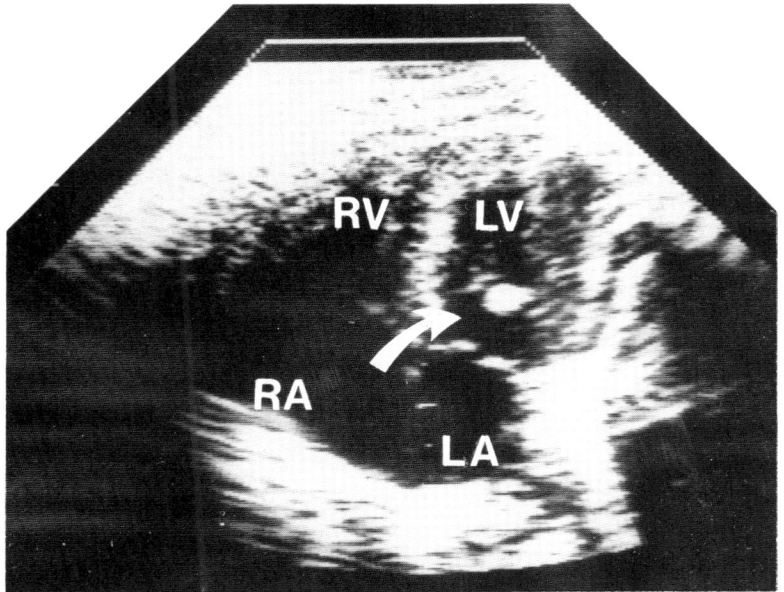

Q60

At birth this child had a markedly distended abdomen and large kidneys were found. After an ultrasound study an IVP was performed.

- What is the diagnosis?
- What is the inheritance?
- What is the prognosis?

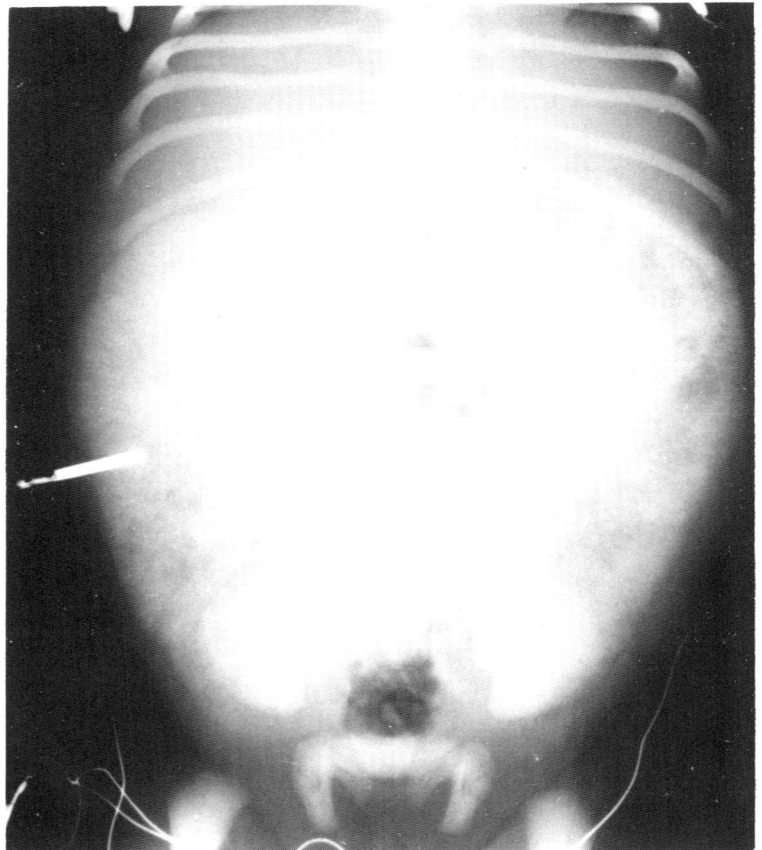

A59

A vegetation of bacterial endocarditis is seen in the left ventricle (LV) associated with the papillary muscles. A heart murmur was noted two days later. Treatment with antibiotics for 6 weeks was curative.

It has been suggested that if a neonatal patient has evidence of septicaemia, skin pustules, positive blood cultures and haematuria, an echocardiogram should be performed to exclude bacterial endocarditis, even when a heart murmur is not present.

A60

This baby has the severe form of infantile poly-cystic disease presenting at birth. This IVP shows the nephrogram phase which may be very late in appearing and shows the typical striated appearance of the enlarged kidneys. Inheritance is autosomal recessive and severely affected children often die within the first months of life.

Infant polycystic disease may present at birth with gross renal enlargement. It may present in childhood with renal failure. Older children may have minimal renal disease but have hepatic fibrosis with portal hypertension as the pre-dominant feature.

Post-mortem examination showed that both kidneys were grossly and evenly enlarged. The anterior surfaces showed marked cystic change in both cortex and medulla which histologically was due to marked dilation of the collecting tubules. The liver also showed large areas of cystic change. These changes are consistent with infantile polycystic disease.

A characteristic of infantile polycystic disease is that the kidneys are echo bright and large on ultrasound examinations (Film B). Overall the large kidney is hyperechoic (large arrow) in comparison with the liver, which is seen deeper in the scan (small arrow).

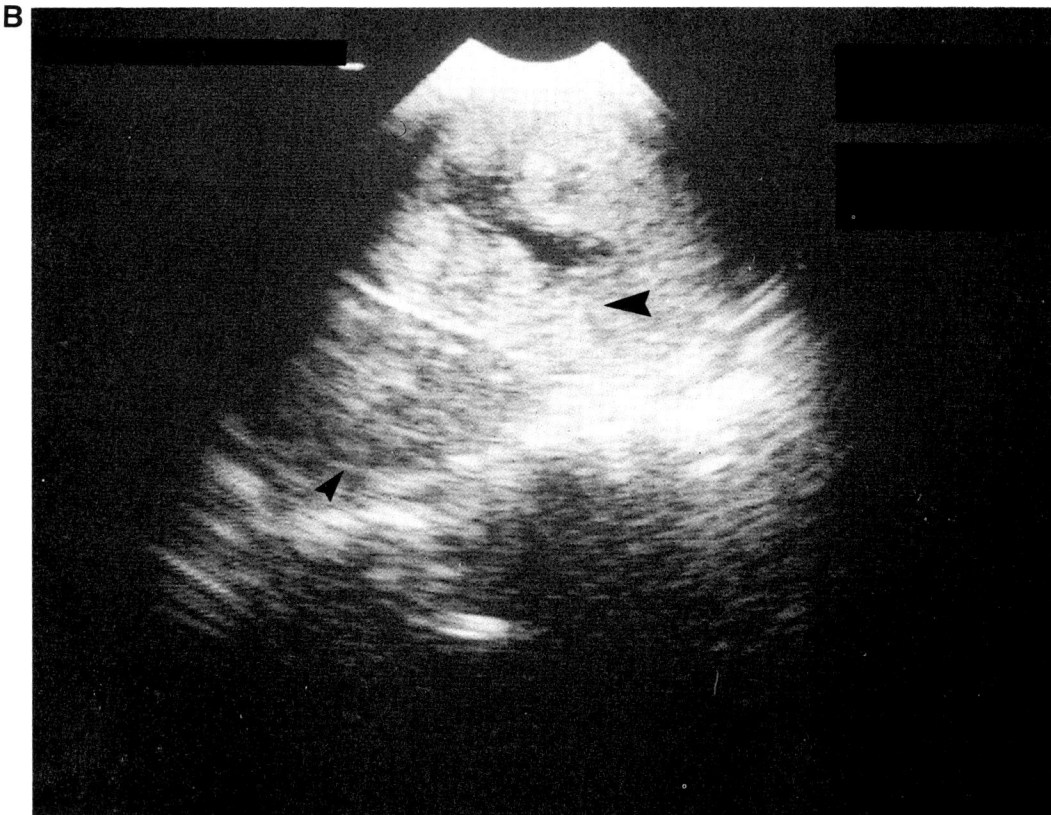

B

What examination has been performed in these patients?

- Explain the radiological findings shown in Films A and B.

- What complications may arise?

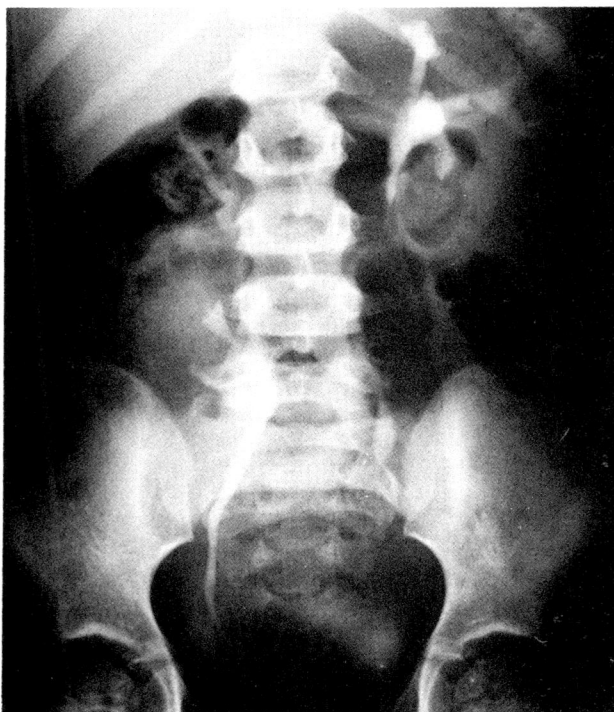

A

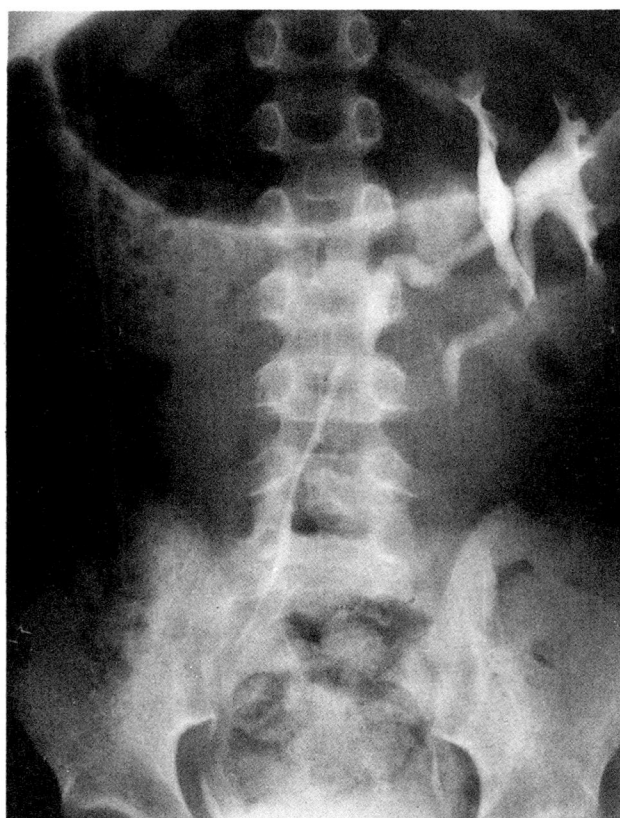

B

A61

The intravenous urograms show patient A to have a malascended kidney. Patient B has cross renal ectopia.

During early foetal life the ureteric bud ascends to connect with metanephric tissue. The consequence is the normal position of each ureter and kidney.

When the ureteric bud makes a low connection with the metanephric tissue the kidney develops in a low position; it may be in the presacral position or, as here, slightly higher.

When the ureteric bud ascends and crosses the midline a double kidney forms on one side, as in patient B.

When the ureteric bud ascent is not normal it is often the case that the origin of the ureteric bud is not normal either. The ureter may connect with the vagina, bladder neck or ectopically elsewhere in the urinary tract. Kidney tissue associated with such ureters often functions poorly.

Q62

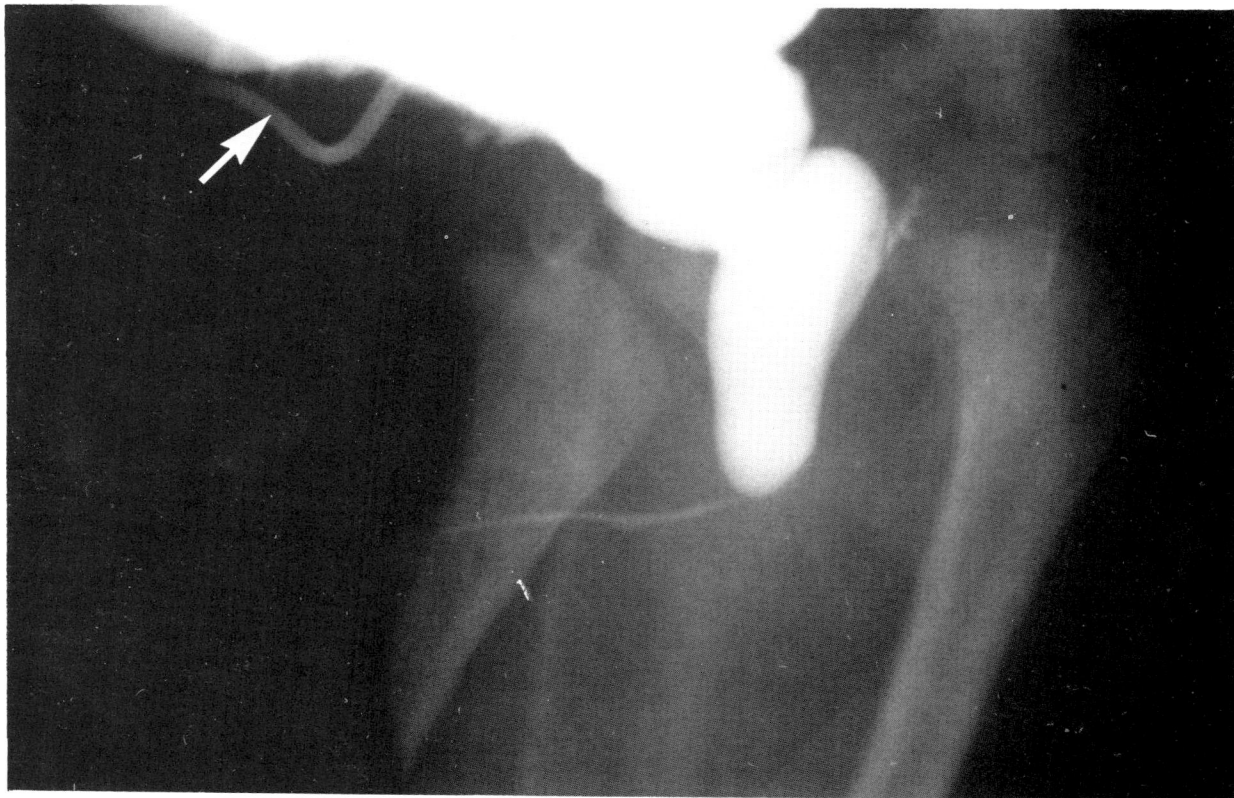

On routine post-natal examination this baby was found to have a distended bladder.

- What investigation has been performed?

- What is the diagnosis?
- What initial investigation would you have performed?

- What is the diagnosis?

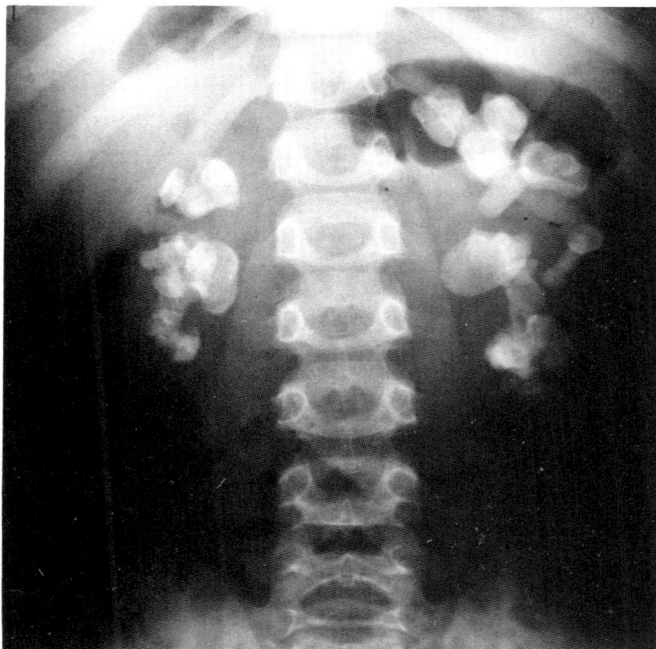

Q64

This small baby was admitted because of the presence of a patent urachus through which urine was draining. He had a thin abdominal wall with wrinkled skin and defective abdominal musculature. Both kidneys were palpable. Urine was flowing from the sinus at the umbilicus and the testes were undescended.

- What examination has been performed?
- What does it show?
- What is the diagnosis?

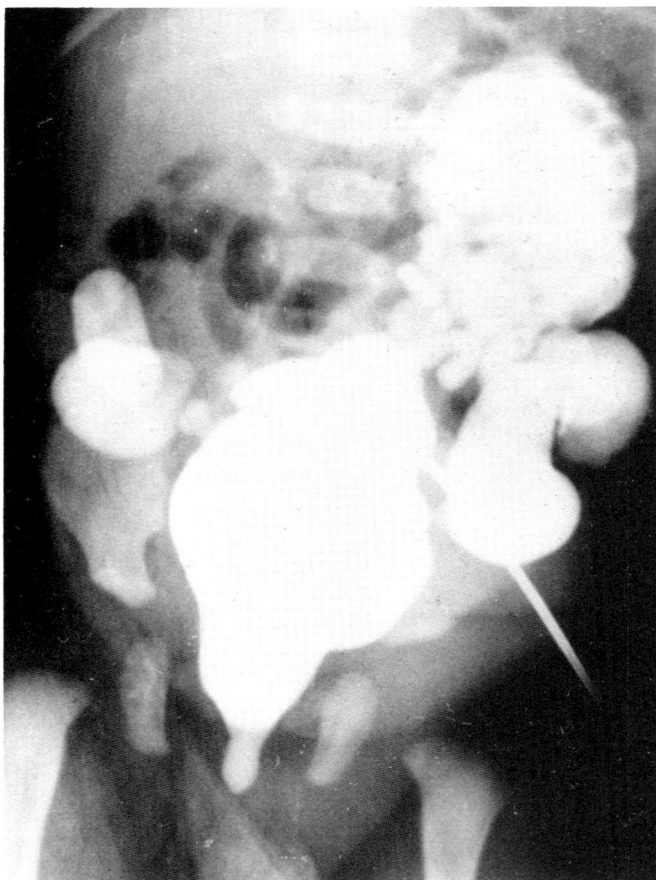

A62

A micturating cystogram has been performed via a suprapubic catheter (arrowed) and demonstrates obstruction due to posterior urethral valves. There is a substantial dilatation of the posterior urethra which is seen to terminate abruptly in a convex border formed by the valves. The distal urethra is usually collapsed but otherwise normal. A small amount of contrast is seen in this patient's urethra.

Posterior urethral valves occur in boys and are composed of folds which obstruct the urethra. Presentation is usually in an infant with a distended abdomen which on examination reveals a large palpable bladder. There may be nonspecific signs such as failure to thrive and vomiting. The urinary stream is poor. Prenatal ultrasound scanning may lead to the suspicion of obstructive uropathy due to valves. Urinary infection in infants and children may be a presenting feature.

An ultrasound examination of the renal system should be the initial investigation. It will show the thick bladder wall, the hydronephrosis and hydroureter.

Even with early diagnosis and resection of valves, the long-term outlook is often poor.

Paediatric urologists will find 'ablation of the valves' easy, but all the problems over the longer term lie in the upper tract.

A63

The plain film shows calcified staghorn calculi in both kidneys. Calcium phosphate stones are particularly prone to form staghorn calculi in the renal pelvis.

Nearly all urinary calculi are calcified and appear partly or totally opaque. Many calculi are associated with urinary infection and deposition of calcium phosphate.

Purely metabolic stones such as uric acid stones in leukaemic patients under treatment and xanthine stones are non-opaque.

A64

Radiology shows retrograde filling through a catheter in the urachus. Grossly dilated ureters and hydronephrosis are shown because of gross reflux. The child has 'prune belly' syndrome (triad syndrome). This comprises (1) hypoplasia or absence of abdominal wall musculature, giving the abdomen a wrinkled 'prune' like appearance, (2) undescended testes, (3) urinary tract anomalies. Lower limb deformities and malnutrition are occasional associations.

In the 'prune belly' syndrome the kidneys and urinary tract are affected. Renal dysplasia is a common feature with poor renal function.

Urinary tract infection can be particularly difficult to treat because of the undrained urine.

A child with a pigmented naevus over the lumbar spine and club foot was referred from the orthopaedic clinic. He had developed incontinence of urine of increasing severity during childhood.

- What investigation has been performed and what does it show?

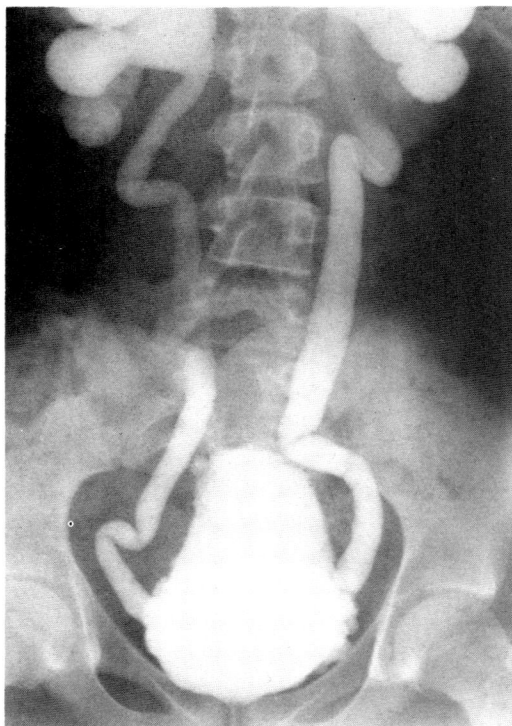

Q66

This child underwent left ventricular angiography for a ventricular septal defect. Plain abdominal films following angiography revealed a right sided hydronephrosis.

- What investigation has been performed and what does it show?

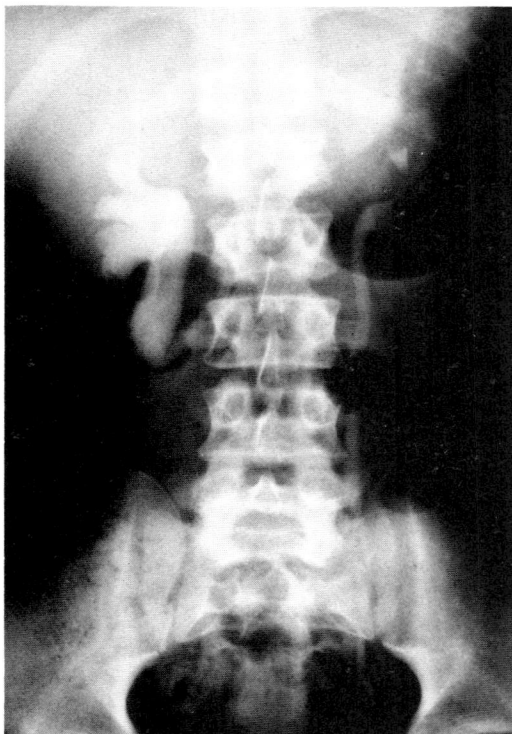

A65

A cystogram has been performed. The child has a neurogenic bladder with numerous sacculations and trabeculations.

The bladder is thick walled. It does not show normal emptying with a normal detruser contraction and there is no sphincteric control. All these features account for the incontinence. In neurogenic bladder there is often a disturbance in function at the vesico-ureteric junction which causes a reflux into the ureters.

A66

The IVP shows dilatation of the upper right ureter and mild hydronephrosis on this side. This is caused by a retrocaval ureter. In this condition the ureter turns abruptly medially and upwards and is obstructed behind the vena cava. It is found on the right side and has an incidence of approximately one in 1,000 births. Many patients with this disorder are asymptomatic. Symptoms may occur with increasing age. These may include continuous or intermittent right loin pain, dysuria, haematuria, and problems with calculi and urinary infections.

Q67

A

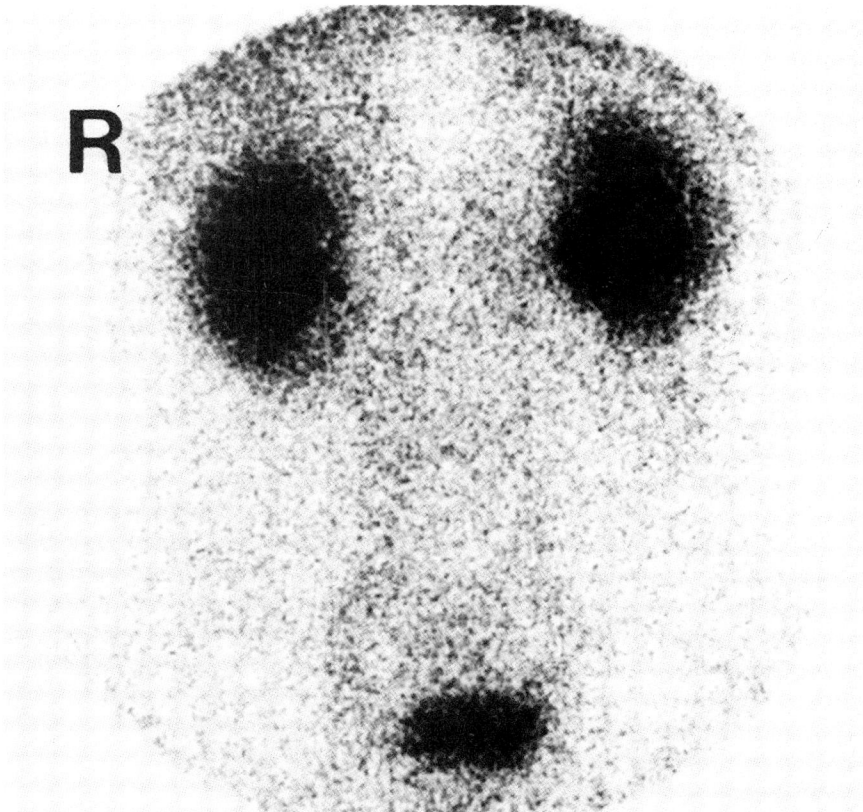

R

B

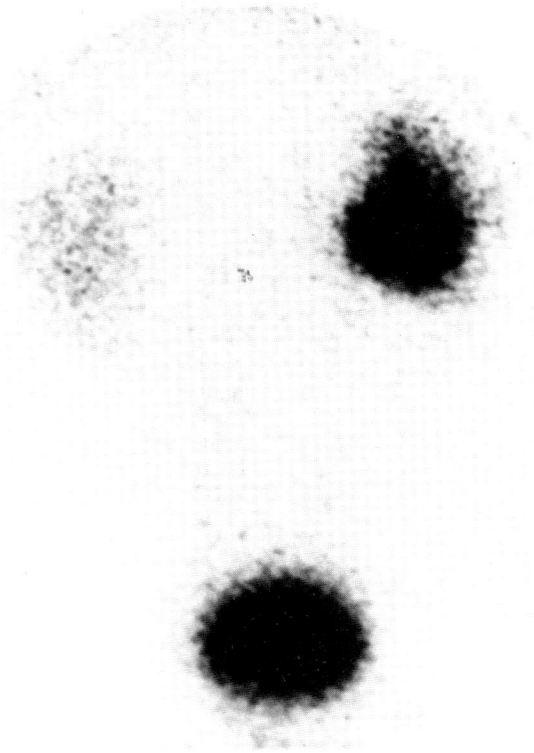

R

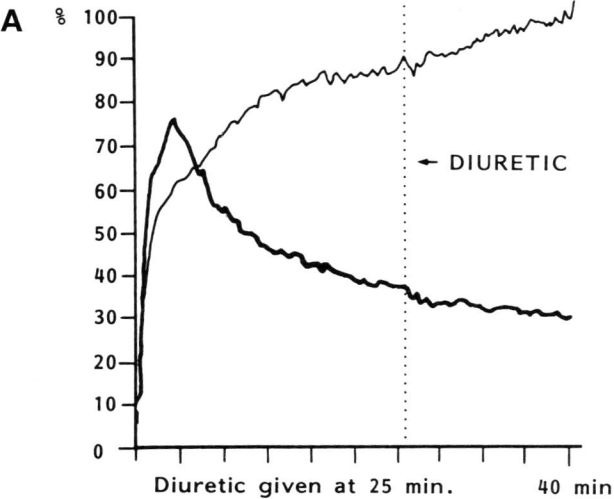

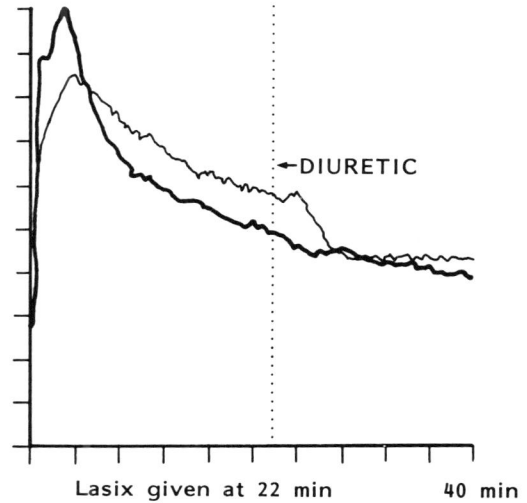

A

B

This child had intermittent left loin pain. An intravenous urogram recorded a left sided PUJ obstruction. A ^{99m}TcDTPA scan was performed. Film A was taken before and Film B after diuretic was given.

• What do they show?

The graphs show the diuretic renogram before and after surgery.

• What do they show?

Film A and Graph A show a prolonged transit time for the left kidney which does not respond to a diuretic. These are the appearances of obstructive uropathy. Both kidneys contribute equally to the glomerular filtration rate (GFR). Following a left pyeloplasty the renogram curve of the left kidney has returned to normal (Graph B). Excretion occurred well before the injection of diuretic was given. The left kidney contributes 43% to the total GFR. The right kidney has a normal renogram curve.

The ^{99m}TcDTPA scan is a dynamic study of the renal tract.

After injection, isotope arrives in the kidney in the glomerular capillaries at a rate proportional to its plasma concentration. The isotope is then cleared. The first 2-4 minutes after injection represent transfer from the blood through the nephrons to the collecting tubule. The excretory phase into the calyces begins around 3-5 minutes. The ascending part of the curve represents the uptake phase then later both uptake and early excretion. The curve descends as more isotope is leaving the kidney than is being taken up. The uptake phase of ^{99m}TcDTPA reflects pure glomerular filtration. Differential renal function may be analysed during the uptake phase. If a blood sample is taken at 20 minutes the individual kidney filtration rate (GFR) estimation is possible. Transit time is the time taken for isotope to pass through the kidneys.

After a diuretic is given a normal kidney will show a sharp fall in the number of counts in the renal area because of clearance of isotope into the lower urinary tract. When obstruction is present a sharp fall is not observed and a build up of counts may occur (see Graph A). There is no rapid clearance from the left kidney and the pelvicalyceal system (see Film B) after a diuretic was given.

Gross dilatation of the collecting system or poor renal function both result in a poor response to a diuretic. With dilatation the urine pool in the upper tract is so large that it cannot be cleared. When renal function is very poor excretion is reduced, fixed and not changed by the diuretic.

Indications for the ^{99m}TcDTPA scans include:
— Measurement of parenchymal function.
— Suspected obstruction.
— Evaluation of medical or surgical treatment.
— Screening for renovascular hypertension when a renal artery stenosis delays the arrival and diminishes the amount of isotope reaching the parenchyma.

This child was investigated for a recent urinary tract infection. Ultrasound facilities were not available and an IVP was performed.

- What does it show?

- What problems may be associated with this anomaly?

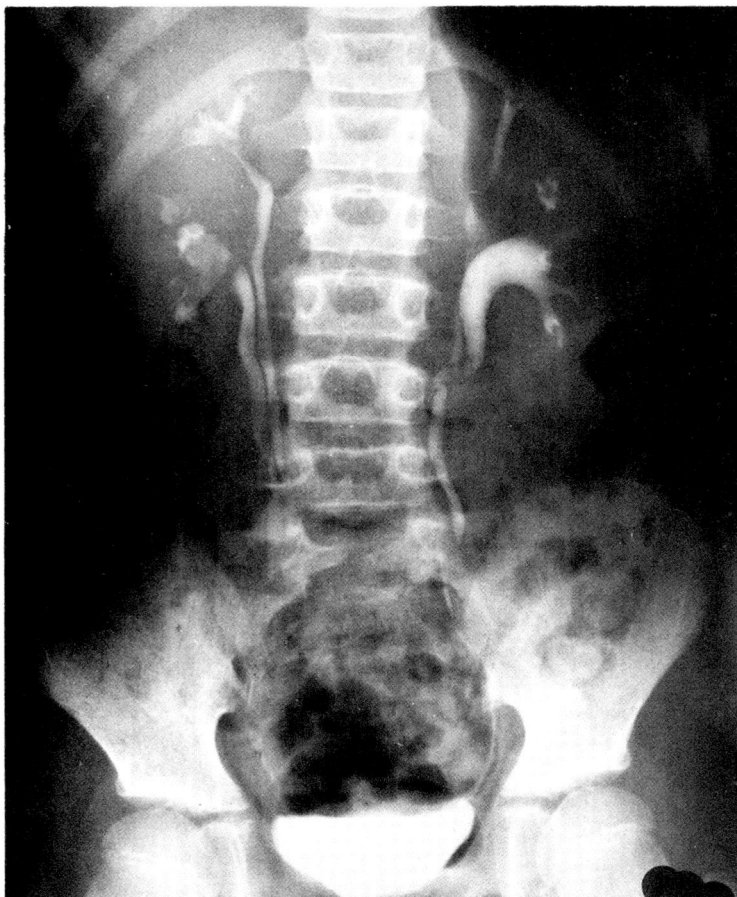

Q69

A micturating cystorethrogram (MCU) was performed to investigate a proven urinary tract infection. Vesico-ureteric reflux was demonstrated on the left side. Three years later she was noted to be hypertensive.

- What investigation has been performed?

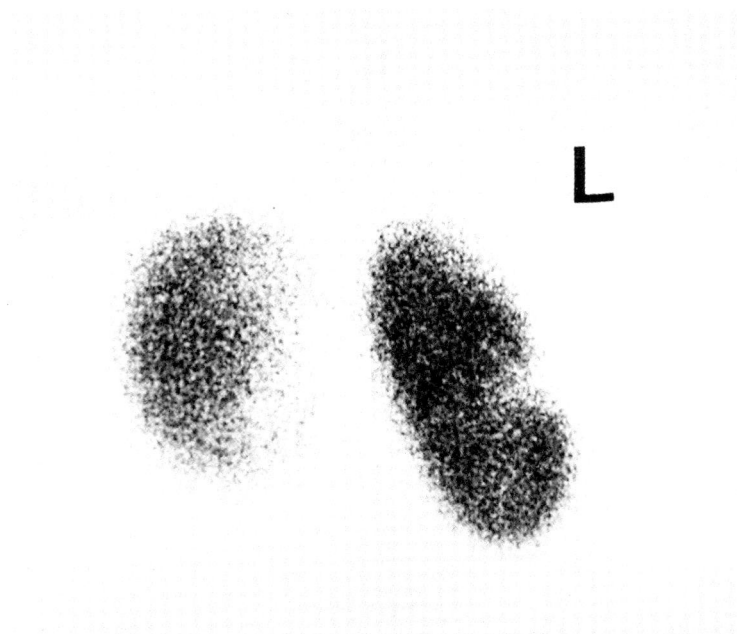

L

A68

The child has normal bilateral duplex kidneys and ureters. All ureters are of normal calibre, open into the bladder and there is no reflux.

An ectopic ureter may pass submucosally beyond the bladder and urethral sphincters and be responsible for urinary incontinence.

If a ureter from an upper pole enters the lower urinary tract near the bladder neck its orifice is often obstructed. The distant end of the ureter then dilates and produces a filling defect at IVP in the base of the bladder – the ectopic ureterocoele.

Prolapse of an ectopic ureterocoele into the urethra obstructs bladder emptying. Large ureterocoeles may affect most of the bladder base and produce obstruction of the ureters which enter the bladder.

In a girl an ectopic ureterocoele may be visible in the perineum.

A69

A ^{99m}TcDMSA scan has been performed. There is a wedge-shaped defect laterally in the left kidney indicative of a scar, i.e. a pyelonephritic scar. This is an oblique projection with the left kidney nearer the camera.

With vesico-ureteric reflux, the ^{99m}TcDMSA scan is the most sensitive technique for the detection of renal scarring.

In a patient with hypertension a normal ^{99m}TcDMSA scan excludes most renovascular causes with the exception of bilateral main renal artery stenosis. The ^{99m}TcDMSA scan will also demonstrate a small kidney due to any cause.

^{99m}TcDMSA administration gives a static renal scan. The isotope attaches to the proximal convoluted tubules. Images obtained after 2 hours represent renal cortical mass.

Indications for a ^{99m}TcDMSA scan include:
— When only one kidney has been found: is there another?
— Detection of an occult duplex kidney.
— Hypertension and vascular disease.
— Infection of the kidney during acute pyelonephritis and for some time afterwards.
— Renal scarring; as here.

This 4 week old child presented with a 5 day history of projectile vomiting. A pyloric tumour could not be felt and visible peristalsis was not seen.

- What investigation has been performed and what does it suggest?
- What biochemical abnormalities suggest the diagnosis?

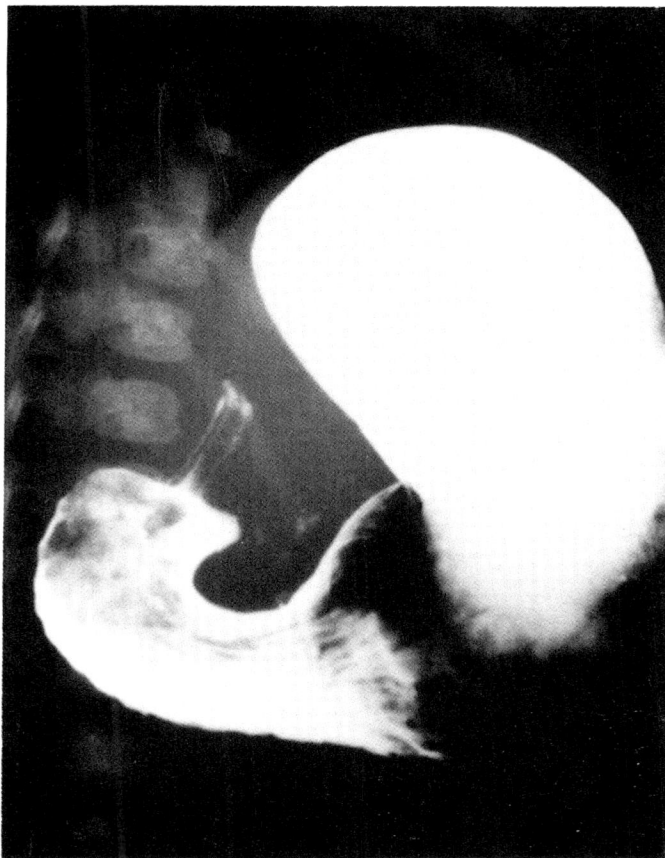

Q71

This young girl had been complaining of dysphagia for the last 2 weeks.

- What is the diagnosis?

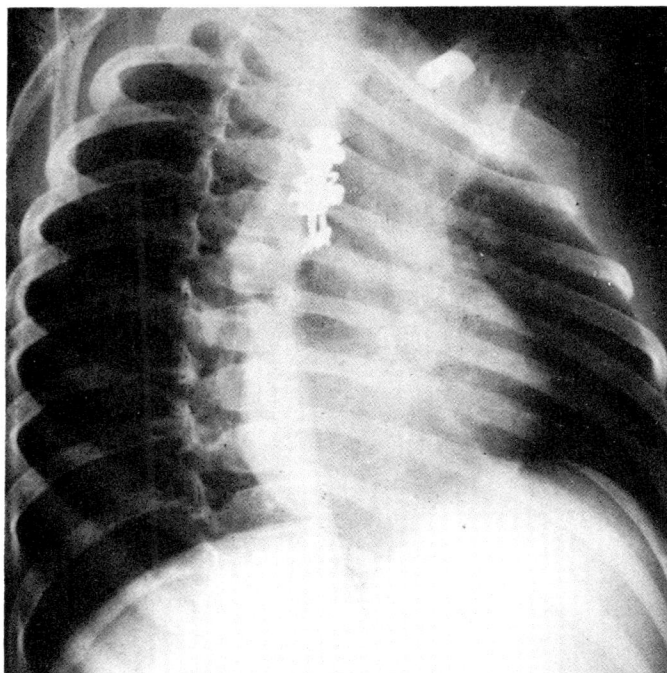

A70

The diagnosis of pyloric stenosis may be difficult. It is usually made clinically by feeling the pyloric tumour. Plain films may show dilatation of the stomach with little or no distal gas in the intestine. Barium by mouth will establish the diagnosis when the tumour is not felt with certainty. The tumour is recognised in this case by narrowing of the lumen of the pylorus at the site of the tumour, which is represented by 2 or 3 lines of barium in the clefts between the mucosal folds. The pyloric canal is narrowed and elongated. Although not well shown here, there is often a crescentic indentation of the barium in the antrum of the stomach and the first part of the duodenum due to the muscular tumour compressing the lumen from the outside.

The vomiting due to pyloric stenosis may cause:
— hypochloraemic alkalosis
— hypokalaemia
— haemoconcentration and mild uraemia due to fluid loss.

The term 'pyloric tumour' often frightens the parents. Describing the problem as pyloric stenosis due to muscular hypertrophy is preferable.

Ultrasound examination will show muscle thickening and canal lengthening.

A71

Her Minnie Mouse badge was lodged in her oesophagus. Her dysphagia resolved on removal of the animal.

Q72

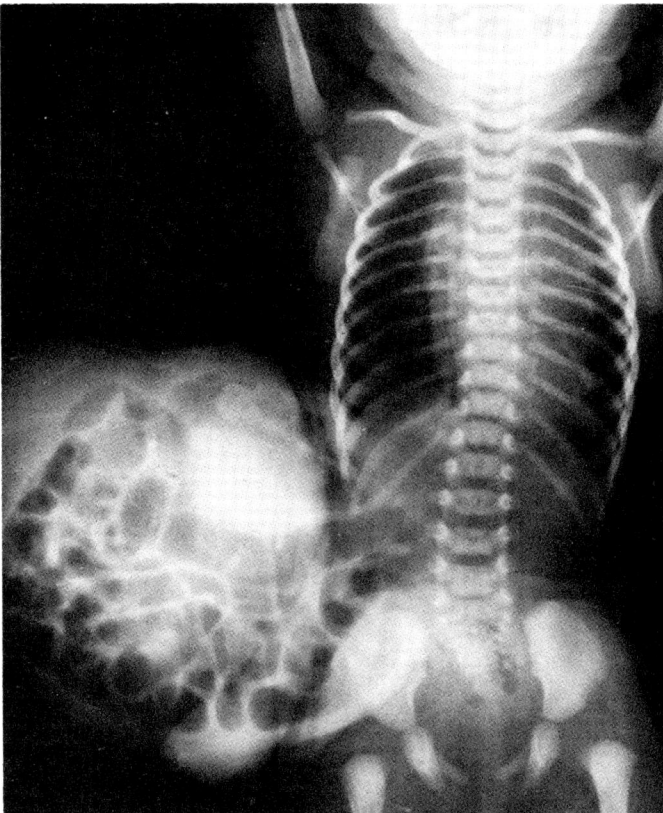

• What is the diagnosis?

The inferior vena cava of this child has been catheterised from the groin and contrast medium injected.

- What does investigation show?
- What may cause this syndrome?
- How may such children present?

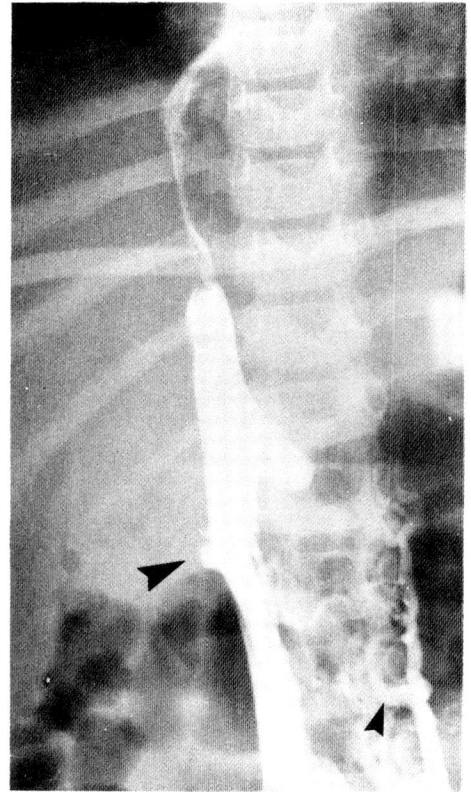

Q74

This child presented to casualty with right sided abdominal pain.

- What is the most likely diagnosis?
- What other problems might this child have?

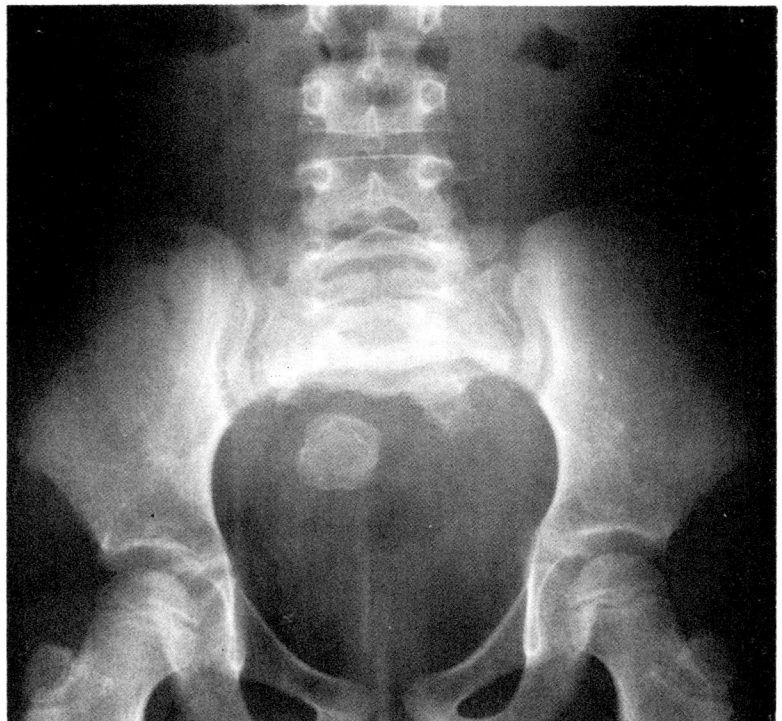

A72

The patient has an exomphalos. This is a herniation of intra-abdominal contents through the umbilical ring into the base of the umbilical cord. The defect may be very small or, as in this case, a very large defect is present through which the stomach, all of the intestines apart from the distal colon, the liver and spleen may bulge. The contents are enclosed by an intact membrane composed of fused amniotic membrane and peritoneum, but this may rupture after or during delivery.

Infants with exomphalos frequently have other major anomalies. They may succumb from a cardiac malformation or other anomaly.

A73

This child has thrombosis of her inferior vena cava and hepatic veins, known as the Budd-Chiari syndrome. This is produced by obstruction of the hepatic vein. In this patient there is external compression of the inferior vena cava with reflux of dye into the renal veins (arrowed) and filling of left ascending lumbar veins (small arrow) by collaterals.

Thrombosis may be associated with polycythaemia, hepatomas, leukaemia, infection and trauma. The syndrome may also arise from membranous obstruction of the inferior vena cava and from veno-occlusive disease of the liver.

Presentation may be acute or chronic. In the latter case splenomegaly may occur and distended superficial veins, oedema of the legs and albuminuria are features. In acute cases there may be abdominal pain and vomiting. Hepatomegaly is marked and ascites and jaundice are seen.

Catheterisation of the inferior vena cava is necessary to exclude inferior vena caval webs.

A74

The patient had appendicitis. A calcified faecalith is seen in the right iliac fossa. There is a strong relationship between this finding and appendicitis. Up to three quarters of such cases may have perforated. The faecalith may cause obstruction, which, in addition to the inflammation results in perforation.

The faecalith must be removed at operation to prevent abscess formation.

The child also has sacral agenesis. This is a rare condition, but is more common in infants of diabetic mothers. Sacral level lower motor neurone paralysis is present to varying degrees, affecting bladder and bowel function and the extensors and abductors of the hip. It is not associated with hydrocephalus.

These chest X-rays were taken 1 month apart in this child whose abdomen increased in girth by 6 cm during the course of the day and returned to normal during the night.

- What syndrome does this child have?
- What is the prognosis?

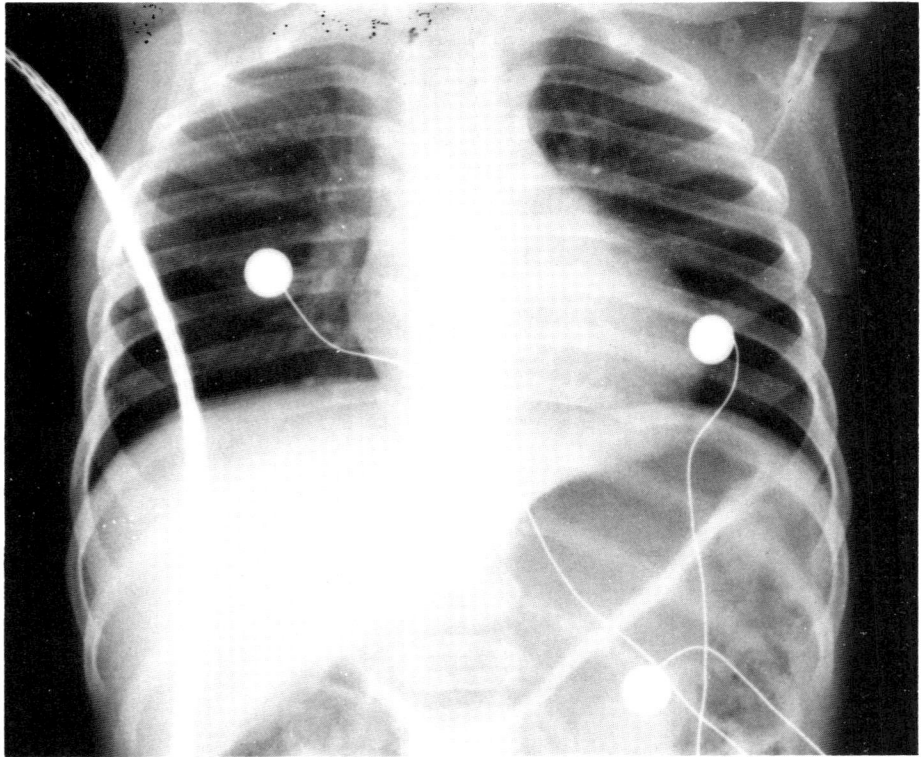

A

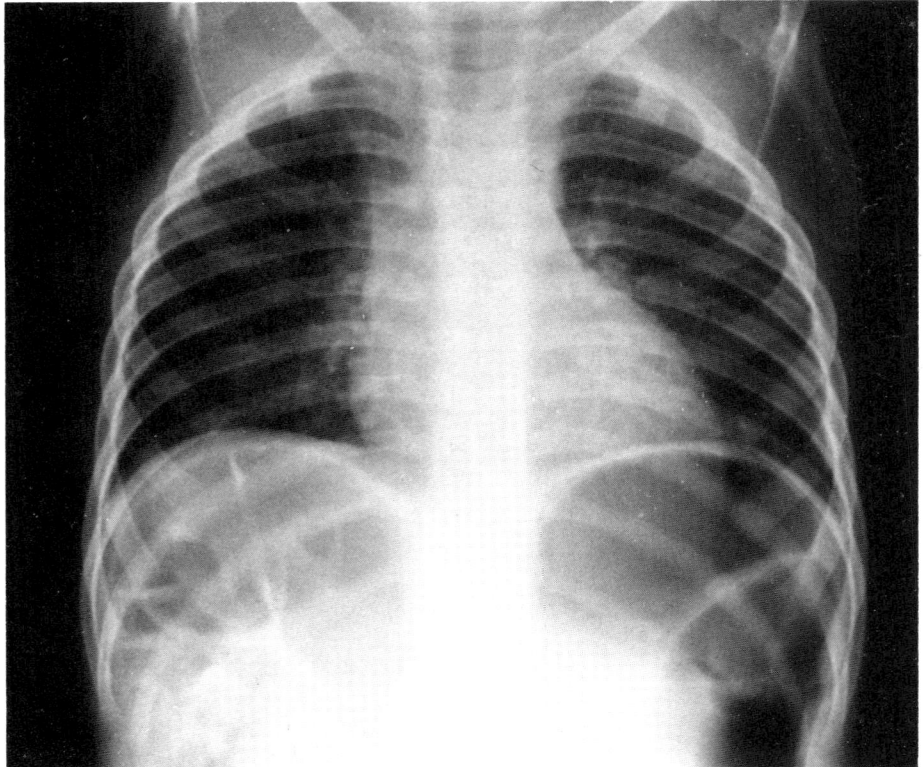

B

A75

This patient has Chilaiditi's syndrome. Film A is normal but a lot of gas is seen in the gut (stomach and colon). In film B there is obliteration of the hepatic shadow by gas-distended intestines interposed between the liver and diaphragm. An X-ray taken 1 month later was again normal. This patient is an habitual air swallower. The term Chilaiditi's syndrome describes the interposition between the diaphragm of gas-filled gut.

To the unwary the hepatodiaphragmatic interposition of colon may simulate free gas under the diaphragm or a gas-containing right subphrenic abscess.

This usually asymptomatic syndrome was first described by Beclere in 1899, but since Chilaiditi described 3 patients in 1910 it has been known as Chilaiditi's syndrome. It has an incidence of between 0.02% and 0.22%.

Q76

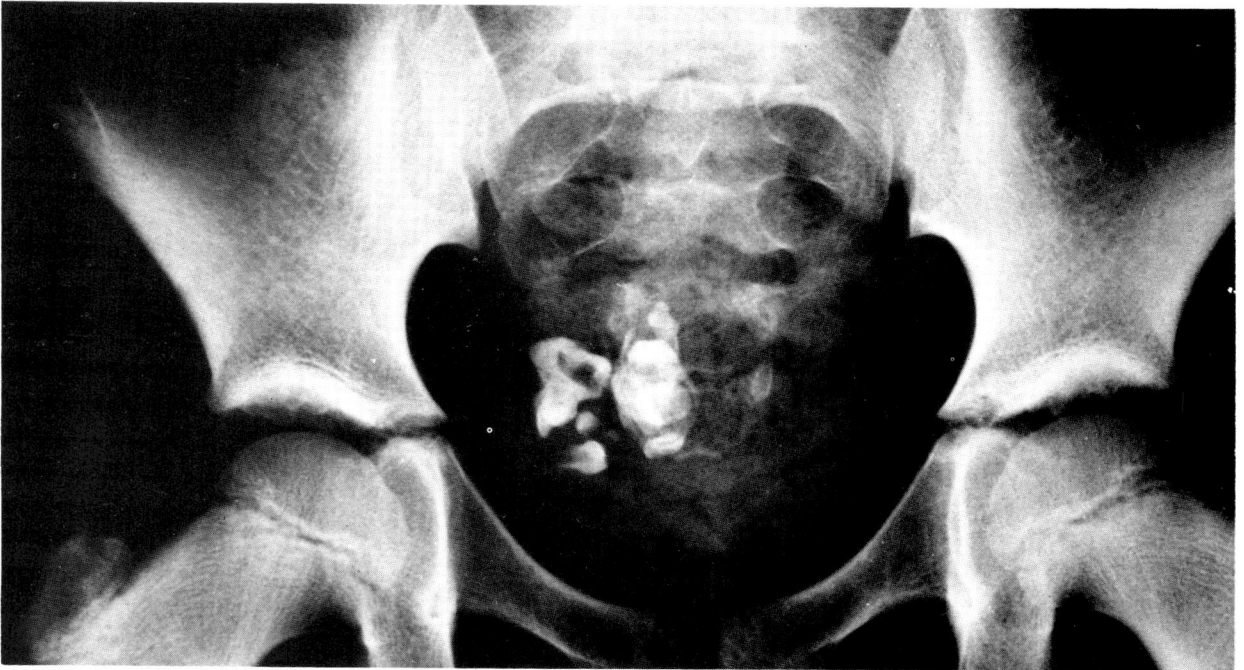

This is the plain X-ray of a young girl.

- What is the diagnosis?

The condition of this premature baby deteriorated (Film A).

- Describe the features seen on the radiograph of the chest and abdomen that contribute to his deterioration.

Later he developed a tension pneumothorax (Film B). A chest drain was inserted.

- How could you improve ventilation further?

Ventilation improved following intervention, but the child's metabolic acidosis worsened.

- What is causing this deterioration?

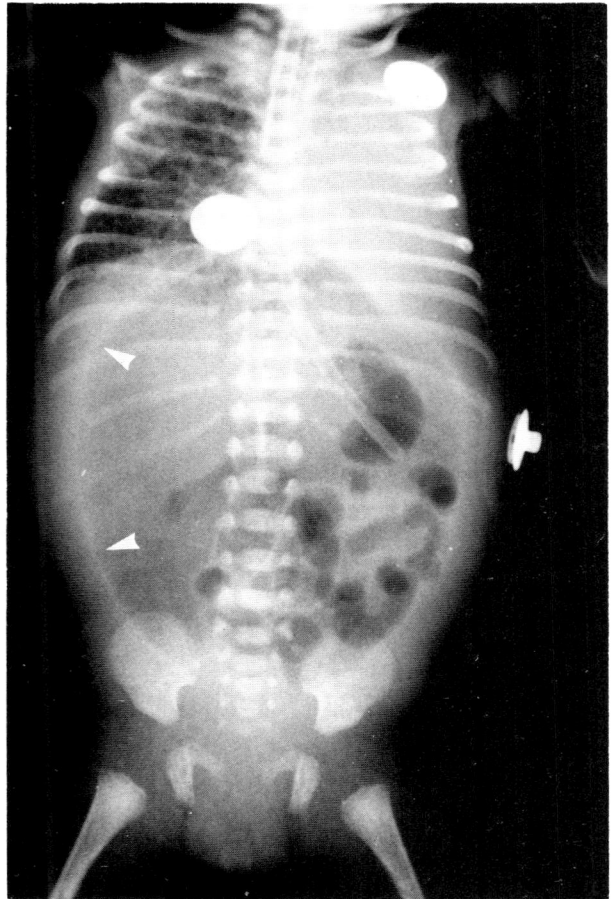

A

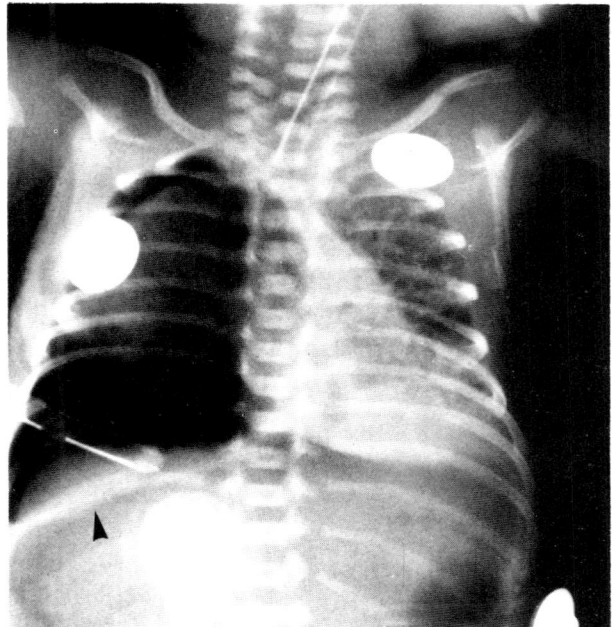

B

A76

The girl has a dermoid cyst (teratoma). There are dense calcified opacities representing bone and dental elements within the tumour. Ovarian cysts in children are most frequently dermoid cysts. They may present as pelvic masses, and X-ray may show them to be outlined by a thin translucent fat line.

Malignant ovarian tumours commonly cause hypergonadism and sexual precocity. If this is the case bone age may be significantly advanced. In the case of the benign dermoid the bone age is normal since the dermoid has no endocrinological activity.

A77

In film A the endotracheal tube has been inserted too far. The left lung collapsed but re-expanded when the endotracheal tube was withdrawn by 1-2cm. Lung disease is seen as diffuse patchy shadowing in the right lung. The oval more translucent area overlying the abdomen is due to free air (arrowed) in the abdominal cavity. This is the appearance of a pneumoperitoneum when the patient is supine. This collection of air can also be seen on the chest X-ray (Film B, arrowed).

Film B shows a tension pneumothorax despite the presence of a chest drain which is not draining. Repositioning of the chest drain or insertion of an extra one is needed to drain the pneumothorax. Aspiration of air from the chest with a needle and syringe may rapidly improve ventilation before formal drainage.

The metabolic acidosis was due to the child's necrotising enterocolitis. Perforation of his jejunum was responsible for the pneumoperitoneum.

Free air under the diaphragm was confirmed, by the referring hospital, (Film C) by holding the patient upright to demonstrate gas under the diaphragm. This should never be done to a critically ill neonatal patient. A lateral decubitus view of the abdomen, with horizontal beam, demonstrates free air.

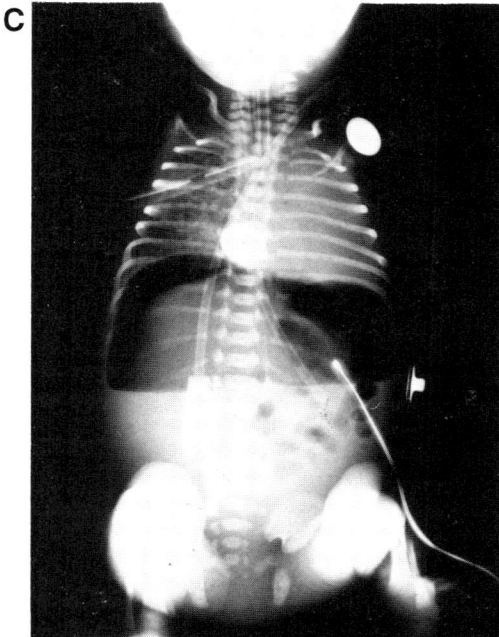

C

Both of these neonatal patients had abdominal distension and a metabolic acidosis.

- What is the diagnosis?
- What are the radiological features of this condition?

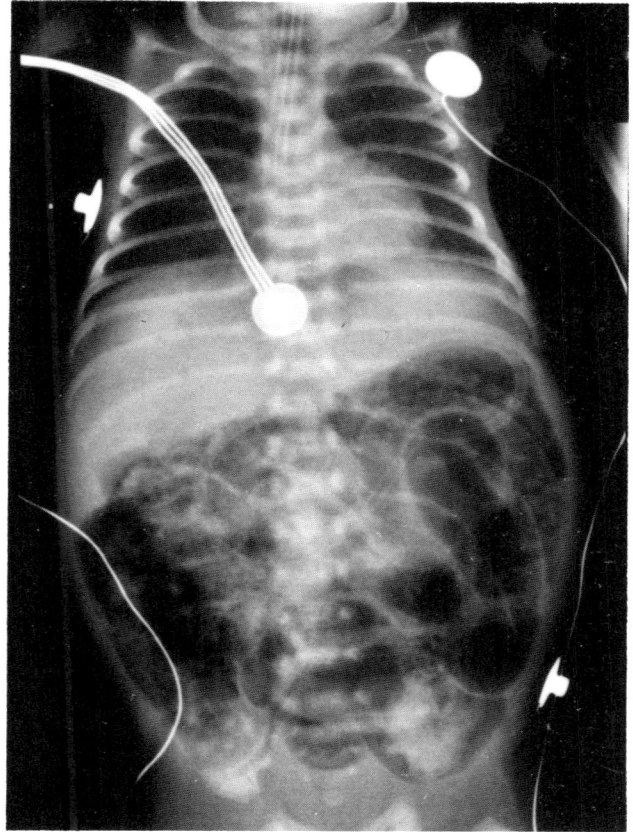

A

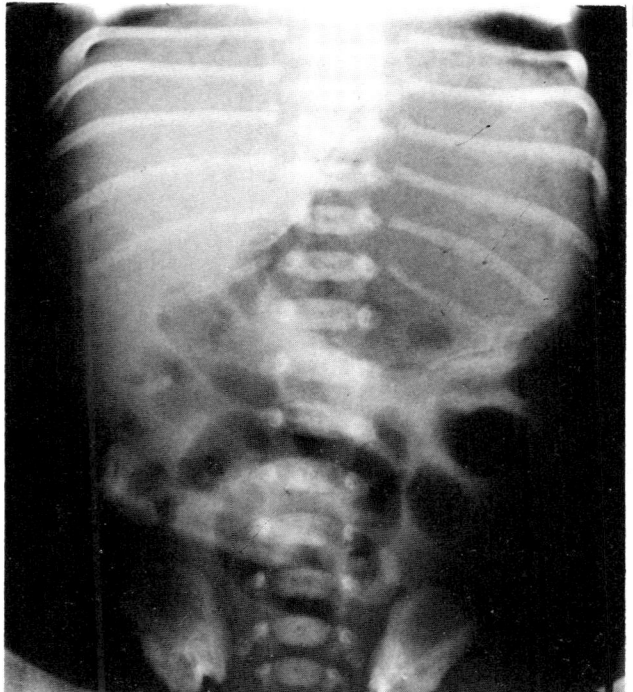

B

A78

Both patients have necrotising enterocolitis. Patient A has pneumatosis intestinalis, which is presence of gas in the bowel wall in sufficient quantities to be seen on a plain abdominal X-ray. The gas is seen as linear translucent streaks parallel to the lumen of bowel, and separated from it by the shadow of the mucosa. There is also gas in the portal vein, another classical sign of necrotising enterocolitis. A pneumoperitoneum was demonstrated on a lateral decubitus film, confirming the presence of free gas as suspected in the subhepatic region and centrally in the abdomen beneath the electrode. In necrotising enterocolitis radiological signs may be nonspecific and consist only of intestinal distension.

Patient B developed necrotising enterocolitis involving the wall of the stomach where intramural air is clearly seen.

The endotracheal tube has been inserted too far in patient A.

Q79

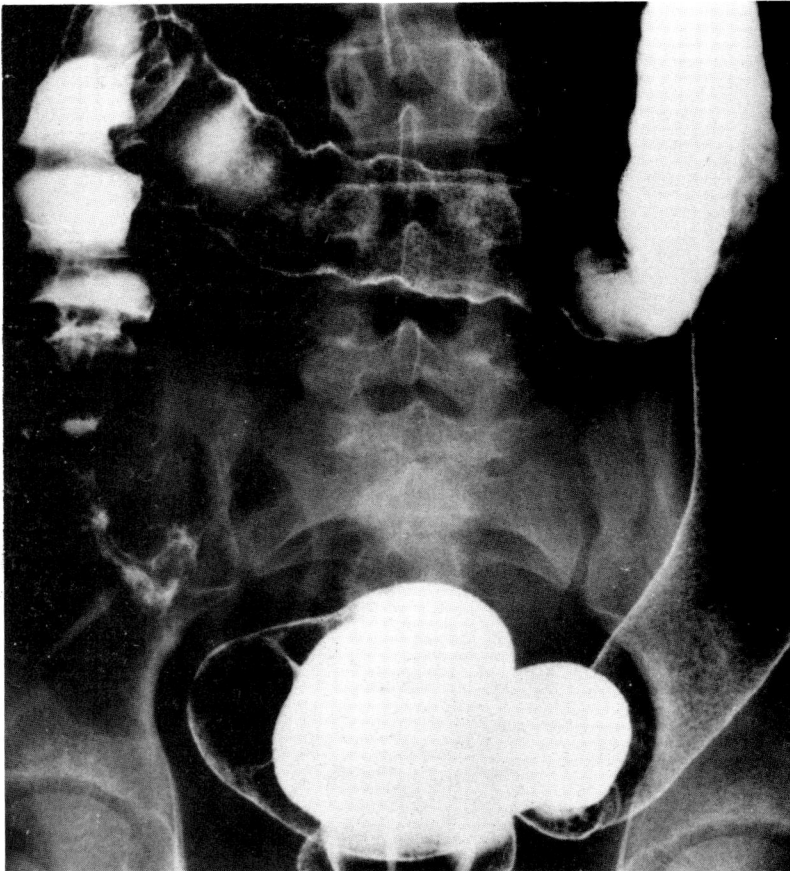

This 12 year old girl presented with a long history of weight loss, pallor and muscle wasting and diarrhoea.

- Rectal examination and sigmoidoscopy were performed. What might these examinations reveal?

- A barium enema was then carried out. What is the diagnosis?

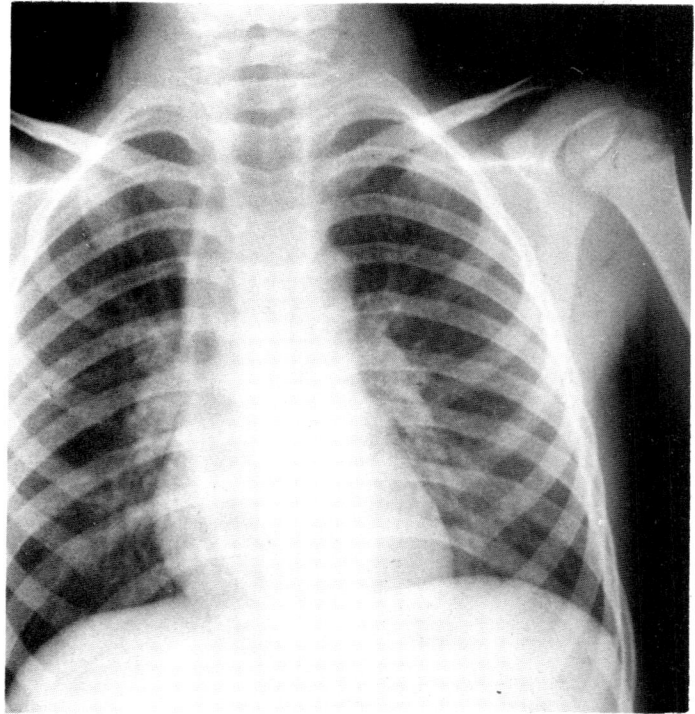

A

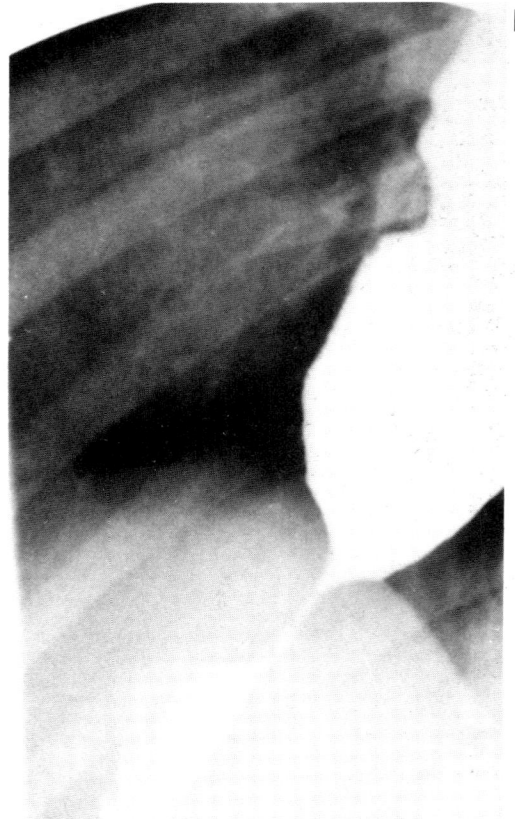

B

These are the plain chest X-ray and barium swallow of an English child being investigated for dysphagia.

- What is the diagnosis?

A79

This patient has severe ulcerative colitis. There is loss of the haustral pattern and the colon has a granular appearance due to superficial ulceration. While the radiological features are well seen in this case it has been estimated that between 10% and 30% of children with ulcerative colitis may show no radiological findings up to 2 years after the clinical onset of the disease.

On rectal examination and sigmoidoscopy a granular friable bleeding and ulcerated mucosa was seen. Colonoscopy is probably the most valuable investigation. The extent of the disease can be assessed and numerous punch biopsies will confirm the histological diagnosis and indicate the severity of inflammation at various levels. The histology report will read 'consistent with ulcerative colitis', for there is no pathogenic lesion. It is imperative to exclude bacillary dysentery, amoebic colitis and specific entero-colitis for these can be cured.

Barium enema should be carried out for a defined purpose. In this patient it was done to demonstrate the length of continually affected intestine.

Malignancy is a long term complication.

A80

The child is suffering from achalasia. The plain film shows marked dilatation of the oesophagus and lack of gas in the stomach.

Barium is retained in the oesophagus, the lower end of which is symmetrically tapered and this is characteristic of achalasia.

In this condition there is degeneration of the myenteric plexus. This results in failure of the gastro-oesophageal sphincter to relax on swallowing and causes abnormal oesophageal motility.

A history of difficulty in swallowing, especially solid foods, regurgitation of retained oesophageal contents and occasional substernal discomfort is usual.

This child presented with constipation and an associated lumbar lordosis.

- What are the two diagnoses on this barium enema film?

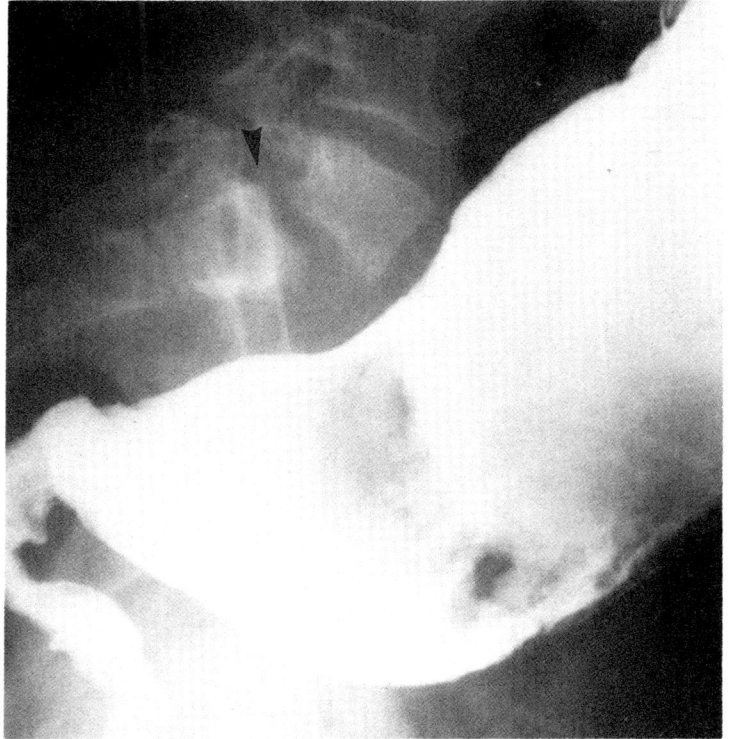

Q82

This child had bile stained vomiting.

- What investigation has been performed?

- What is the diagnosis?

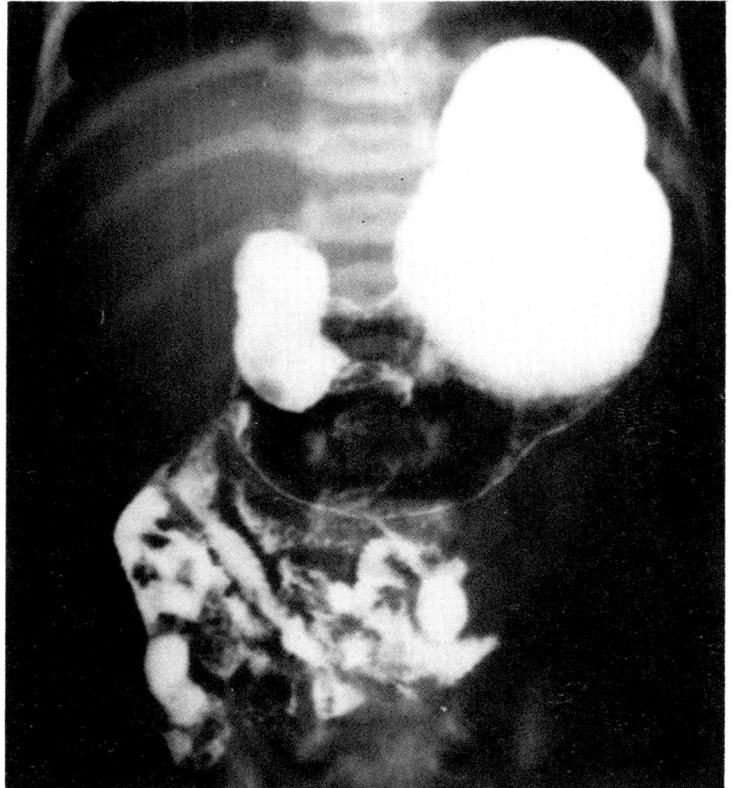

A81

This young lad is suffering from Hirschsprung's disease. There is an absence in a segment of distal gut of the ganglion cells of both Auerbach's plexuses and Meissner's plexuses with an increase in number and size of the mesenteric nerve fibres. It is a congenital condition and in childhood leads to problems with chronic constipation and complications of the faecal stasis. In infancy diarrhoea may be the presenting complaint.

In this X-ray the aganglionic segment is seen distally affecting the rectum and sigmoid colon which are narrow. More proximally the sigmoid is grossly dilated and between this dilated and narrow segment is a transition zone.

If the patient had simple constipation the distended bowel would extend as far as the anal canal.

Hirschsprung's disease is now the commonest cause of intestinal obstruction in the newborn. The classical signs in neonatal patients are:
— delay in passage of meconium
— bile stained vomiting
— abdominal distension and absence of gas or content in the rectum on plain film.

He also has a spondylolisthesis grade I (arrowed)

Diagnosing Hirschsprung's disease on the basis of a barium enema examination in a young infant depends on the level of skill locally. Now, diagnosis based on acetylcholinesterase histochemistry and on a rectal manometry is well over 90%. In Hirschsprung's disease there are abundant nerve fibres in the bowel wall; these are rich in acetylcholinesterase, which stains deeply. A small suction biopsy specimen of mucosa can be evaluated accurately by an experienced pathologist using this technique.

A82

The barium meal confirms the child's malrotation with barium entering the duodenum which passes downwards and towards the right where the jejunum lies. Normally the duodenum passes across the spine to the left of the spine and the duodeno-jejunal junction.

The ill effects of malrotation are produced by partial or complete blockage in the passage of intestinal contents along the alimentary tract. This causes vomiting which is almost always bile stained. Because the obstruction is high and partial the abdomen is distended in only half of the cases.

When a plain film of the abdomen is taken a volvulus is present with gas in the stomach and only a small amount of air in the small intestine. Stenosis of the duodenum may cause this picture.

In cases of malrotation a barium meal or a barium enema can show the nature of the problem. On the barium enema the large intestine is not fixed in the usual position, rather it lies towards the left part of the abdomen. In general when the small bowel lies to the right of the lumbar spine and the large bowel to the left malrotation is present.

- What examination is being performed in film A?

- What is the diagnosis?

Contrast medium was injected directly into the distal limb of patient B's colostomy.

- What does the examination reveal?

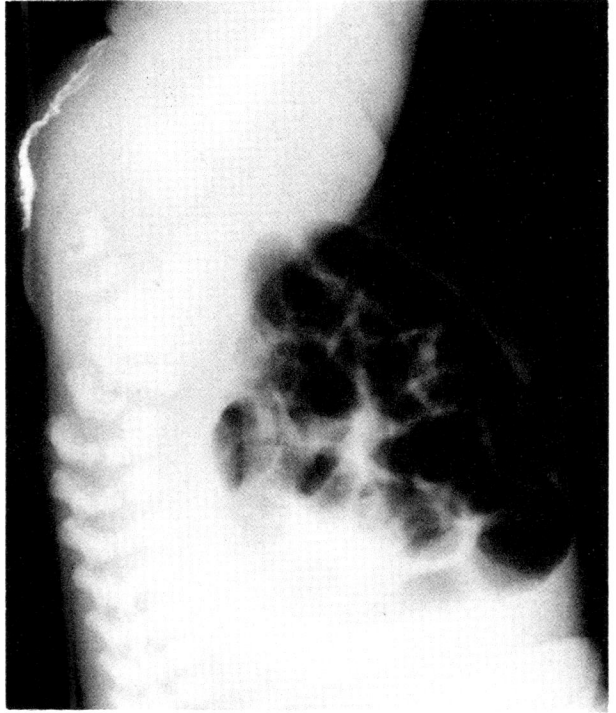

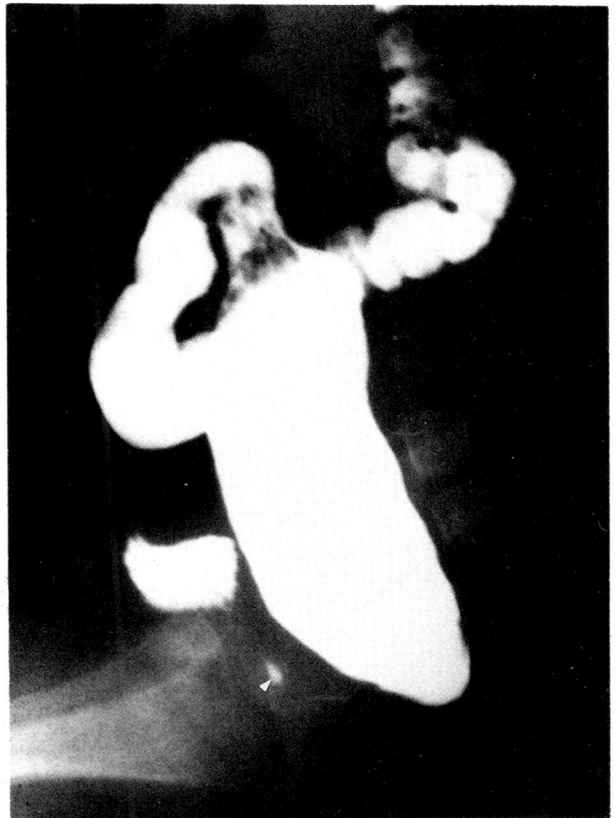

A83

Both children have an imperforate anus.

A lateral film of the abdomen has been taken with the infant inverted and a radio opaque swab placed on the expected site of the anus (Film A).

Gas rises to the apex of the blind bowel, and its level may be compared with various skeletal landmarks, which in turn correspond to the level of the puborectalis sling.

It is now thought that this examination may contribute little to determining the level of the lesion, though it may show air in the bladder confirming the presence of a recto-vesical fistula or the presence of sacral agenesis. The level of the anomaly is important. If it lies above the levator ani and the bowel has not passed through the puborectalis sling repair entails bringing the bowel through the sling.

Film B is of a patient with an imperforate anus with contrast agent spilling anteriorly through a fistula (arrowed) to the urethra and then upwards to the bladder.

Note the abnormalities of segmentation with vertebral body fusion etc.

Following resuscitation this 24 hour old infant did not pass meconium.

- What does the X-ray show?
- What is the most likely diagnosis?

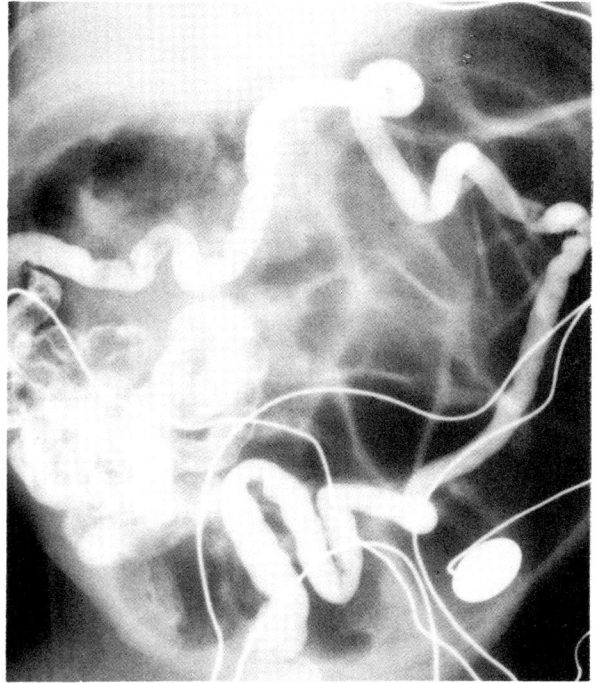

Q85

This child presented with weight loss, poor growth, pyrexia of unknown origin and retardation of skeletal maturation.

- Describe the X-ray.
- What is the diagnosis?

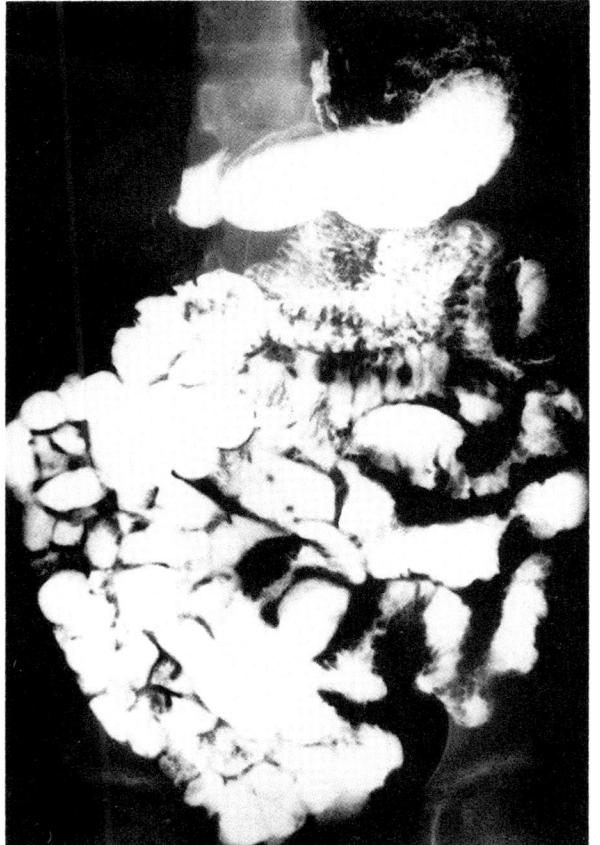

A84

This infant has cystic fibrosis. He developed abdominal distension and had not passed meconium. Injection of water soluble contrast medium showed a normally rotated microcolon and an undilated terminal ileum containing meconium. Much of the terminal ileum was filled but contrast medium did not reach the dilated bowel. Towards the right of the midline the distal ileum is seen to contain meconium, in quantity, outlined by gastroffin. Meconium obstructs the bowel and plugs the ileum. Small bowel proximally is gas-filled and wide.

Meconium ileus is the earliest gastro-intestinal lesion in patients with cystic fibrosis and is present in 5-25% of cases. Meconium ileus is an intestinal obstruction with thick, dark, sticky meconium lodged in the terminal ileum. The bowel distal to the obstruction is collapsed and narrow. Volvulus, small bowel atresia, and perforation, with meconium peritonitis, occasionally occur antenatally.

After a water-soluble contrast enema the patient cleared meconium and did not require surgery. Surgery is required when volvulus or perforation are present.

A85

This patient has Crohn's disease. The barium meal and follow through shows multiple narrowed jejunal loops with separated loops and irregular mucosa. The terminal ileum was radiologically normal.

Crohn's disease is a chronic inflammatory disorder affecting the full thickness of the bowel wall. It may occur at any age, but is rare in infancy. Diagnosis is confirmed by large and small bowel barium studies. Over half of the lesions are found only in the small intestine. The terminal ileum is most commonly affected. In only 10% is the colon alone affected. In Crohn's disease short segmental lesions are common with normal bowel in between; these are known as skip lesions.

Fistula may develop from one piece of bowel to another. The mucosal surface of the bowel is said to resemble cobblestones. This appearance is created by oedema and longitudinal fissures. Stenoses of the bowel may occur and may be multiple. The 'string sign' appearance is a consequence of narrowing of the lumen of the bowel over a considerable distance and when this lumen fills with barium it gives the appearance of a white string.

In the colon, radiological features are often similar to ulcerative colitis. The haustral pattern is increased in early stages. It is lost in later stages and shortening of the colon may occur. Ulcers undercutting the mucosa may create a 'collar stud' effect.

A

B

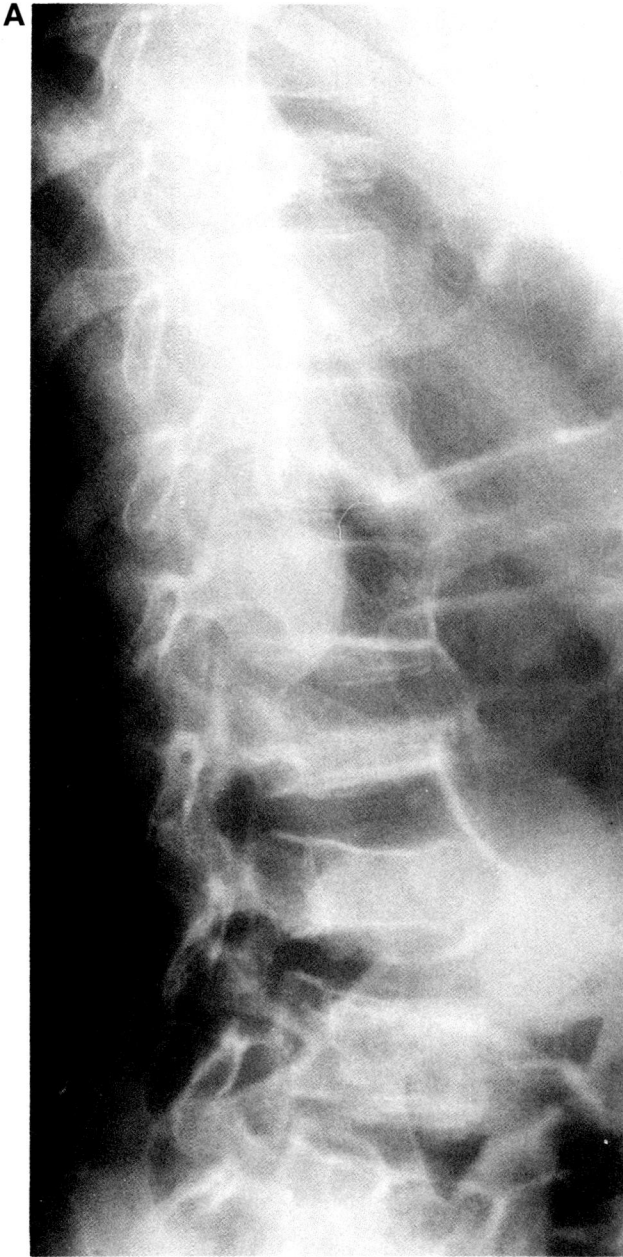

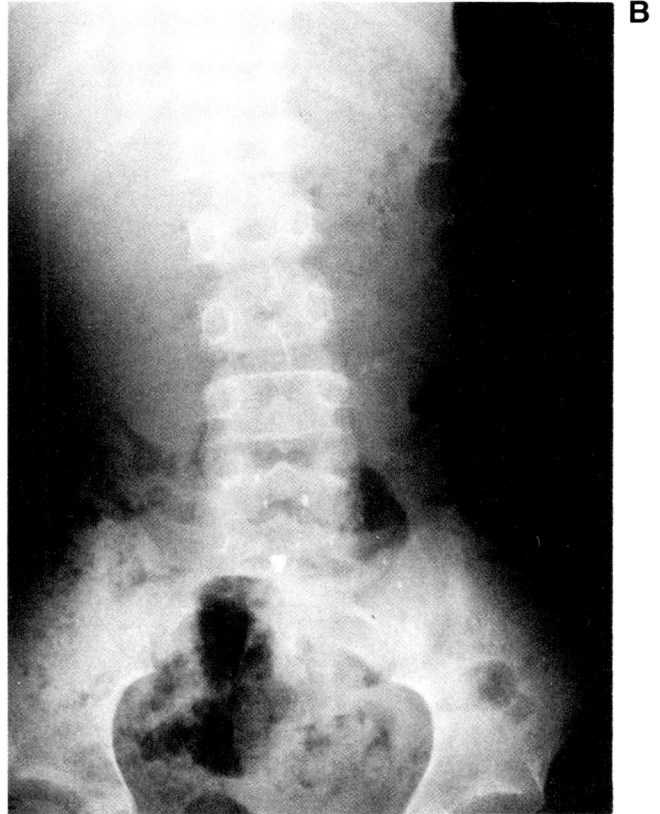

These are the X-rays of a patient presenting to casualty with malaise, back pain and a palpable abdominal mass. Examination of her urine confirmed the diagnosis.

- What did analysis of her urine reveal?

- What radiological features support the diagnosis?

A86

A 24 hour urine collection showed a greatly increased urinary concentration of vanillylmandelic acid (VMA) and homovanillic acid (HVA). The increase of these urinary catecholamines supports the diagnosis of neuroblastoma. The plain abdominal X-ray shows calcification in the neuroblastoma of her sympathetic chain (Film A). This was found anteriorly and below the inferior pole of the left kidney. Radiology of the spine reveals bone metastases with complete collapse of a lower thoracic vertebra with flattening of the lumbar vertebra (Film B).

Neuroblastoma accounts for 7% of childhood cancer. Neuroblastomas originate in tissues derived from the neural crest and may occur along the sympathetic chain, most frequently in the adrenal glands.

The usual radiological findings are a mass on straight X-ray of the abdomen, with calcification, which may extend across the midline. IVP may demonstrate displacement of a kidney that still excretes.

In contrast to some other childhood cancers, neuroblastomas have not responded dramatically to modern antitumour therapy.

Q87

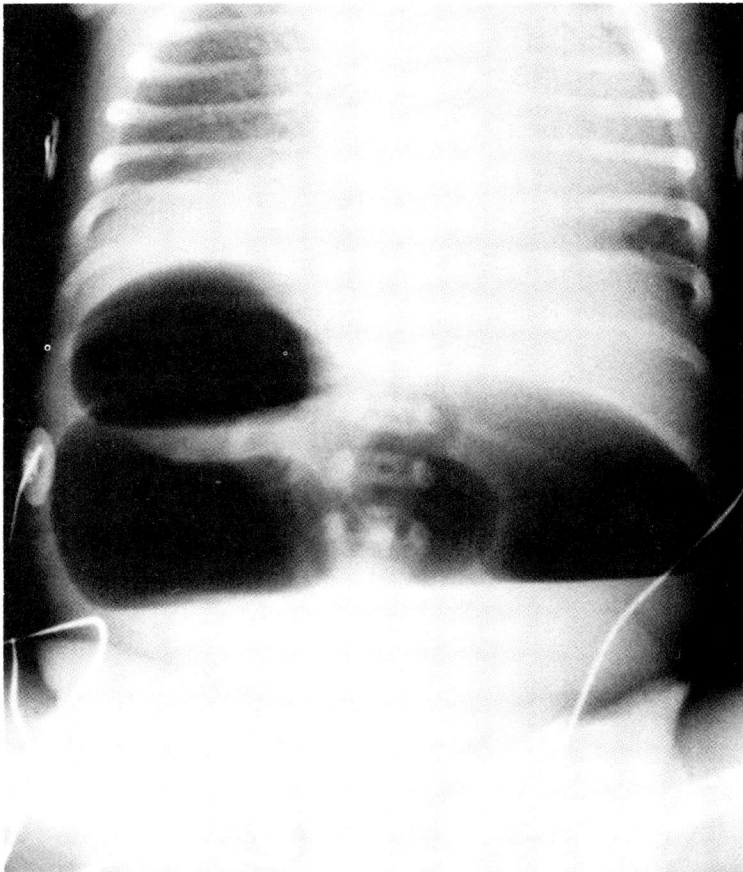

This is the X-ray of a one day old neonatal patient with bilious vomiting.

- Describe the abnormalities seen.

Q88

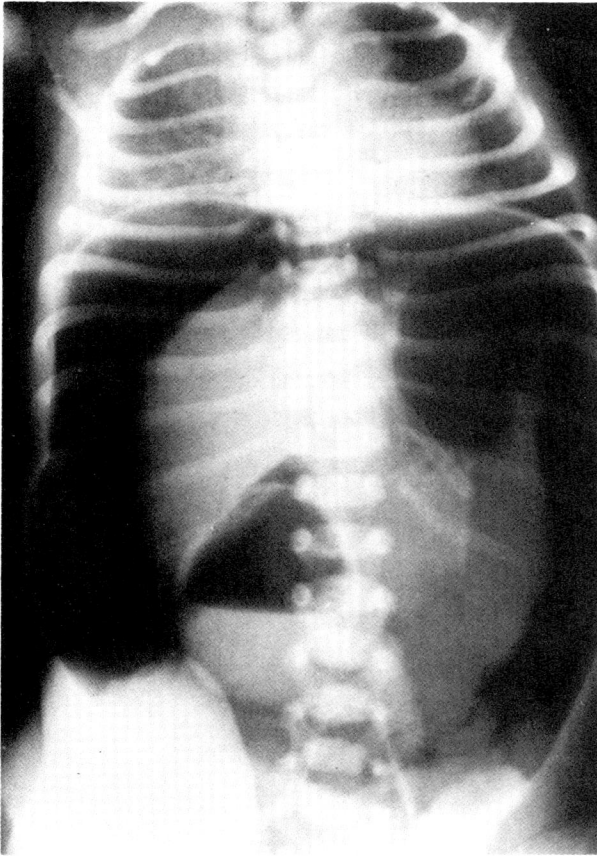

This neonatal patient had a recent history of blood stained faeces, distended abdomen and respiratory distress.

- What does this X-ray show?

His respiratory distress increased despite intubation and ventilation.

- What would be your emergency management?

Q89

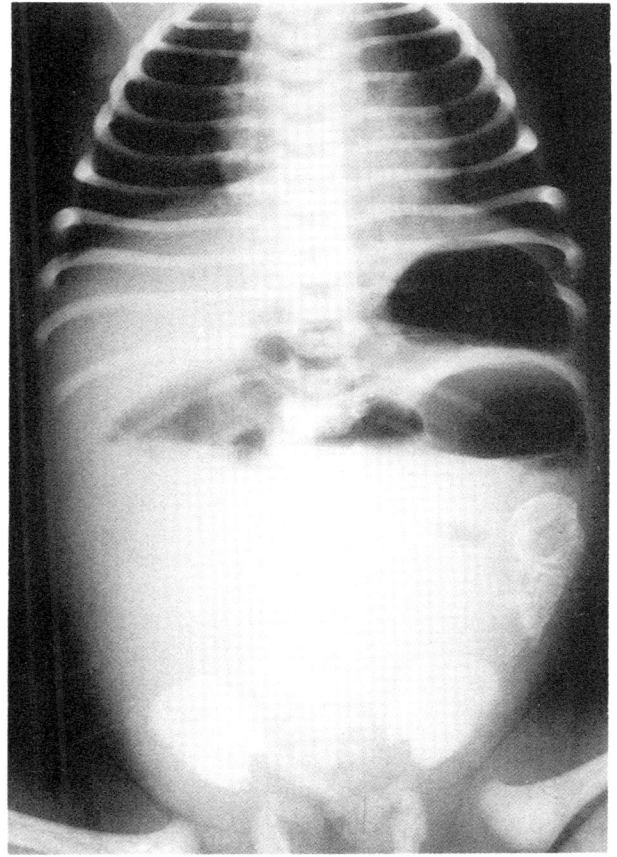

This patient began to vomit bile 12 hours after delivery and was noted to have mild abdominal distension. Meconium had not been passed. The patient's one year old brother had no problems at birth but was now failing to thrive and suffered from frequent chest infections.

- Describe the findings on the abdominal X-ray.

- What may have caused the calcification seen?

- What is the likely association between this child and his brother?

- What test would you use to confirm this? What may cause a false positive result?

A87

This neonatal patient has a high jejunal atresia. The stomach bubble is on the right side and the upper small bowel is dilated. There is absence of gas in the lower abdomen. The infant was noted to have cardiomegaly on chest X-ray which was due to an atrio-ventricular canal defect.

Surgery revealed multiple jejunal atresias which were excised and an enterostomy was performed. The infant died shortly afterwards.

Autopsy revealed situs ambiguus. Both liver and stomach were situated on the right side. A large spleen and multiple small spleens were also seen on the right side.

Infants with jejunal atresia present with gastro-intestinal obstruction in the neonatal period. Vomiting occurs but abdominal distension may not be obvious in jejunal lesions if stenosis is proximal. However, with distal lesions abdominal distension may be gross causing ventilatory problems.

A88

This neonatal patient has a pneumoperitoneum which appears to be under tension. Free gas within the peritoneum is usually due to perfora-tion of some part of the gastrointestinal tract. Visceral rupture may be secondary to necrotising enterocolitis, neonatal volvulus, intussusception, meconium ileus, intestinal atresia and imperforate anus. In a small number of cases no cause can be identified.

It is of interest that any air introduced into the peritoneal cavity at laparotomy is rarely seen radiologically more than 24 hours after operation. Some regard the presence of air as evidence of leak from an anastamosis 24 hours after laparotomy. Tracking of air from a pneumomediastinum may also result in a pneumoperitoneum.

Emergency management of a tension pneumo-peritoneum requires aspiration of peritoneal air to improve ventilation and subsequent surgical intervention.

A89

There is dilatation of the proximal small bowel, with fluid levels and no gas in the distal small bowel or in the large bowel. A mass of calcifi-cation is seen in the lower half of the left side of the abdomen.

The most common cause of such calcification is intra-uterine perforation of the bowel which allows the escape of sterile meconium into the peritoneal cavity. The meconium undergoes rapid calcification. Most cases are due to meconium ileus. Such calcification can occur in any situation where intestinal obstruction with perforation is present before birth such as with volvulus and congenital bands.

Meconium ileus is the earliest clinical mani-festation of cystic fibrosis.

The history of failure to thrive and recurrent chest infections in the sibling also suggests screening for cystic fibrosis should be carried out.

The diagnosis of cystic fibrosis is made by finding increased sodium and chloride levels in sweat obtained by pilocarpine iontophoresis. Con-ditions causing a false positive sweat test include ectodermal dysplasia, Addison's disease, nephrogenic diabetes insipidus, glucose-6-phosphatase deficiency, hypothyroidism, muco-polysaccharidoses and malnutrition. Meconium peritonitis can occur without cystic fibrosis being present. Therefore it is imperative to check a positive sweat test.

This child presented with rectal bleeding.

- What examination has been performed?
- What do the arrows reveal?
- What may you find on inspection of the oral region?
- What complications are associated with this syndrome?

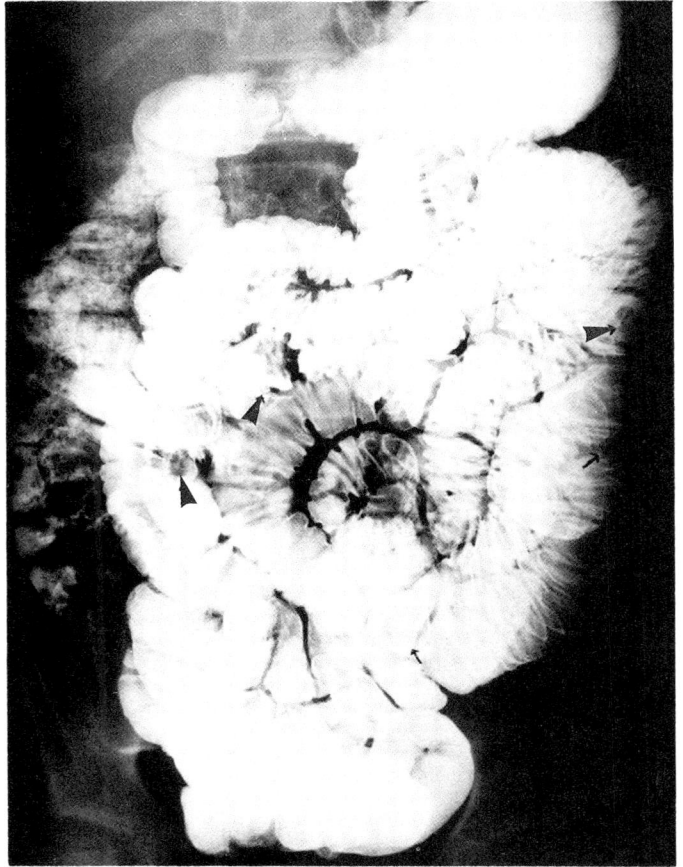

Q91

This child presented with fullness after eating, and occasional upper abdominal pain.

- What has the barium study revealed?

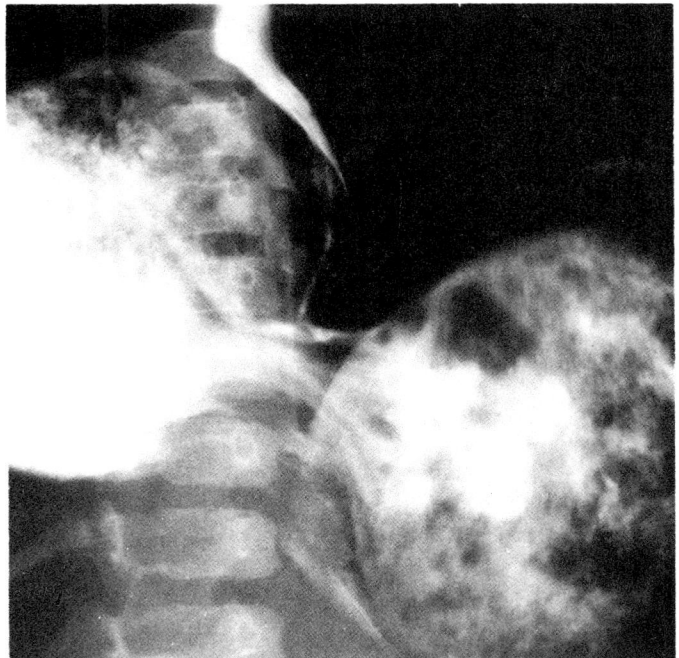

A90

A barium meal and follow through examination has been performed and shows a number of rounded filling defects due to polyps (arrowed). Some patients with polyps have pigmented freckles on the mucocutaneous margins of their lips and anus. This is known as the Peutz-Jeghers syndrome. The polyps, which may be found anywhere in the gastrointestinal tract, may give rise to massive bleeding, intussusception, or intestinal obstruction. Rarely a polyp may become malignant.

A91

The child has a para-oesophageal hiatus hernia. Herniation of part of the stomach into the thorax through the oesophageal hiatus is para-oesophageal in some patients and sliding in others. In the former type the gastro-oesophageal junction is positioned normally, but a portion of the stomach herniates through a patent oesophageal hiatus. With a para-oesophageal hiatus hernia gastro-oesophageal reflux seldom occurs and there are frequently no symptoms. The lesion is often first diagnosed by an air/fluid level being seen on the chest film (Film B).

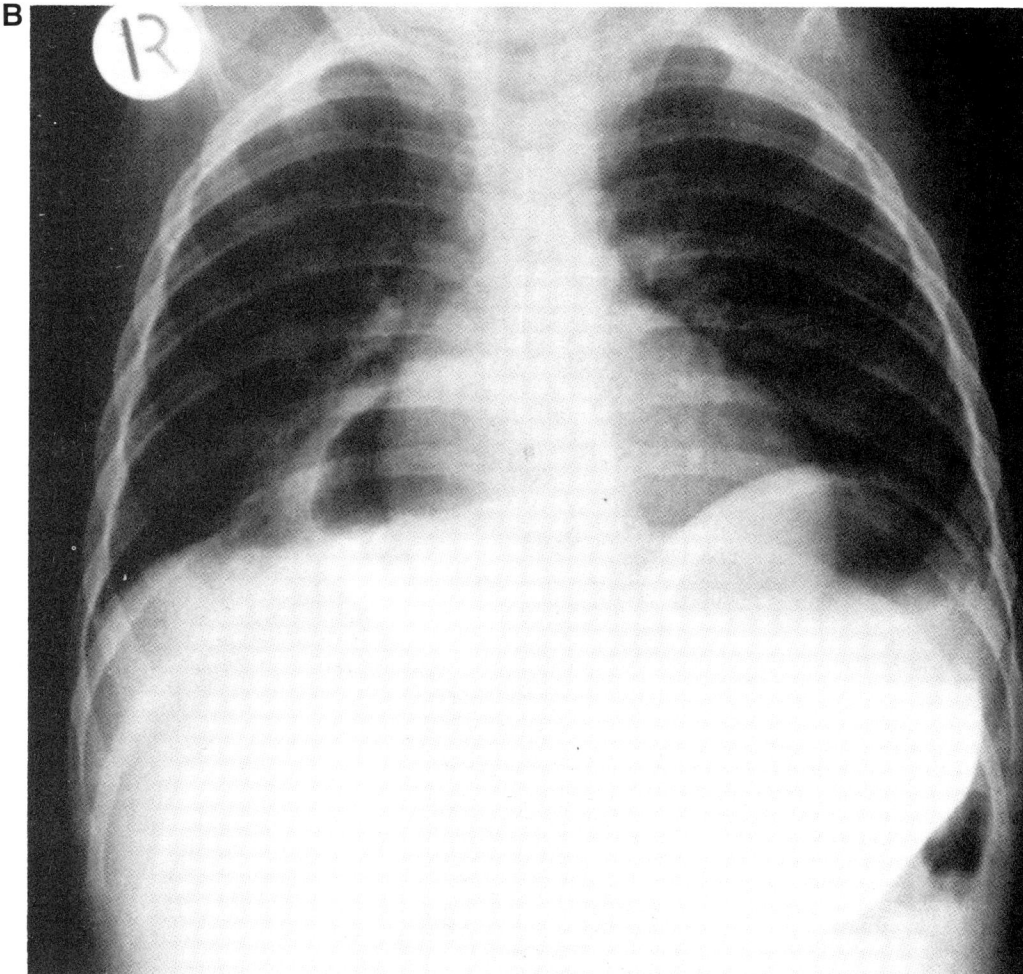

B

This child was noted to have asymptomatic splenomegaly. There was no clinical evidence of liver disease.

- What investigation has been performed and what does it show?

- What major problem may the child encounter?

- If the study above was repeated after this major problem had occurred what might it show, and how may the physical findings change?

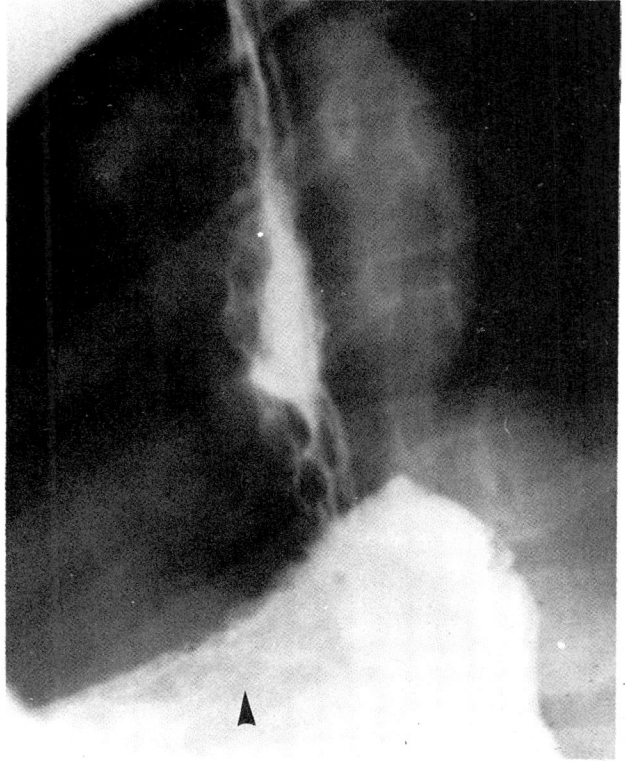

Q93

This child had recurrent abdominal pain.

- What is the diagnosis?

- What treatment is required?

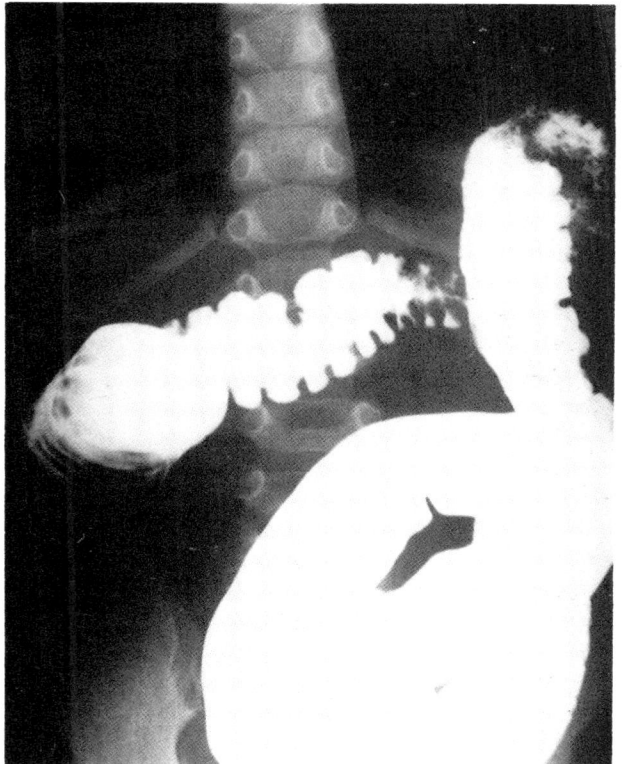

A92

A barium swallow has been performed and shows multiple filling defects in the lower part of the oesophagus. These defects are caused by large oesophageal varices secondary to extra-hepatic portal hypertension. Varices are rarely found except in the inferior portion of the oesophagus. Best visualisation of the dilated veins is obtained in the partially filled oesophagus when they are outlined by a fine layer of contrast agent which adheres to the mucosa. There are also gastric varices present in the fundus of the stomach (arrowed).

Patients with extra-hepatic portal hypertension present with asymptomatic splenomegaly, as in this case, or with alimentary bleeding. Less commonly children may present with ascites or failure to thrive.

The major problem is bleeding from the varices which is a contributory factor in the early death of up to 12% of patients. Following marked blood loss the spleen contracts and may be impalpable, so it has been said. Barium studies of the oesophagus after bleeding may fail to show varices because of the reduced vascular volume.

Following an acute bleed the diagnosis is best made by emergency endoscopy which defines both the site and the cause.

A93

This child has an intussusception. This is the invagination of one segment of bowel within the lumen of an adjoining segment. It most commonly begins in the region of the ileo-caecal valve. As barium passes along the large intestines it demonstrates the concave defect at the head of its column: that is the barium demonstrates the lead point of the intussusception.

The peak incidence is in infants 4-6 months old, and 70% of patients are under 1 year of age. In older children there may be an abnormality of the bowel which becomes the leading point of the intussusception, such as a polyp, a sub-mucosal cyst, a Meckel's diverticulum, or a lymphosarcoma of the ileum.

Hydrostatic reduction by means of a barium enema or insufflation of air, is usually attempted in patients who are fit. Indications for operative reduction include: children outside the typical age group (2 months to 2 years), moderate abdominal distension, multiple fluid levels on plain abdominal X-ray, signs of peritonitis, collapse and failure of hydrostatic reduction.

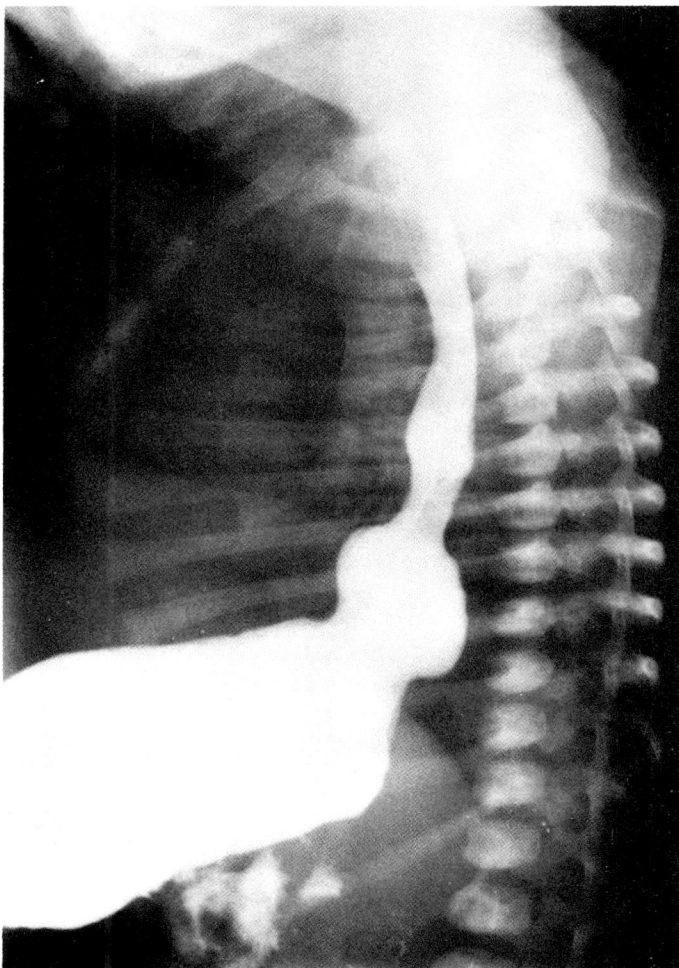

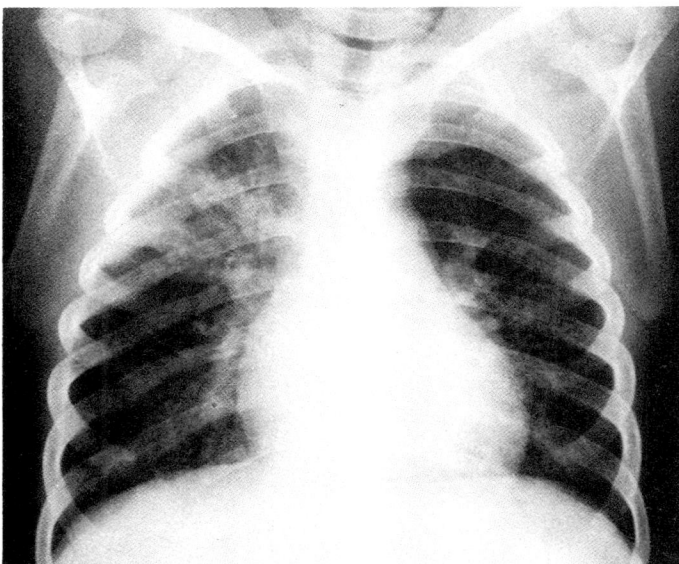

This child had recurrent cough and wheeze. A barium swallow (Film A) was performed because of recurrent vomiting and choking.

- What does the barium swallow show?
- Comment on the distribution of changes seen on the chest X-ray.
- How may you improve this child's chest symptoms?

A94

The barium swallow shows an episode of marked gastro-oesophageal reflux and a sliding hiatus hernia.

Acute and chronic lung disease frequently follows the aspiration of foreign material into the lower respiratory tract. Aspiration in children occurs as a result of disorders of sucking and swallowing, gastro-oesophageal reflux, abnormal connections between the airways and the alimentary tract and accidental aspiration. Aspiration may cause a range of lesions in the lungs including acute bronchitis, bronchiolitis, broncho-pneumonia, chronic bronchitis, obliterative bronchiolitis, interstitial pneumonia and pulmonary fibrosis.

The clinical features are a combination of the features due to the primary cause such as reflux and vomiting and secondary respiratory symptoms. Respiratory symptoms depend on the amount and duration of aspiration but include cough, rattly and wheezy breathing and tachypnoea. Wheeze and crepitations may be heard over the lung fields. Extensive inhalation may give recurrent pneumonia with fever, cough and tachypnoea. Continual inhalation may give chronic interstitial pneumonia, failure to thrive, cough, recurrent fever, malaise and tachypnoea. Mentally retarded children with chest disease may have a swallowing problem as a cause. Organisms retrieved may include aerobic and anaerobic organisms and fungi.

Chest X-ray findings tend to depend on age and gravity appears to be the determining factor. Infants usually fed in a supine or recumbent position often show evidence of inhalation into the posterior parts of the upper and lower lobes (Film B), whereas in the upright child the lower lobes and right middle lobes are commonly involved.

A normal barium study does not exclude the diagnosis of significant gastro-oesophageal reflux and pH monitoring may provide the answer. Demonstration of fat-laden macrophages on tracheal aspiration is highly suggestive of recurrent aspiration.

Q95

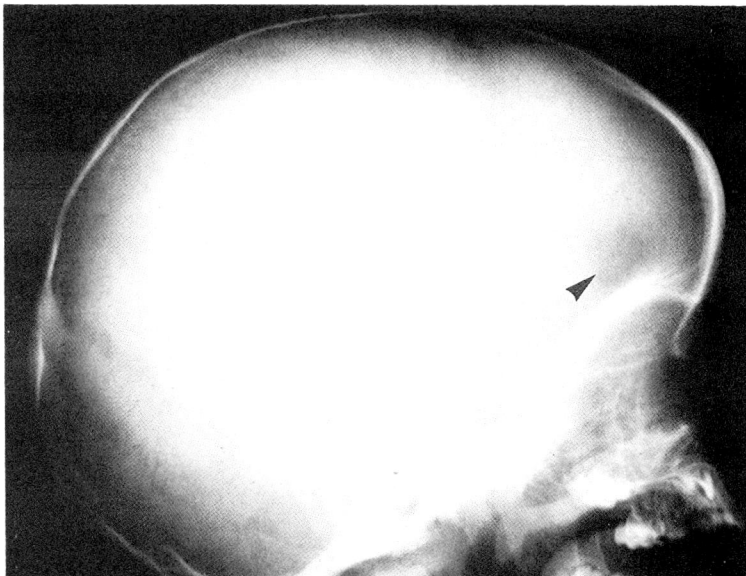

This boy presented with polyuria and polydipsia. He was noted to have exophthalmos on physical examination. A skull X-ray was taken.

- What abnormality is seen?
- What is the diagnosis?

A

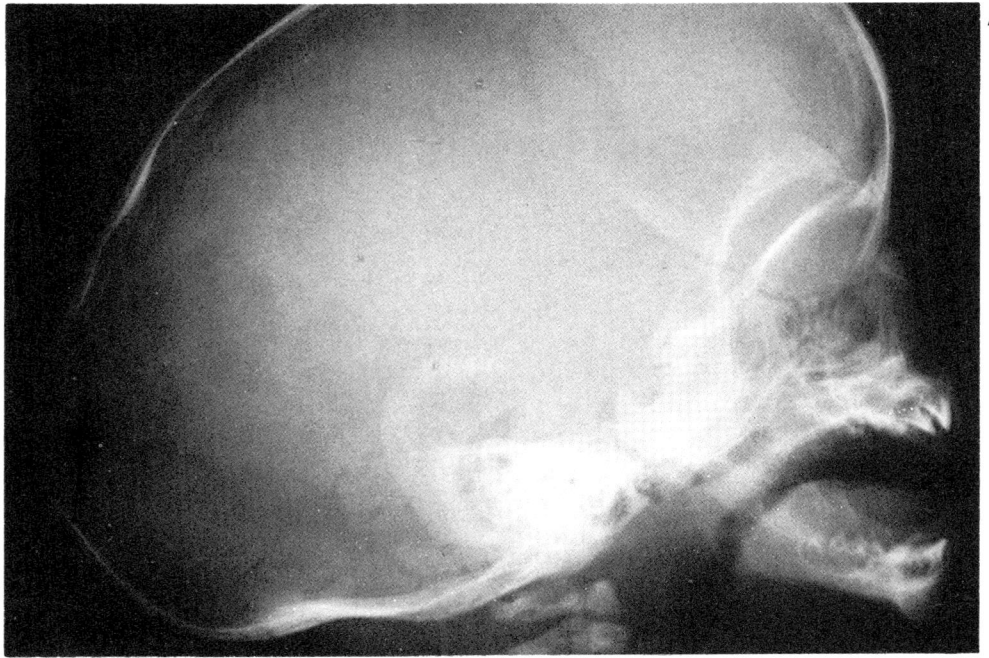

B

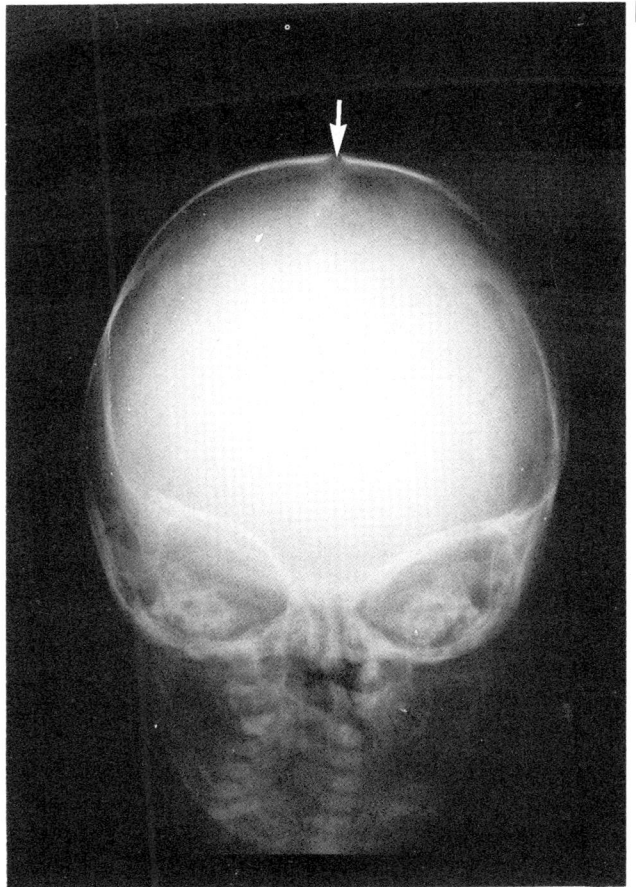

This is the skull X-ray of an infant with an abnormal head shape.

- What is responsible for the abnormal skull shape seen?

A95

The skull X-ray shows a round translucent destructive lesion (arrowed). The combination of skull defects, exophthalmos and diabetes insipidus suggests the diagnosis of Hand-Schüller-Christian disease. This combination is rarely seen. Children under 5 years of age are most frequently affected. The disease is characterised by loose teeth and soreness of the mouth, due to deposits in the gum and jaw and classic skin lesions.

Translucent areas of bone destruction with sharply defined margins are seen on X-ray. They tend to be numerous and commonly affect flat bones. In the skull they tend to coalesce resulting in the so called 'geographical skull'. The prognosis is good, as spontaneous remission, possibly accelerated by radiotherapy occurs in the majority of cases.

A96

This child is suffering from craniosynostosis, in which there is premature closure of the sutures between the bones of the vault. Closure restricts the development of the region affected because compensatory growth occurs at other suture lines, usually in a parallel direction to the fused suture.

This child has fusion of the sagittal suture.

Continued growth at the coronal and lambdoid sutures has resulted in a cranial vault which is long and relatively diminished in height ('scaphocephaly'). The sagittal suture is not visible throughout its length on the AP view. Indeed, only a tiny segment of the suture is visible in the vault (arrowed) with some density along its margin.

This child was referred when microcephaly was noted. Ultrasound revealed calcification of the ventricular walls.

- What is the most likely diagnosis?
- What ophthalmological problems may occur?

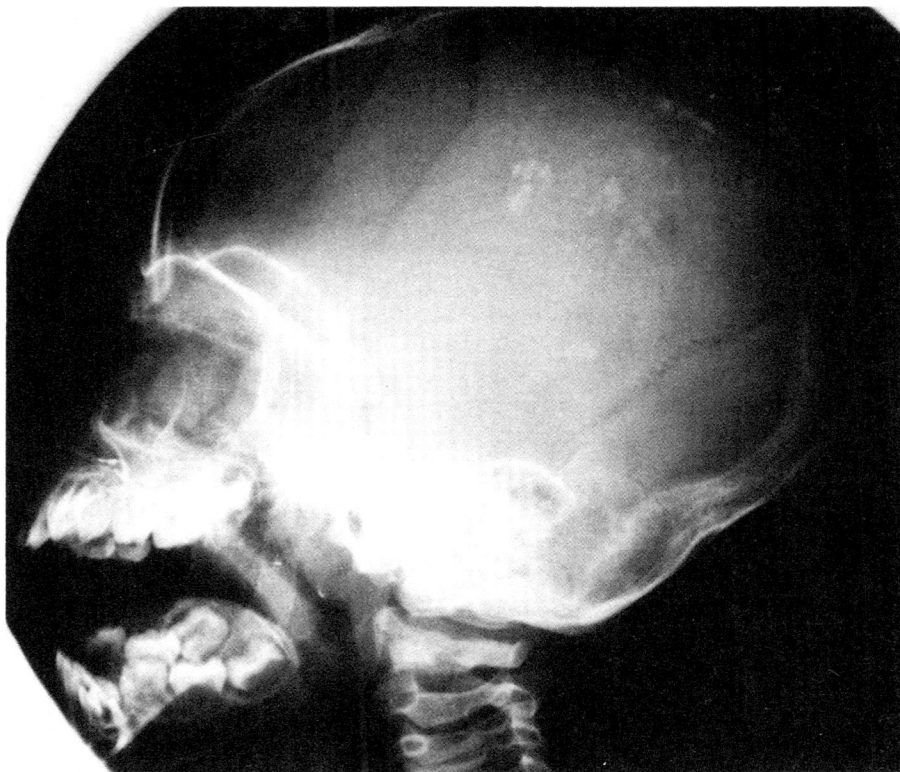

Q98

This is the skull X-ray of a child with epilepsy.

- What is the diagnosis?
- What ophthalmological problems may be encountered?

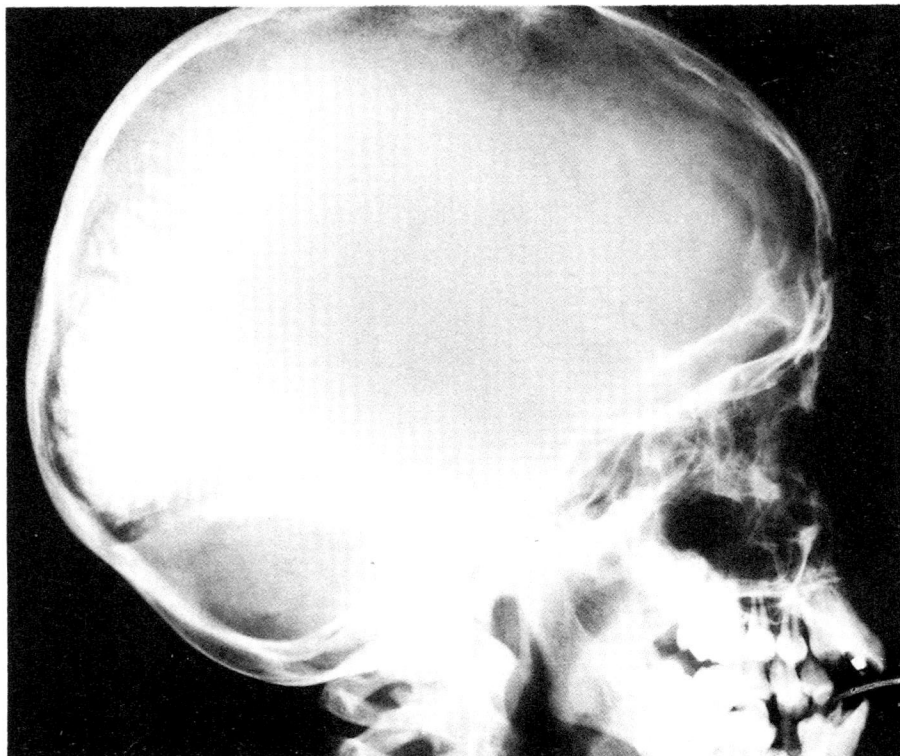

A97

There is intracranial calcification. Note the small size of the vault of the skull, especially the anterior fossa. Cytomegalovirus infection is the most likely cause. Cytomegalovirus infection may produce necrosis of the ventricular walls which later calcify. This form of calcification may occur in toxoplasmosis infection but is less common. However, microcephaly is usually seen in cytomegalovirus infections whilst hydrocephalus is often seen in toxoplasmosis infections. Chorioretinitis, conjunctivitis and uveitis may occur.

A98

This child has Sturge-Weber syndrome. The angiomatous malformation of the skin usually overlies one of the branches (usually ophthalmic) of the trigeminal nerve, and a similar vascular anomaly of the occipital area of the ipsilateral cerebral hemisphere.

Calcification is seen on the surface of the cerebral hemisphere. There is a curvilinear pattern and parallel lines which are due to convolutions and sulci outlined by the superficial layer of calcium deposited.

Ophthalmological problems include congenital glaucoma, buphthalmos, telangiectasia of the conjunctiva, and varicosities of the retinal vessels. The fundus may be dark red and the retina may detach.

The resultant cerebral ischaemia may give rise to mental retardation, epilepsy and hemiplegia.

Q99

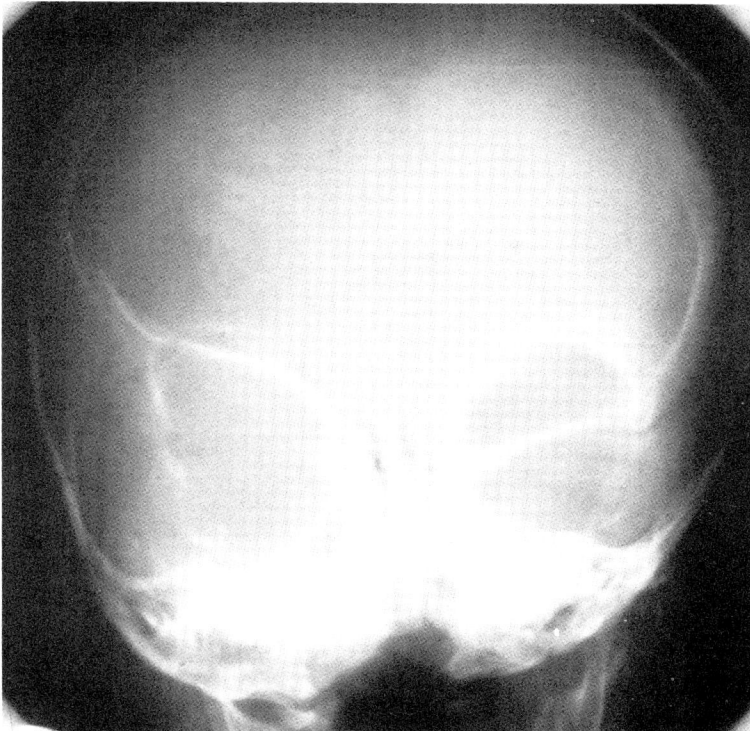

This child had an abnormal head shape.

- What abnormality is seen in this skull X-ray?
- What is the cause?

This child has a cranial meningocoele.

- Describe the abnormalities seen on this skull X-ray.

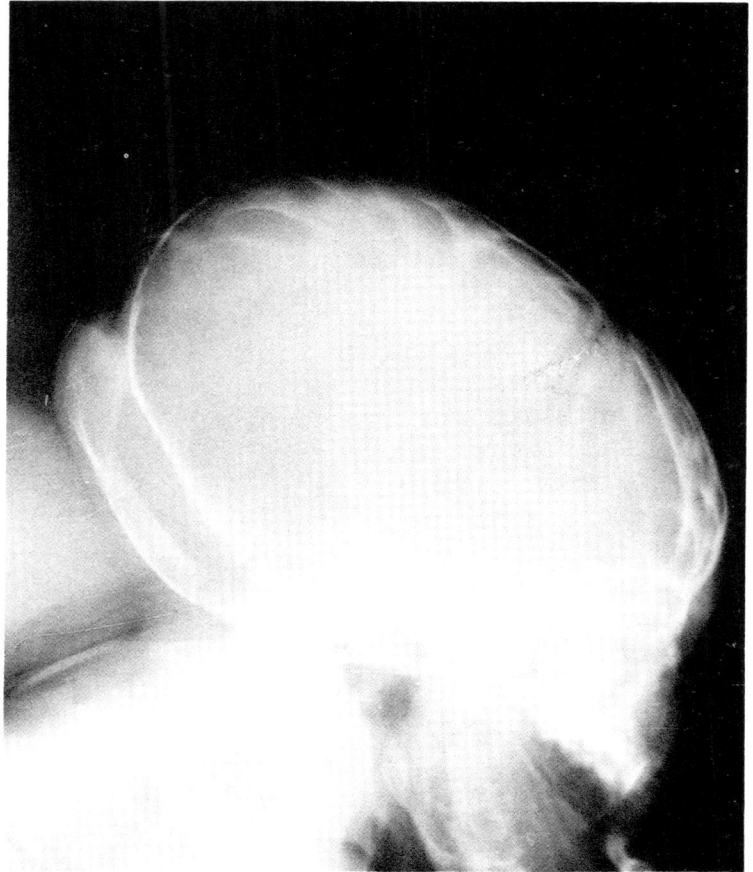

Q101

This child was delivered by forceps. A swelling developed over the parietal bone some hours later. After one week it began to diminish in size, but a hard protrusion remained near the midline.

- An abnormality was seen on the skull X-ray taken at 8 weeks of age (arrowed). What has caused this abnormality?

- What is the natural history of this lesion?

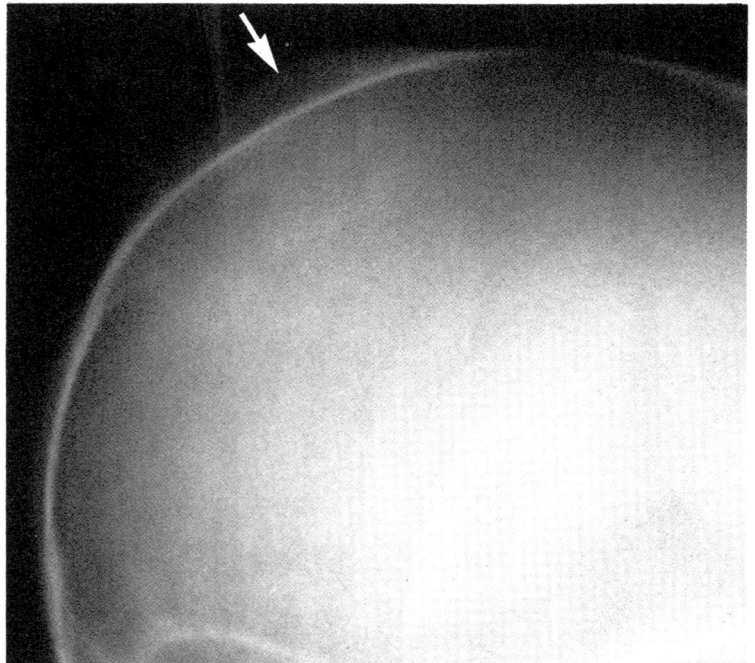

A99

The child has plagiocephaly. The roof of the right orbit is lifted into a more oblique position as is the right wing of the sphenoid. Obliteration of the sutures, commonly the coronal and occasionally the lambdoidal, is limited to one side of the skull and is a unilateral cranio-synostosis. This is known as plagiocephaly.

Premature fusion results in decreased volume on the affected side with compensatory increase in size of the opposite side.

In this child additional views confirmed the absence of the right coronal suture, and she required cranioplasty to correct the synostosis.

A100

This child has craniolacunia which is an anomaly of the skull characterised by multiple large areas of thin poorly mineralised bone separated by strips of normal bone. These lesions are often associated with hydrocephalus and meningo-myelocoele. Encephalocoeles are common in this region also. In this child there is a large cranial meningocoele. Cranial meningocoeles are typically located near the median sagittal plane in the occipital region. Frontal lesions may also occur. The hernial sac may be covered with skin and contains meninges only.

A101

This child has an ossified cephalhaematoma. New bone formation develops from the elevated periosteum with the effusion of blood beneath.

Cephalhaematomas in new born infants are accompanied by a fracture in 25% of cases. In most cases they resolve without sequelae. Only occasionally does ossification occur, and may persist for several months before resolving.

- Describe the abnormalities seen.
- What is the diagnosis?
- What is the inheritance of this condition?

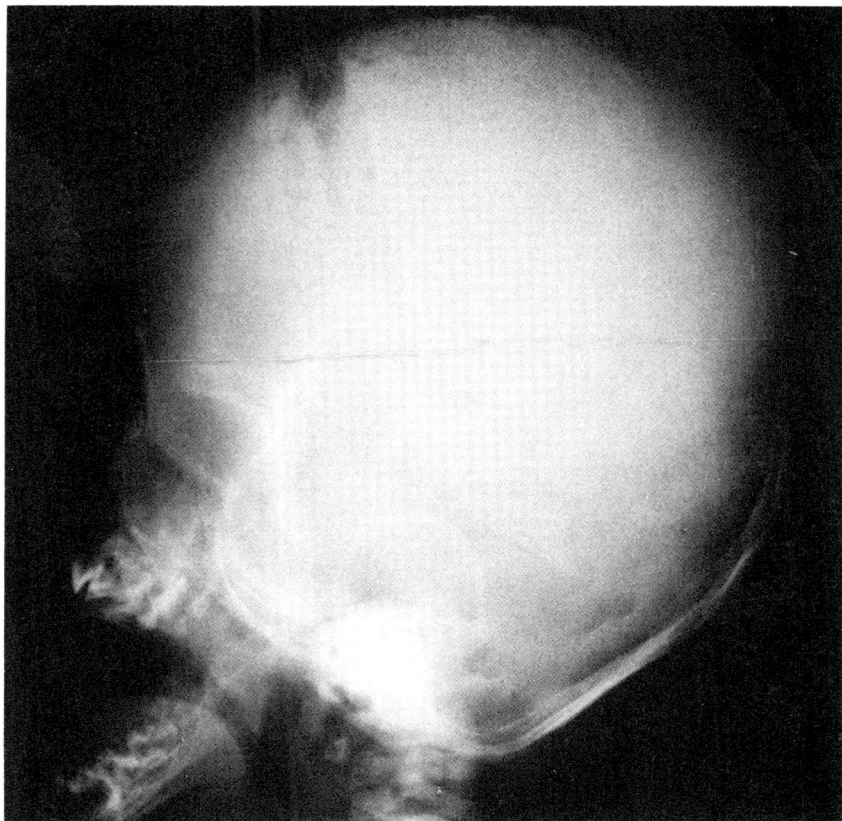

A

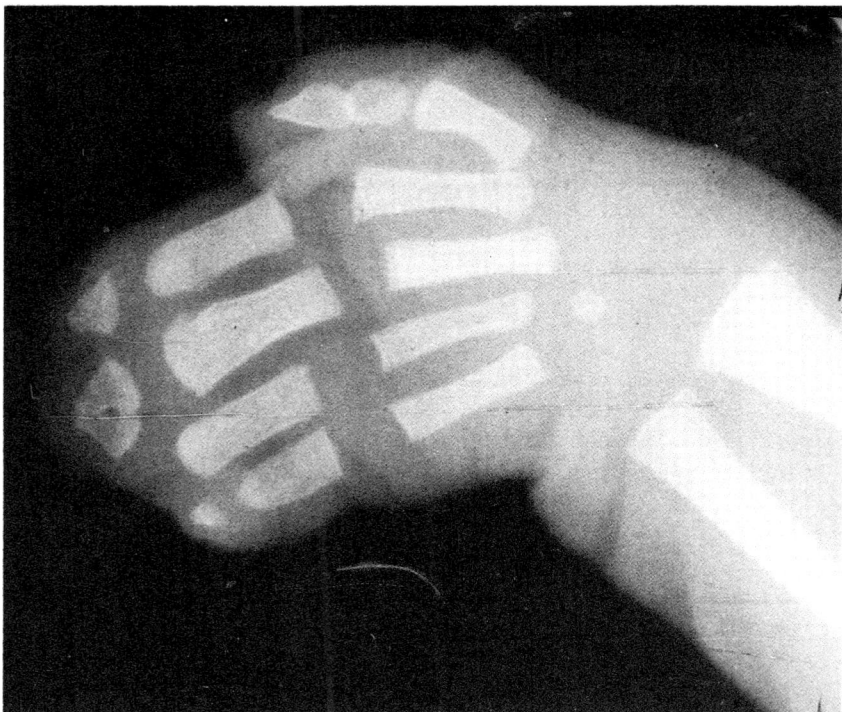

B

A102

The lateral view of the skull shows the cranial vault to be abnormally tall and short from back to front (turricephaly). This is due to fusion of the coronal sutures. The hand shows characteristic syndactyly (the digits are joined). This combination is characteristic of Apert's syndrome (acrocephalosyndactyly).

The facial appearance is bizarre with a steep forehead, hypoplastic middle third of the face, and sometimes asymmetry, hypertelorism, malocclusion and strabismus. There is a risk of mental retardation. Stature may be normal, but marked shortening may be present associated with congenital limb abnormalities. Visceral and genito-urinary anomalies occur.

Inheritance is autosomal dominant. However, the vast majority of cases are sporadic and represent new mutations.

Q103

A

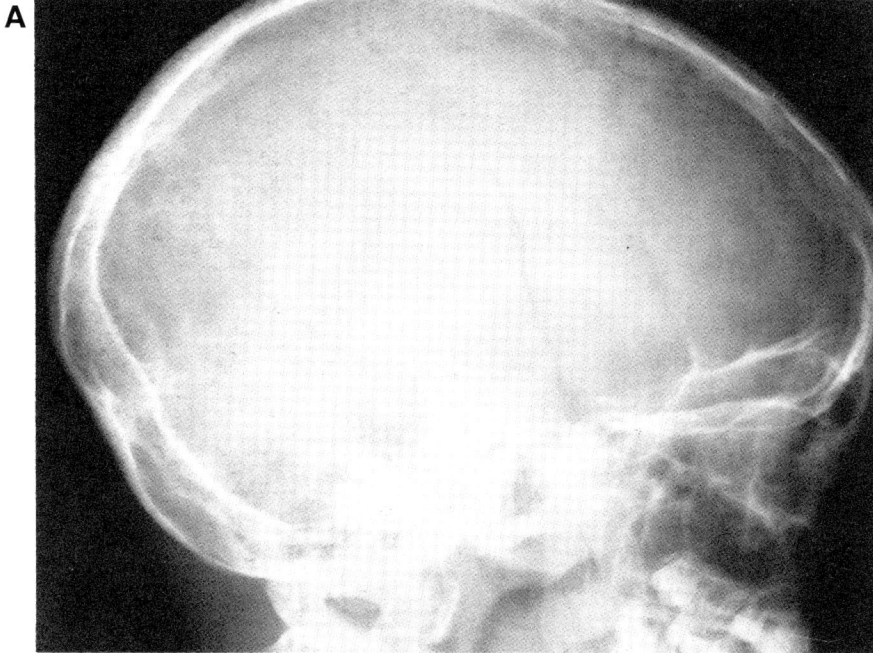

This child presented to hospital following a road traffic accident. The child recovered from his concussion. However, his level of consciousness started to deteriorate and he was admitted to the ward for overnight observation.

• What abnormality is seen on his skull X-ray?

• Why would you be concerned about the patient?

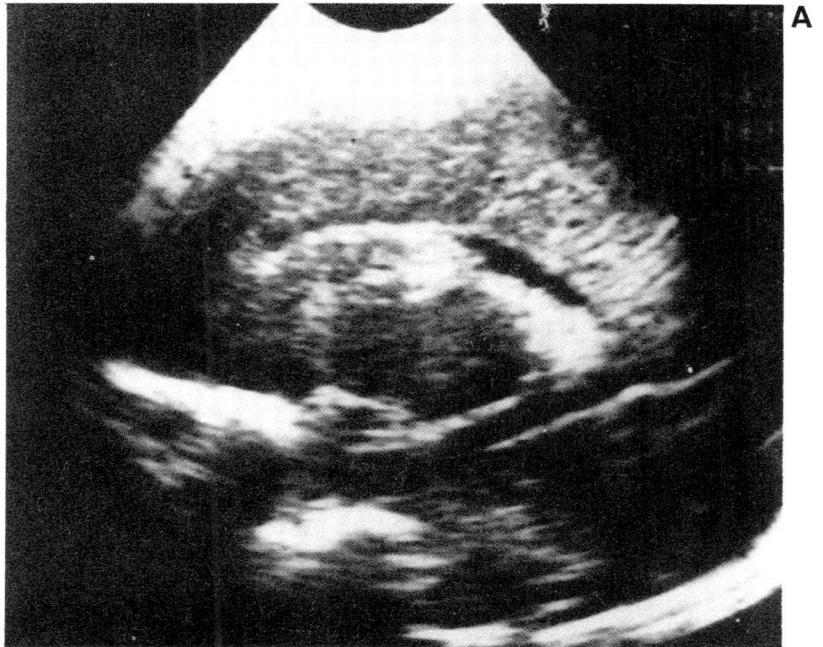

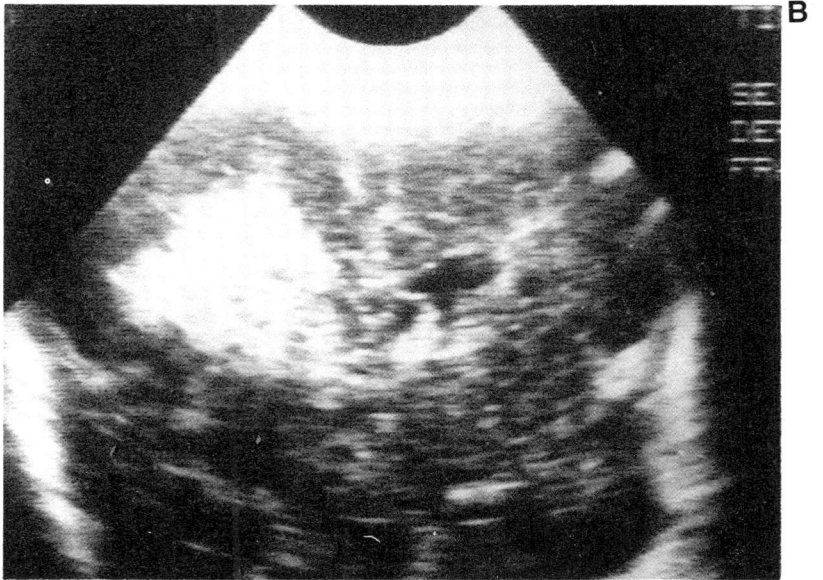

These are the cerebral ultrasound scans of two very premature neonates. Ultrasound scan A was performed after a sudden deterioration in condition. Ultrasound scan B was performed on a routine scanning session.

- What do they show?

A103

There is a linear fracture of the skull in the temporo-parietal region. The child deteriorated rapidly on the ward. The pupil on the side of the fracture was dilated and he developed a contra-lateral hemiparesis followed by respiratory arrest. The sudden deterioration was due to the pressure effects of an extradural haematoma (middle meningeal artery haemorrhage). The history and presence of a fracture in this region should alert one to an extradural haematoma. Once the diagnosis is made immediate evacuation and haemostasis should be secured without delay.

On the CT scan (Film B) the extradural haematoma is visible as a high density area in the frontal region (arrow). The structures normally found in the midline are displaced laterally by the pressure of the haematoma.

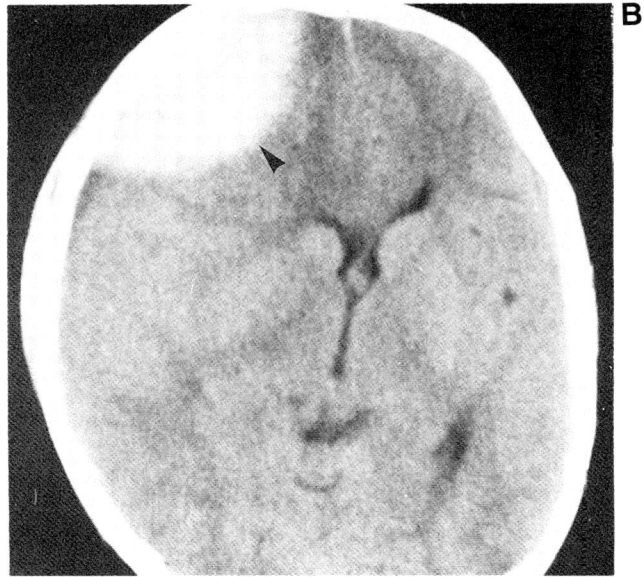

A104

Both neonates have developed a periventricular haemorrhage (PVH) (see diagrams).

Patient A has suffered a parenchymal extension of the haemorrhage. This was responsible for his sudden clinical deterioration. The rich vascular network lying on the floor of the lateral ventricles is prone to rupture and cause periventricular haemorrhage.

PVH is rare in infants over 32 weeks' gestation as the rich vascular network involutes early in the third trimester.

PVH may be divided into 4 grades:
1 Germinal layer haemorrhage.
2 Intraventricular haemorrhage (IVH) – not distending the ventricular system.
3 IVH with distension of the ventricular system.
4 Intracranial extension.

Routine cerebral ultrasound scanning of low birth weight infants has shown that up to 40% of infants less than 1.5 kg will have some form of PVH. Most cases of PVH will be missed if clinical criteria alone are relied upon.

Cerebral ultrasound scanning is the method of choice for detection of PVH and for assessment of ventricular size. The main limitations of real time ultrasound cerebral scanning are difficulties in recognizing small PVH, primary subarachnoid haemorrhages and small laterally placed subdural haemorrhages.

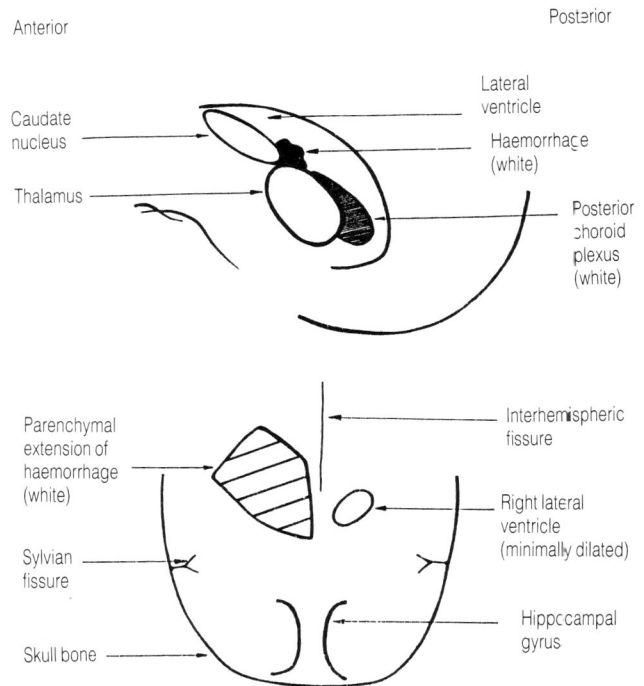

This 3 month old child presented with irritability, fever, pallor and tender soft tissue swellings over his mandible, clavicles and ulnae. The skin over the soft tissue swellings was neither hot nor erythematous.

- What does the X-ray of his jaw reveal?

- What other sites may be affected?

- What is the diagnosis?

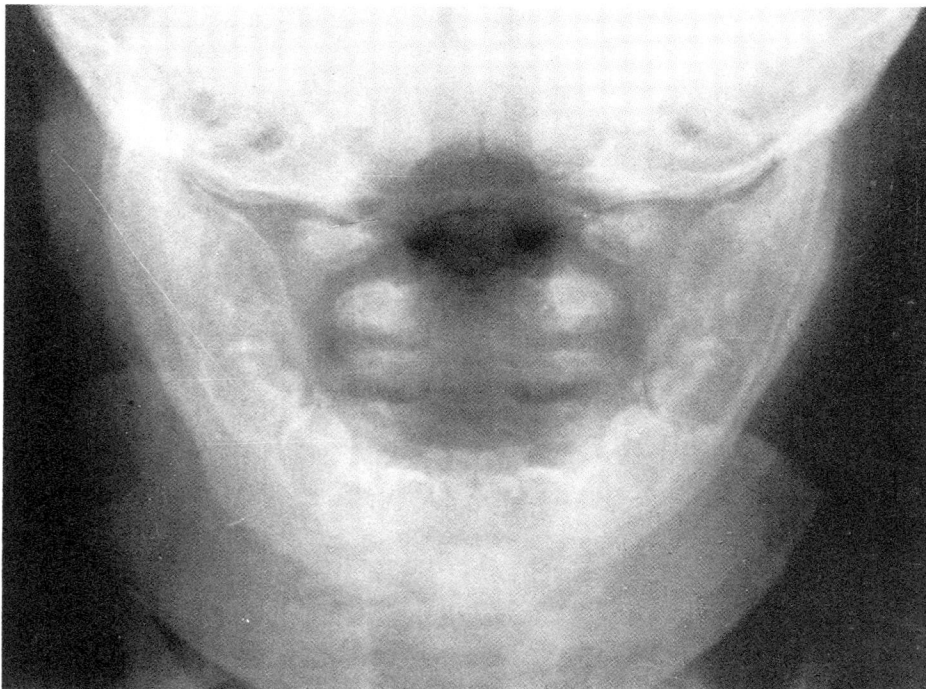

Q106

This is the X-ray of a child with ectopia vesicae. The child also had a rectal prolapse.

- What abnormality is seen on the X-ray and how will it affect the child's gait?

- Is sexual intercourse possible in either sex later in life?

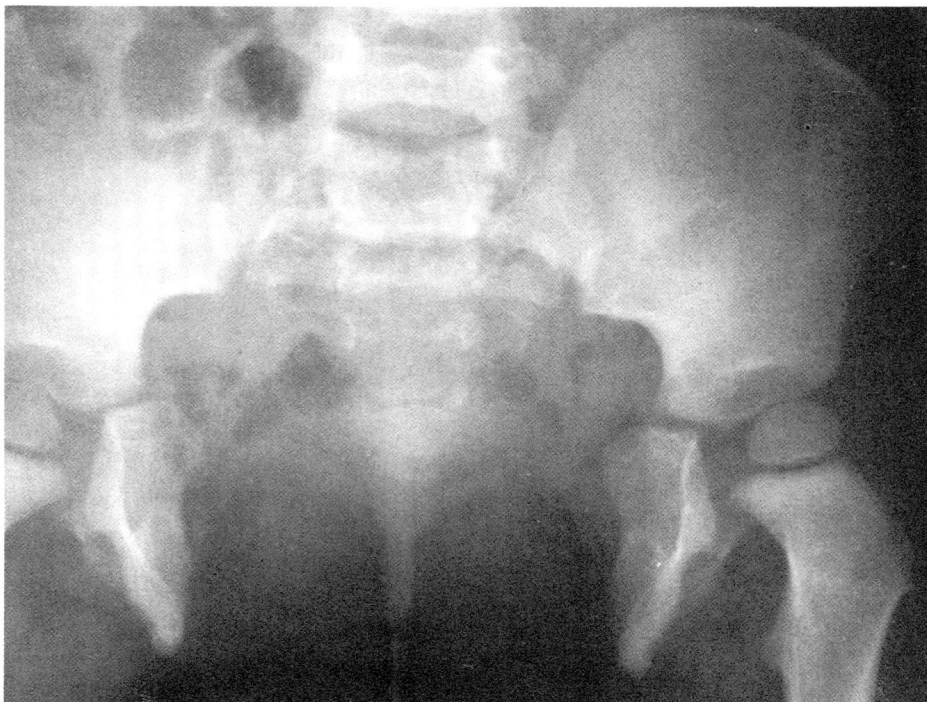

A105

This infant is suffering from Caffey's disease (infantile cortical hyperostosis). It is characterised by systemic disturbance and an acute inflammatory reaction in the periosteum. The onset is always before 5 months of age. The reactive periosteum becomes enclosed in fibrous tissue and periosteal new bone is laid down. The new bone is gradually reabsorbed leaving a normal bone contour. The cause is not known.

The X-ray of his jaw reveals periosteal new bone formation on the external aspect of the mandible, which is always involved at some stage of the illness.

The mandible, ulnae, clavicles and ribs are the most common sites. Most bones may be affected but the spine and round bones are rarely involved. Rib lesions may be associated with a pleural effusion. The disease is usually self limiting with the hyperostosis resolving 3-12 months after swelling and fever have subsided. A chronic monostotic form has been described in children and systemic corticosteroids are indicated providing the diagnosis is certain. Intercurrent infection in an already debilitated infant may be serious.

A106

Ectopia vesicae occurs as part of an abnormality of the abdominal wall, the pelvic girdle, and the pelvic floor. The mucosa of the bladder is exposed and becomes the anterior boundary of a ventral hernia. The deficient pelvic floor leads to rectal prolapse. Extrophy of the bladder produces wide separation of the symphysis pubis which is clearly seen on this child's X-ray. This is often associated with rotational deformities of the pelvic bones around the sacro-iliac joints. These children have a waddling gait.

The condition is more common in males and additional abnormalities include epispadias, deficiencies in the corpora cavernosa, and, frequently, undescended testes and an inguinal hernia. In females the clitoris is separated in two halves and the vagina is often duplicated.

Sexual intercourse is possible in females but may depend on episiotomy. It is sometimes possible in males, but depends amongst other features on the correction of the upward curvature of the shaft of the penis.

The X-ray of patient A was taken before the days of antibiotics. Patient B had presented with septicaemia.

- What are the diagnoses?
- How may this condition present in neonatal patients?

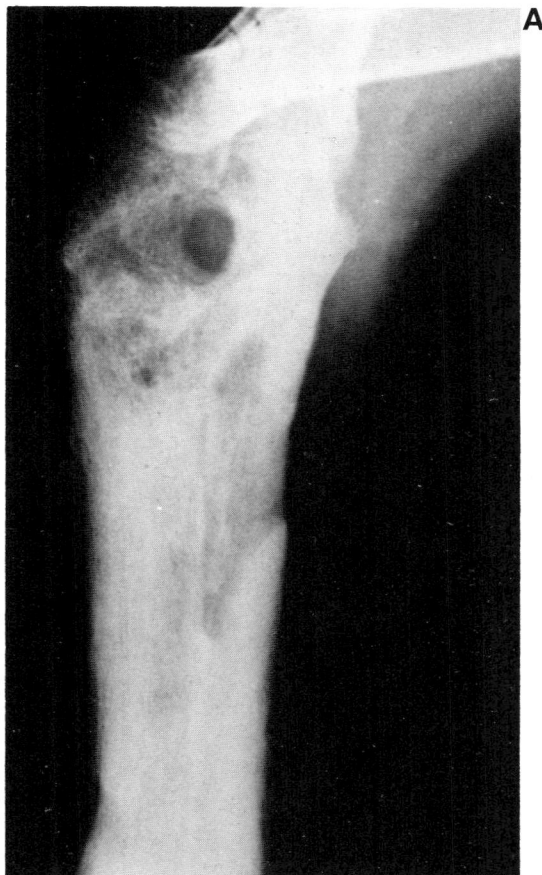

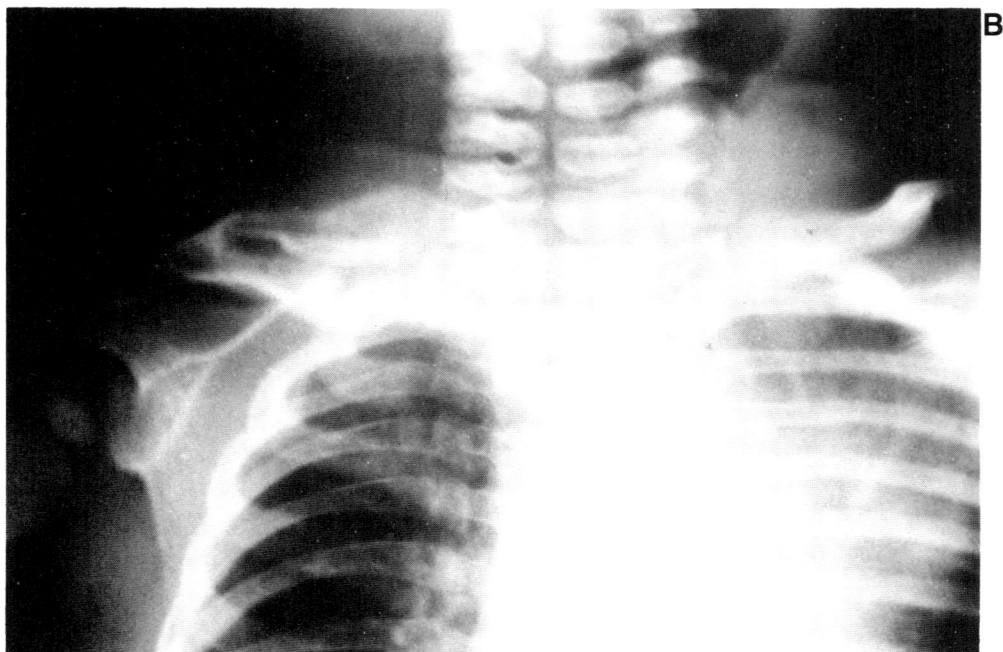

A107

Both patients have osteomyelitis. Patient A has a chronic osteomyelitis which was not uncommon prior to the introduction of antibiotic therapy. Bone changes on X-ray are not visible until 4-14 days after the onset of infection. Changes begin with bone destruction in the metaphysis with a periosteal reaction. This may become extensive and surround the bone to form an involucrum. Part of the original bone may die and form a dense, dead, infected fragment called a sequestrum. In this patient with chronic osteomyelitis the bone has become thickened and sclerotic with loss of differentiation between cortex and medulla. Within the bone there are sequestra and areas of destruction.

The neonatal patient (Film B) has extensive new bone formation around his affected clavicle. Patient B also has infection/collapse of his left upper lobe.

There are two well recognised presentations of neonatal osteomyelitis. Most commonly there is a misleading benign course with virtually no general systemic symptoms and minimal local signs despite destruction of the affected bone. For example an afebrile feeding infant may show pain on moving the hip and X-rays taken at this time commonly show extensive bone damage.

Neonatal osteomyelitis may also present as a life threatening septicaemia with obvious inflammation in a long bone. Multiple sites are often involved.

The initial diagnosis within a few days of onset of osteomyelitis is not dependent on finding an abnormality on X-ray or radioisotope bone scan, both of which may be negative.

This adolescent boy presented with pain in the spine which was aggravated by standing and improved on lying down. His father had a similar condition.

- What radiological features are seen?
- What is the diagnosis?

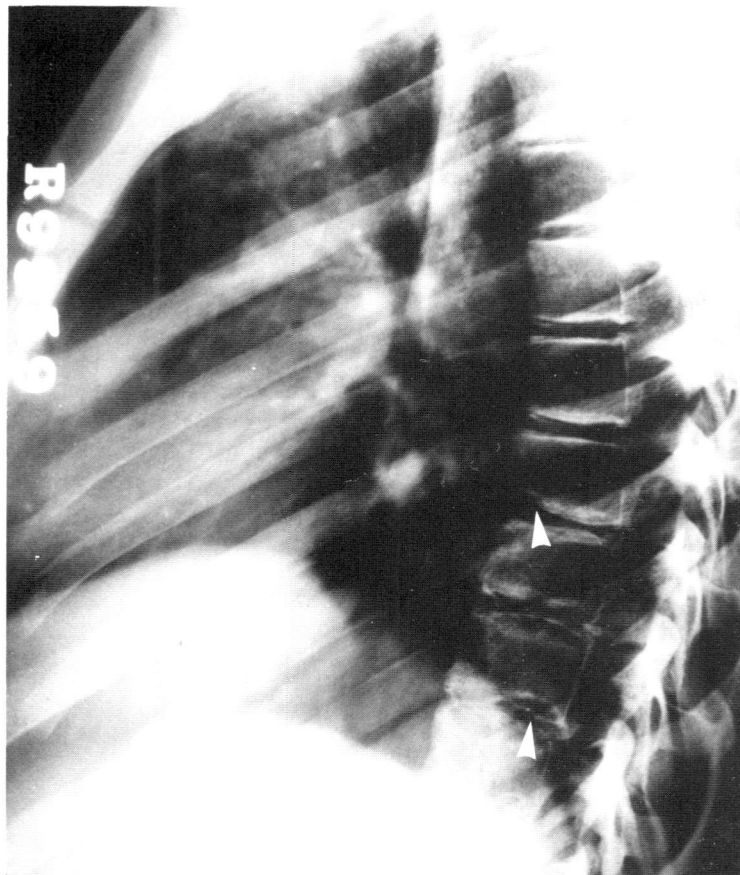

Q109

This child presented with foot pain.

- What is the diagnosis?
- What is the natural history of this condition?

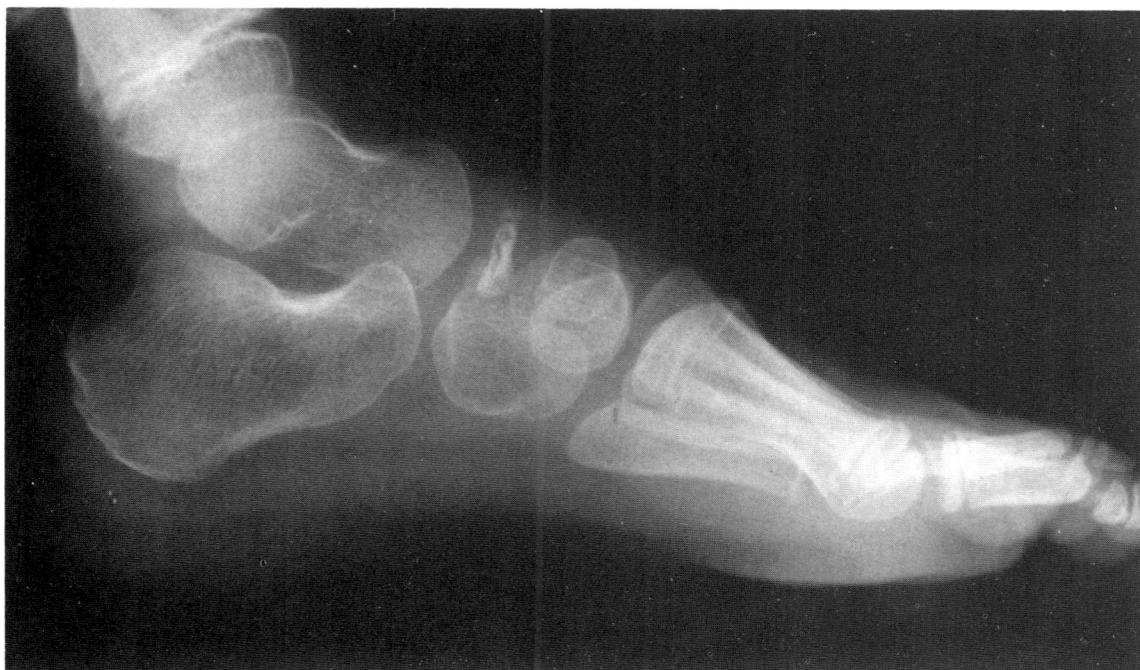

A108

This patient has Scheuermann's disease which is an osteochondritis. Scheuermann's disease is a condition of kyphotic deformity usually in the lower thoracic, upper lumbar and sometimes lower lumbar spine. It is most common in boys in the second decade. At the site of the lesion there is disc height loss with defects of ossification in the anterior third of the vertebral body end plates (arrow).

Lower down there is a Schmorl's node due to protrusion of disc material into the vertebral body which has an indentation in the mid part of the end plate (arrowed).

A109

The child is suffering from Köhler's disease, which is an aseptic necrosis of the tarsal navicular bone. It is usually found in the fifth and sixth year, and it is most common in boys (15-20% are bilateral). Pain, tenderness and limp are common. True Köhler's disease shows progressive destructive changes over several months. Recovery of the shape and texture of the navicular occurs with 2-3 years. These X-ray changes can be an incidental finding in asymptomatic children.

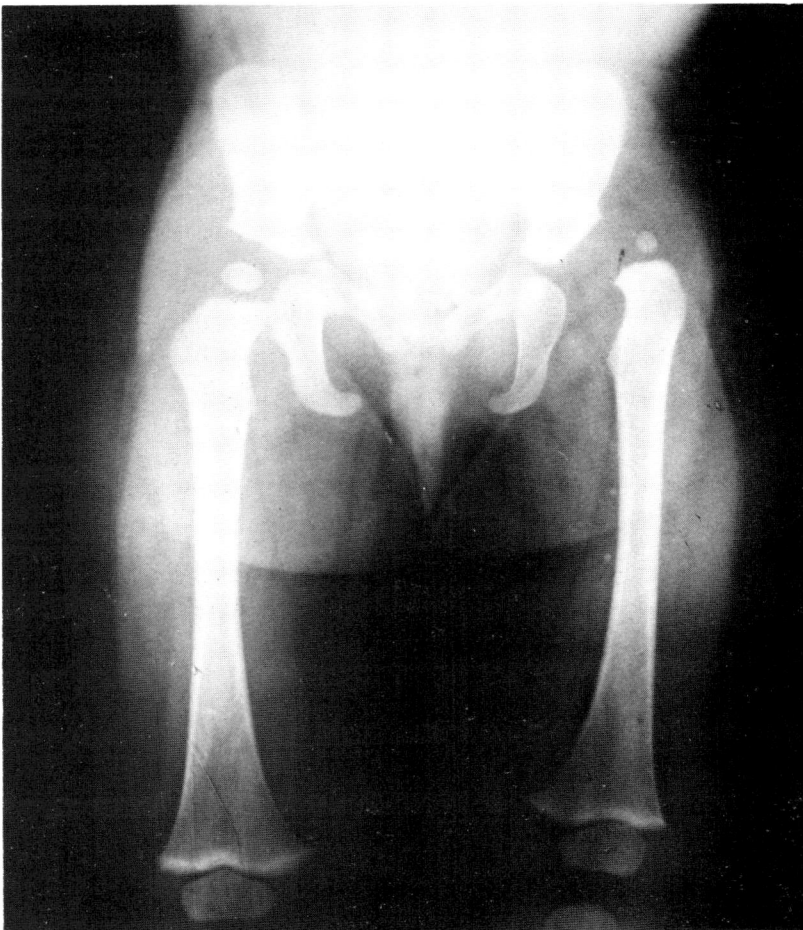

Q110

Describe the radiological features seen.

• What is the diagnosis?

Q111

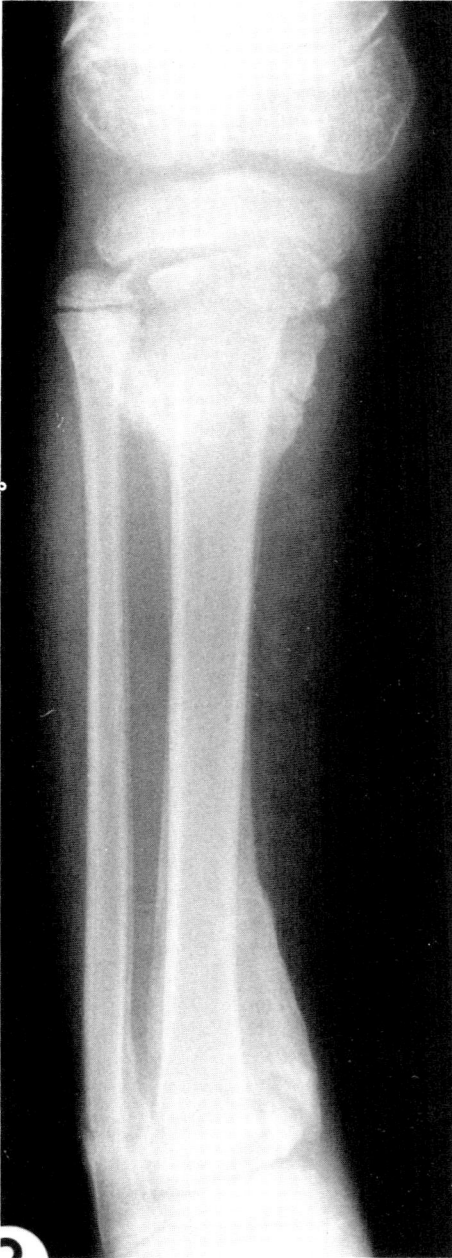

This child had never experienced pain and had not been battered.

- What is the most likely diagnosis?
- What other sensation may be reduced?

Q112

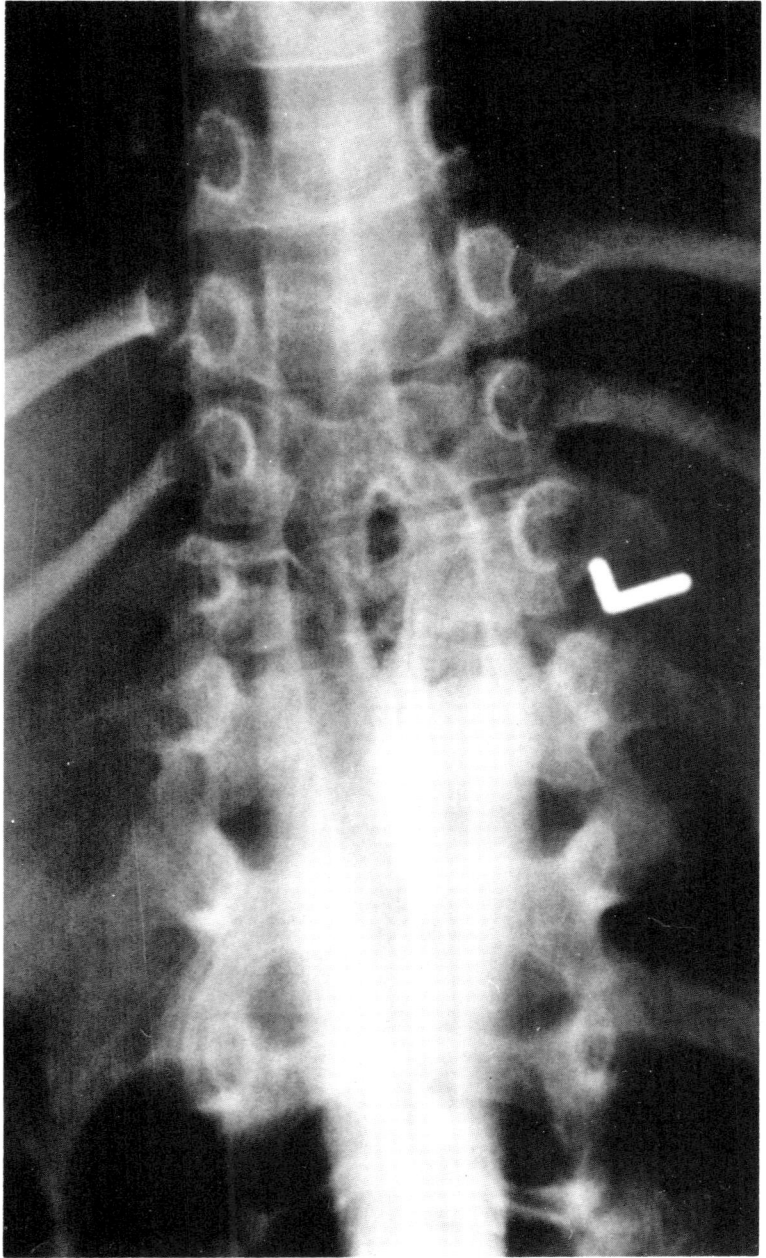

A myelogram has been performed.

- What is the diagnosis?
- What problems may the child encounter?

A110

This child has a congenital dislocation of his left hip. The femoral head of the dislocated hip is small and it is high in relation to the acetabulum. The fossa is shallow with a steep sloping roof. A posterior thigh crease can be seen on the left side. Any infant with additional posterior thigh creases should be suspected of having congenital dislocation of the hip.

On examination the child had a limp, apparent shortening of the left leg and limitation of hip abduction in flexion.

A111

This child has a congenital insensitivity to pain. Temperature sensation may also be reduced. In such children the nervous system is otherwise normal on clinical examination. The cause is unknown. The X-ray reveals fractures of tibia and fibula with extensive callus formation. The lateral femoral condyle is also fractured. Congenital insensitivity to pain is familial and presents in early life with a liability to burns, dental sepsis and bone lesions.

A112

The myelogram shows diastematomyelia. In diastematomyelia a bony cartilaginous spur splits the spinal cord into more or less equal parts for a variable vertical distance. There is also marked increase in the transverse diameter of the spinal canal and the pedicles are wider apart than normal.

The septum usually disrupts the anterior horn cell column. This may result in muscular atrophy, reduction or loss of deep tendon reflexes and weakness of the muscles in the lower legs and feet. Talipes equinovarus or pes cavus are often present. Changes are usually bilateral. Atony of the bladder and weakness of the lower legs are common presenting signs. Skin lesions over the spine include lipoma, soft tissue swelling, a hairy patch, sacrococcygeal sinus and myelomeningocoele. Pain and temperature sensation may be diminished. Cortico-spinal tract disruption with upper motor neurone signs is uncommon.

Consultation with surgical colleagues is imperative once the diagnosis is made.

Often calcification in the spur is delayed and may not be detected until the child is several years old.

This thin infant (A) was found to have RSV positive bronchiolitis. His costochondral junctions were particularly prominent.

- What else is he suffering from?

- Is it possible to monitor his improvement radiologically?

- Patient B was mentally retarded and epileptic. What does the X-ray show?

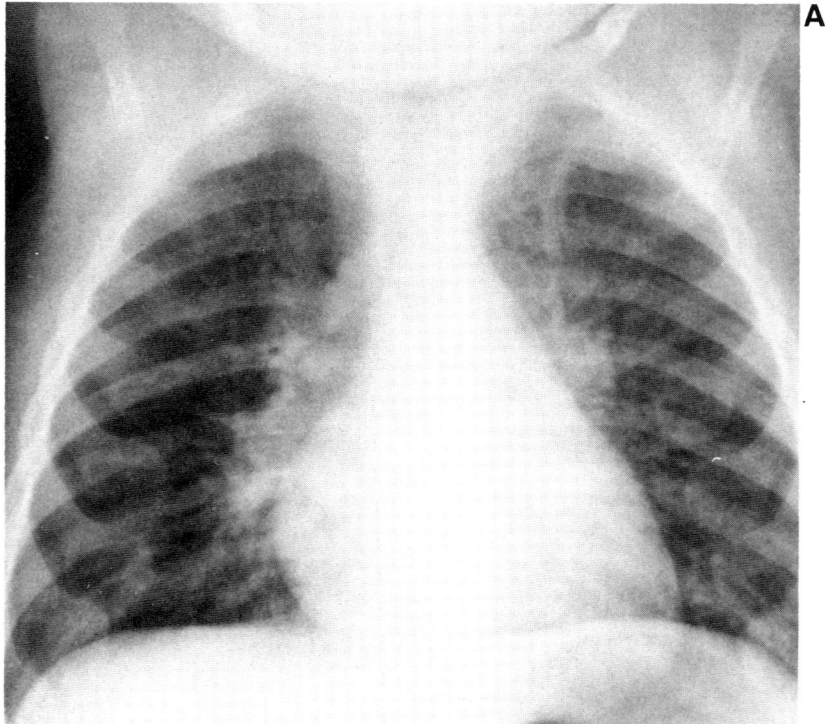

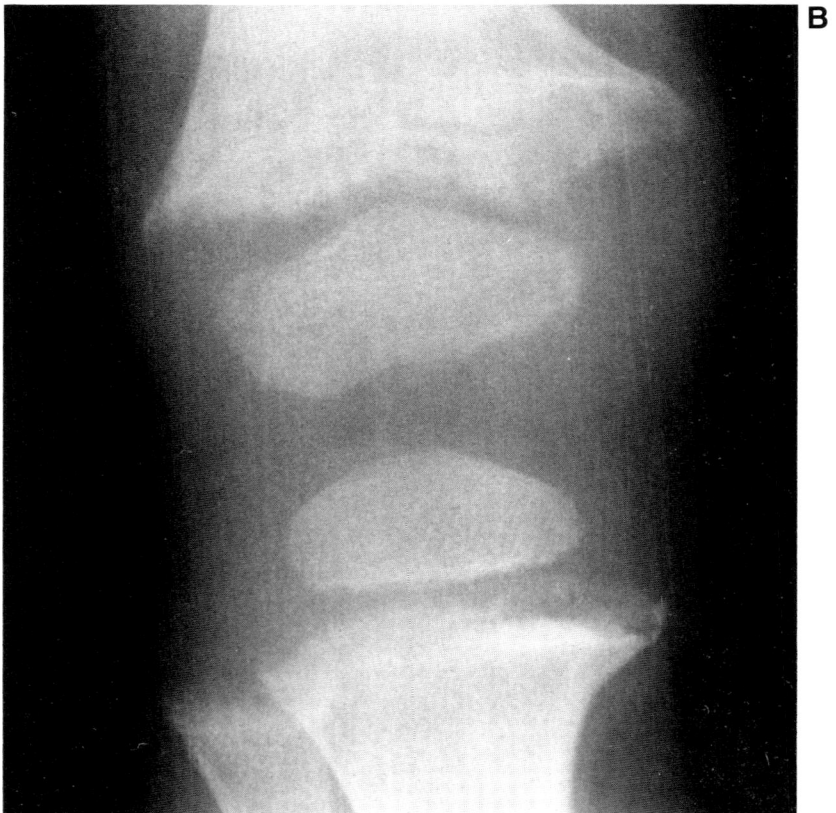

A113

Both children have rickets. The chest X-ray of patient A shows the anterior ends of his ribs to be widened, concave and ill defined at the costochondral junctions.

The severe rickets in patient B was due to prolonged phenytoin therapy. Bones in patients with rickets usually lack minerals. The metaphyses are widened and appear frayed. Cartilage and uncalcified osteoid between the metaphysis and epiphysis result in an increased distance between them (patient B). Consequently the diaphysis appears shortened and may be bowed due to the soft osteoid and change in direction of bone growth.

Changes are best seen at the anterior ends of the ribs, the knees, ankles and wrists where growth is rapid. Skull changes are mild with widening of sutures and fontanelles with ill-defined edges. Skull radiography may be normal.

Healing may be seen radiologically 1 to 2 weeks after treatment starts. The osteoid becomes calcified and may appear as a dense line. If the increased density persists or increases it may be indicative of vitamin overdosage.

Q114

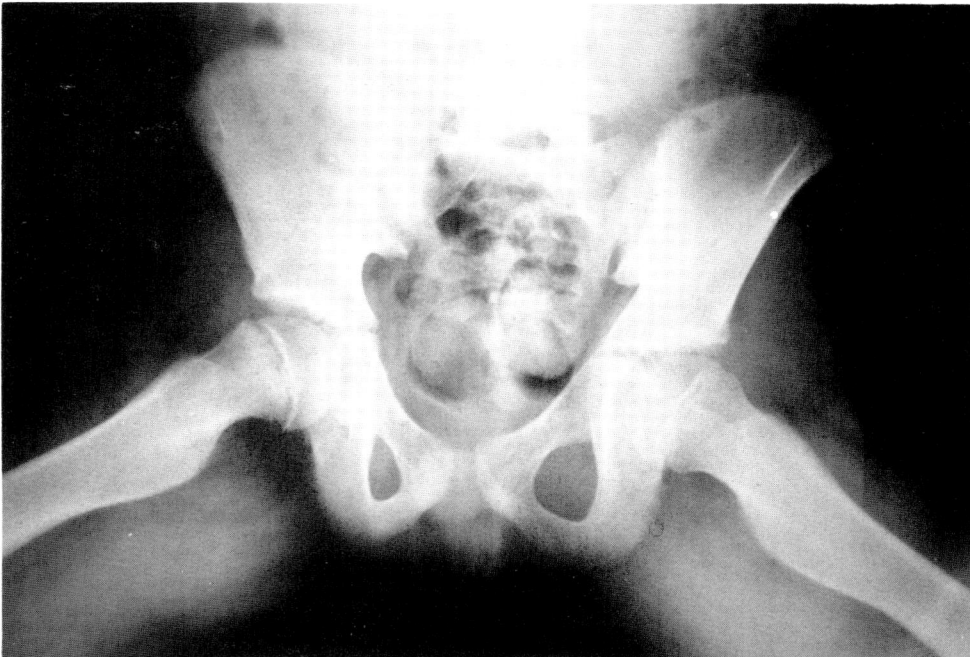

This 11 year old boy presented to casualty with a limp. An X-ray of his pelvis was taken.

- What is the diagnosis?
- What may you find on examination?
- Why is it important to make the diagnosis?

This athletic 15 year old boy complained of pain in his knee. The site of the tibial tuberosity was warm, tender, painful and swollen at the point of insertion of the patellar tendon.

- What is the diagnosis?

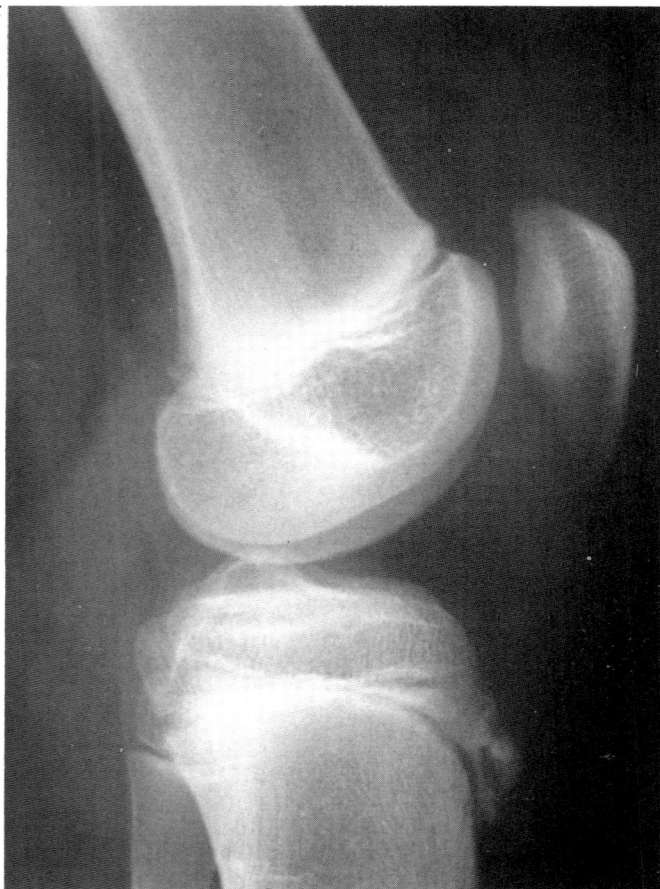

Q116

This adolescent has suffered from juvenile rheumatoid arthritis (JRA) for many years.

- Describe the radiological changes seen.

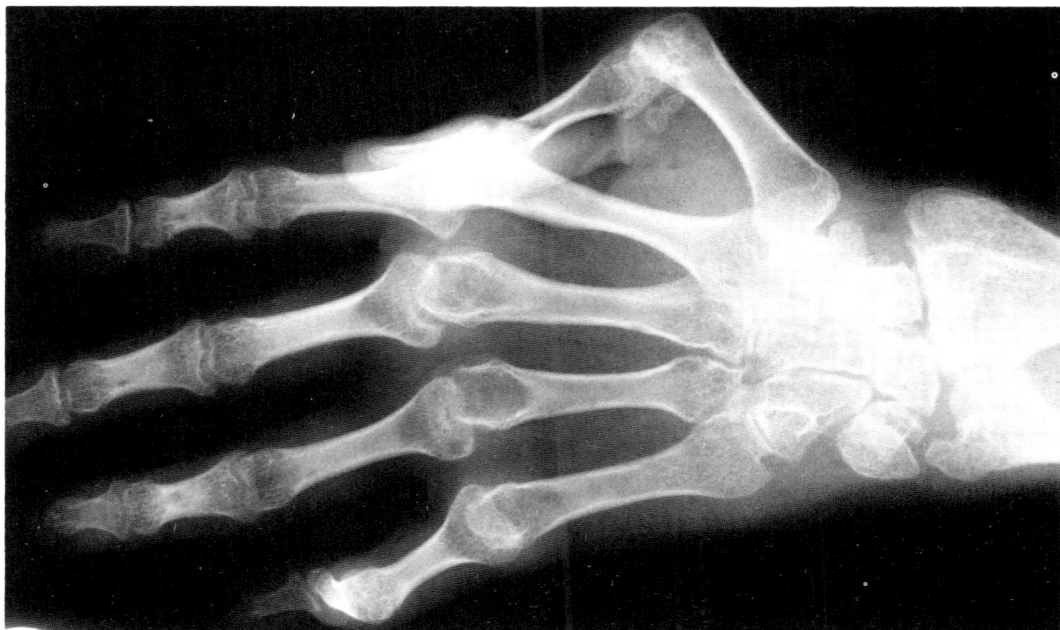

A114

This child has a slipped right femoral capital epiphysis. This tends to be a disorder of adolescence. Aetiology is not known but it usually coincides with the growth spurt of puberty. In 20% of cases both hips are involved.

The radiological appearance is that of displacement of the epiphysis in relation to the metaphysis. This usually occurs in a posterior direction.

This X-ray gives a lateral view of the femoral head and neck. If the condition is suspected both AP and lateral projections are necessary as the condition will not be apparent in at least 10% of the AP radiographs.

The child may complain of pain in the hip or just have a limp, but is otherwise well. Pain in the ipsilateral knee may also be a presenting complaint. Limited internal rotation, abduction and extension are found. Swelling is absent.

As the slip increases the retinacular vessels which supply the capital epiphysis may be damaged as they cross the growth plate, resulting in avascular necrosis, hence the need for early recognition and treatment.

A115

There is fragmentation of the tibial tuberosity at the insertion of the patellar tendon, characteristic of Osgood-Schlatter's disease. This is a traction apophysitis. It must be stressed that Osgood-Schlatter's disease is mainly a clinical diagnosis with the X-ray evidence supporting.

The boy complained of pain in his knee particularly on climbing stairs and after exercise.

Pain could be reproduced by contraction of the quadriceps against resistance.

Osgood-Schlatter's disease is most common in boys between 8 and 14 years of age and resolves spontaneously, usually with no long term problems. A small proportion may need the loose bodies in the epiphysis excised if there is persistent pain.

A116

The cardinal change in JRA is loss of cartilage cover of the articular surface and this occurs at all ages. The 'joint space' then appears narrow. Bone erosions may be seen. Osteoporosis in the bone adjacent to the joint is present. This patient demonstrates the classic ulnar deviation of the

fingers in relation to the metacarpal bones.

Unlike psoriatic arthropathy where the distal interphalangeal joints are affected in classical JRA these joints are spared. JRA may be monarticular, affecting one joint, such as the hip joint.

This is the radiograph of a boy who presented with low back pain and a notable lumbar lordosis.

- Describe the abnormalities seen.
- What problems may this child encounter?

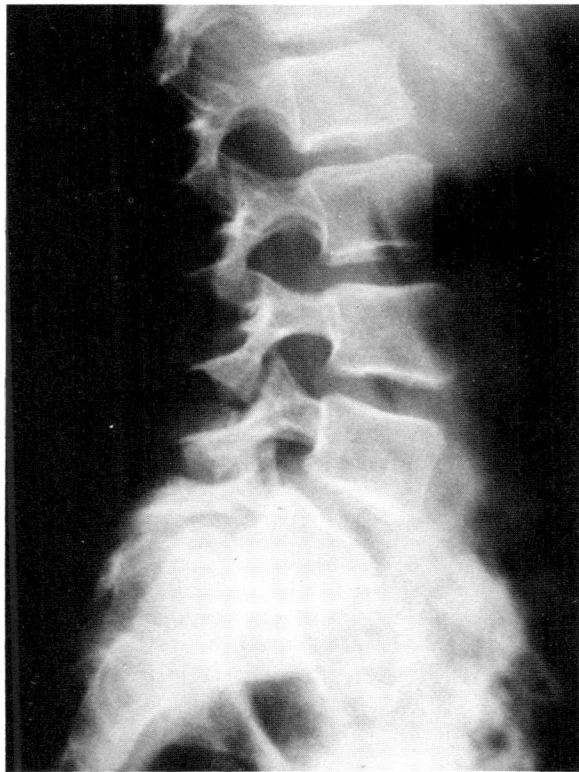

Q118

This patient presented with a new lump close to his knee.

- What is the underlying diagnosis?
- What is the cause of the new bony lump (arrowed)?

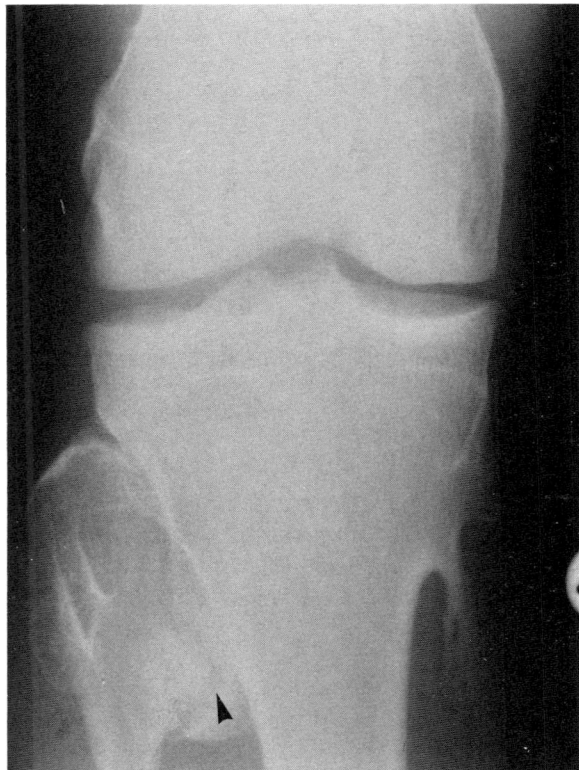

A117

This condition is spondylolisthesis which is the forward slide of one lumbar vertebra on another In this case the fifth lumbar vertebra has slipped forward through the plane of the intervertebral disc below. The disc space is narrowed. Usually, this movement is prevented by intact bone lying between the superior and inferior facets. Often a bone defect can be seen, although not in this case.

The shape of the neural arch may be compared to the silhouette of a Scots terrier in the oblique view. The transverse process represents the nose, the inferior articular process the front leg, and the superior articular process representing the ear. Most of the lesions are due to a stress fracture of the pars interarticularis, the dog's neck (see diagram). These fractures may only be visible in oblique projections in the early stages. The presence of a pars interarticularis defect without forward slipping of the vertebra is known as spondylolysis.

Spondylolisthesis may be due to congenital hypoplasia of articular processes or due to degenerative changes in the posterior intervertebral joints. Large slips tend to occur in the congenital cases.

Because the lamina is left behind in its normal position the anterior displacement of the vertebral body does not cause narrowing of the spinal canal. However, root pressure can occur with sciatica.

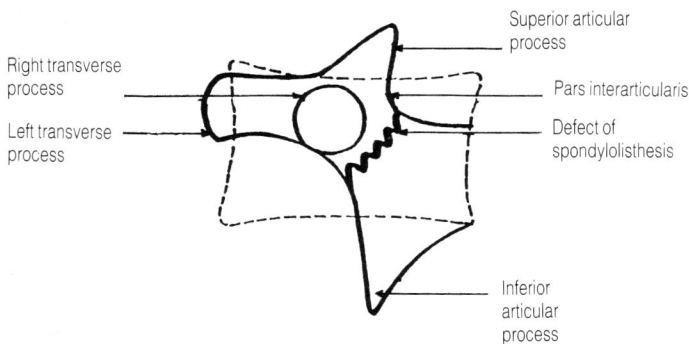

Right transverse process — Left transverse process — Superior articular process — Pars interarticularis — Defect of spondylolisthesis — Inferior articular process

A118

This child has diaphyseal aclasia (multiple exostoses). These are spurs of bone that develop at the growing ends of the long bones. The condition is familial. These osteochondromata are multiple and tend to arise from the metaphyseal region of long bones and grow away from the end of the long bone. They may lead to pressure effects on adjacent structures such as blood vessels, nerves, bones or the spinal cord.

He had developed a chondrosarcoma (arrowed) which is associated with diaphyseal aclasia.

Biopsy of this lesion showed blood and connective tissues with aggregates of giant cells.

- What is the diagnosis?
- What are the commonest sites affected?

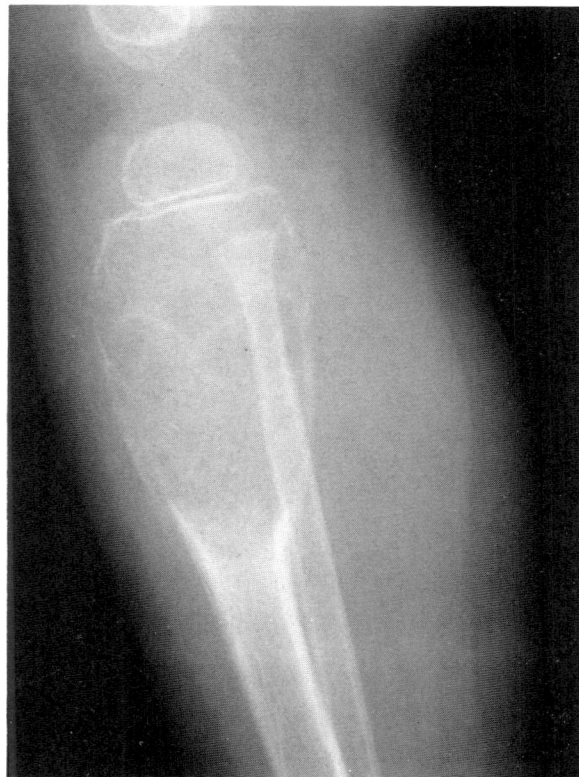

Q120

This child presented with pain in her foot whilst walking. The pain had been present for some time.

- What is the diagnosis?

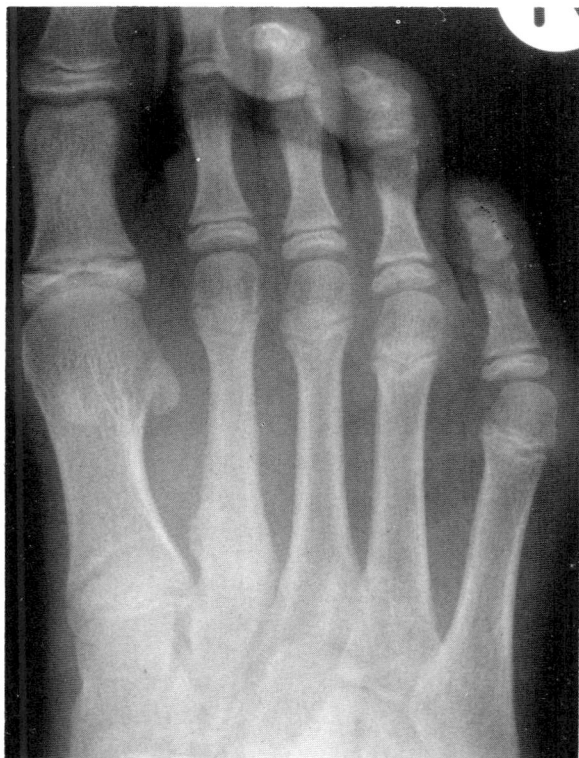

A119

This patient has an aneurysmal bone cyst. These are defined as expanding osteolytic lesions consisting of blood filled spaces of variable size, separated by connective tissue septa containing trabeculae of bone or osteoid tissue, and osteoclastic giant cells.

Aneurysmal bone cysts are destructive lesions, producing an area of well-defined radiolucency with thinning of the overlying cortex and frequently, as in this case, considerable expansion of the bone. Pain and swelling tend to be the presenting symptoms. These tumours tend to present in childhood or early adolescent life and long bones and vertebrae are the commonest sites affected. Treatment includes excision, and bone grafts.

A120

There is a stress fracture of her second metatarsal. This is seen as an undisplaced healing fracture. Stress fractures are usually recognised by the marked periosteal reaction which is evident in this case. Such lesions may occur in the absence of a clear history of injury. These fractures of the metatarsals are known as march fractures and are the most common stress fractures seen. These lesions often produce pain before they become radiologically evident. However, radionuclide scanning may detect the fracture at an earlier stage.

Q121

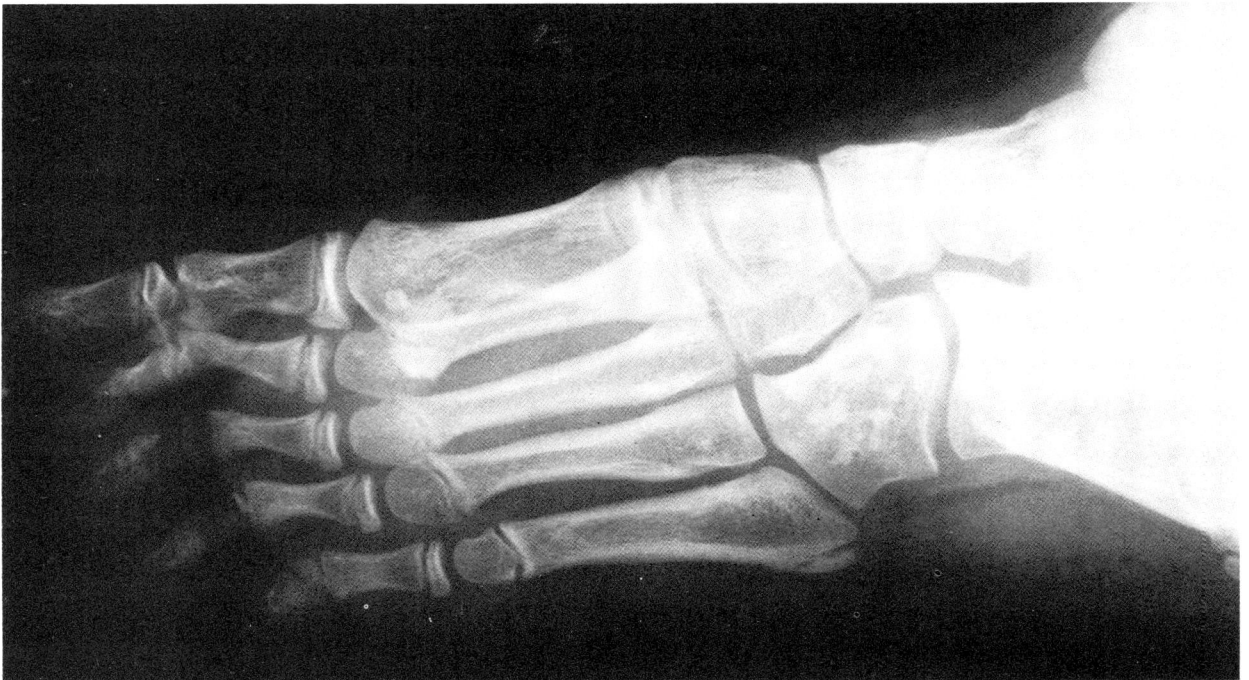

This child presented to casualty with foot pain.

- What can you see on this radiograph?

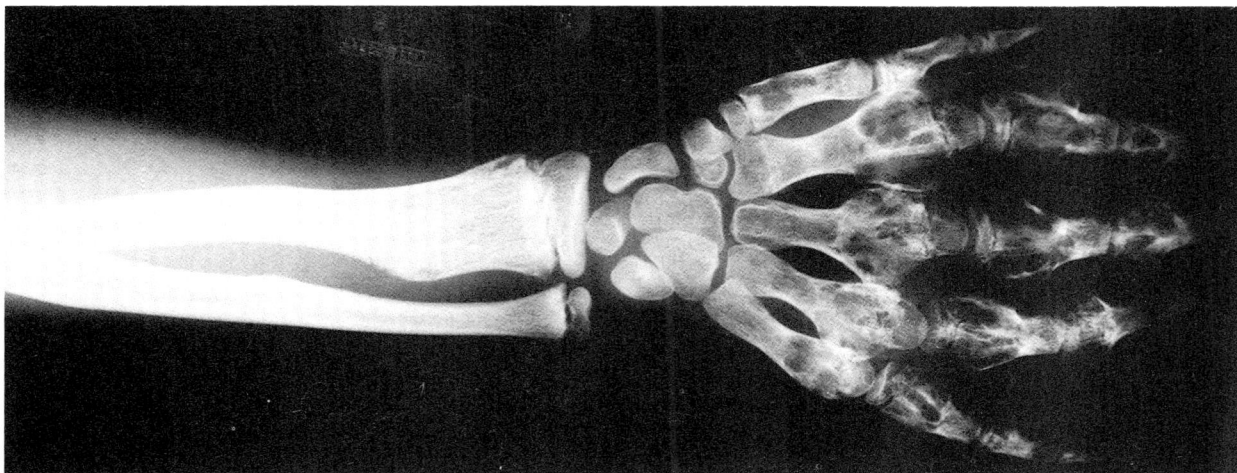

- What is the diagnosis?
- What is the cause?

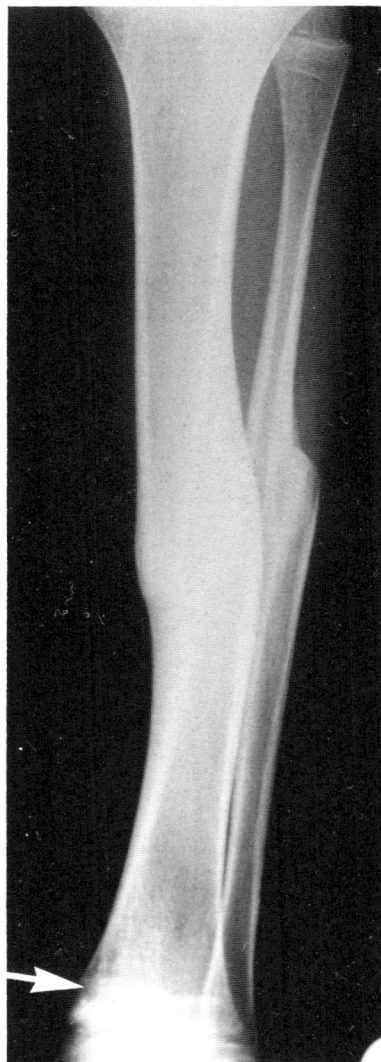

Q123

This young girl has fractured her tibia and fibula which are healing well.

- What is the dense white line (arrowed) due to?

A121

The child has osteopoikilosis (spotted bones). There are multiple sclerotic foci caused by thickening of the spongiosa. The cortex is normal. This condition is symptomless and is usually found by chance on X-ray. Other members of the family may be affected. It requires no treatment and the sclerotic areas often disappear with time.

In practice the dense islands of osteopoikilosis are not mistaken for tuberosclerosis and bony metastases.

A122

This child has gross Ollier's disease. In this condition there is abnormal endochondral ossification leading to persistence of cartilage in the bone, producing expansion of bone. This cartilaginous expansion in the hand bones often results in pathological fractures. The radiograph shows globular lesions expanding the bones and thinning the cortex. It may occur in infancy but is usually detected between 2 and 10 years.

A123

There is a dense transverse line at the lower end of the tibia. These lines are known as Harris' lines, or growth arrest lines. They are found when chondrogenesis occurs more slowly than normal and osteogenesis becomes the more rapid of the two leading to the production of a dense band at the metaphysis. These lines eventually fragment and fade after several years. Slowing of chondrogenesis may be caused by illness, irradiation, or nutritional deficiency. Harris' lines remain at the same distance from the centre of the shaft as when they were formed and move away from the metaphysis as the bone increases in length. They may be multiple and are seen in the tibia and femur especially.

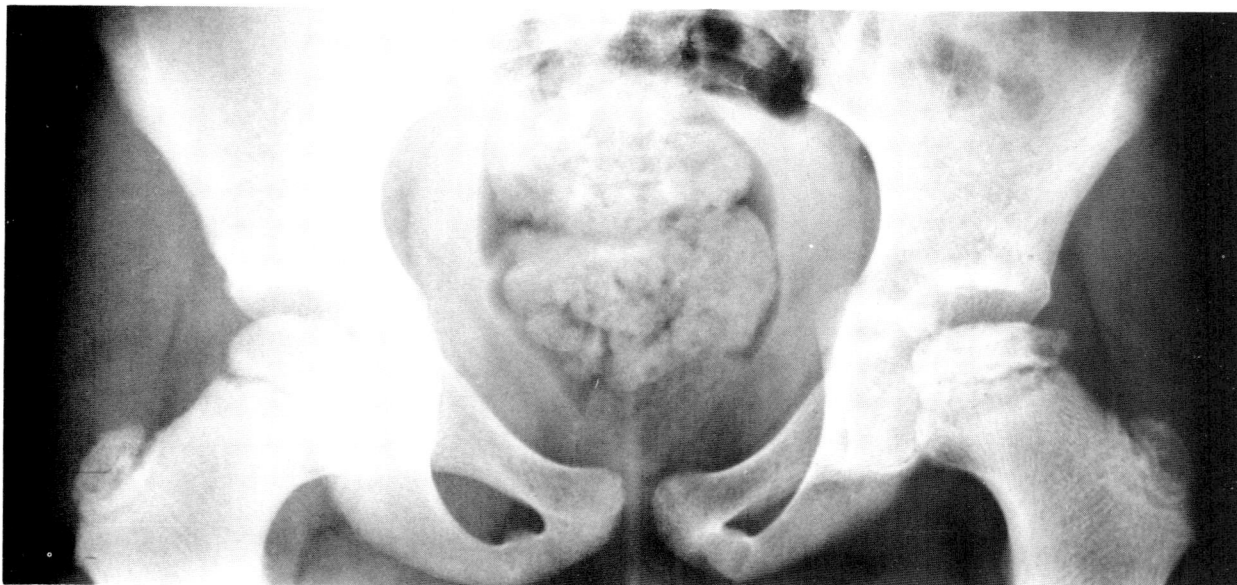

This is the X-ray of a 6 year old boy who presented with a painless limp.

- What is the likely diagnosis?
- What is the radiological course of this condition?
- What may be found on clinical examination?

Q125

This child died shortly after birth.

- What is the diagnosis?
- How may this condition present later in life?
- What is the inheritance?

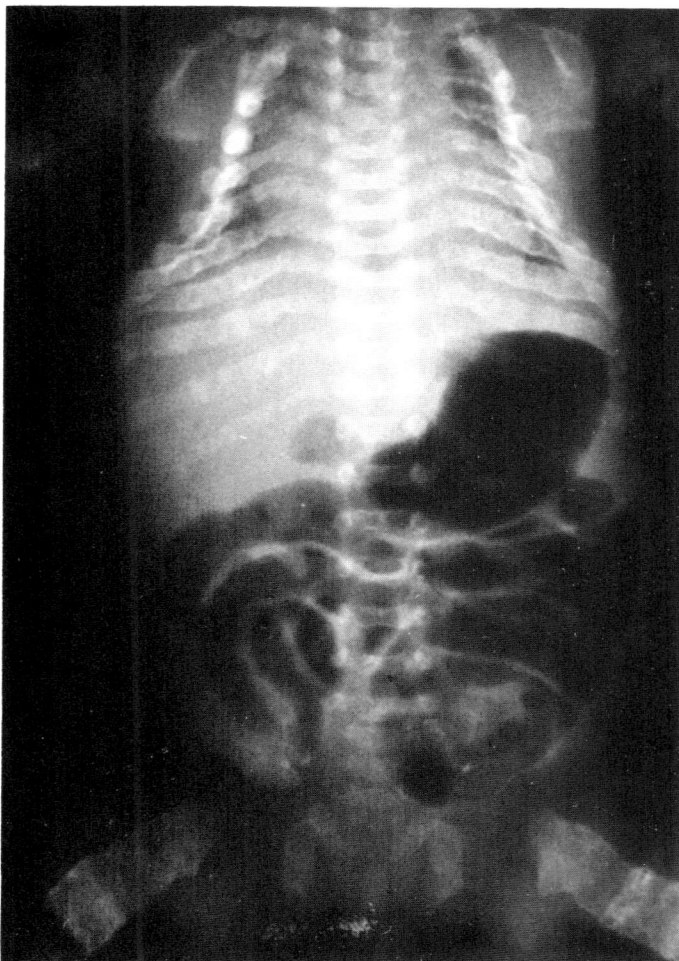

A124

This young lad has Perthes' disease. It is an osteochondritis affecting the head of the femur found mainly in boys between 3 and 10 years of age. In 10% of cases both hips are affected.

The typical radiological features in the early stages are widening of the joint space, decalcification in the metaphysis with the femoral head becoming more dense and flattened. Later, the femoral head becomes fragmented. The end stage of this condition may be a flattened femoral head and coxa vara with a broad femoral neck. There is a risk of early osteoarthritis for those with a poor outcome to the lesion.

Some children have a painless intermittent limp for 1-2 years and can lead a normal life during this period. Examination may reveal slight limitation of hip joint movement, especially abduction in flexion. The buttock may be soft and flat due to wasting of the gluteal muscles and Trendelenberg's sign is positive.

A125

This child has osteogenesis imperfecta congenita which is the most severe form of this disease. Multiple fractures of the long bones and ribs have occurred prenatally. If live-born, multiple fractures are associated with bowing and shortening deformities. Fragility of the skull may lead to brain damage during delivery.

The tarda form of this condition usually presents at some time during childhood. There may be blue sclerae, ocular defects, fine hair, hyperextensible joints, hypoplastic milk teeth, growth retardation, and a family history of fractures. These features are not always present and presentation may be with a succession of fractures.

In infancy radiology may reveal osteoporotic bones with evidence of bending due to the physiological stresses of weight bearing and breathing. The skull may show basilar invagination and outward bulging of the vault over the skull-base together with osteoporosis and multiple wormian bones.

The prenatally occuring condition has a very poor prognosis, but, in the later onset form a reasonably normal life span may be predicted.

The majority of cases are inherited as an autosomal dominant gene occuring as a sporadic mutation. It has been suggested that more severe forms, as in this case, with multiple intrauterine fractures may be transmitted by autosomal recessive inheritance.

Q126

Q127

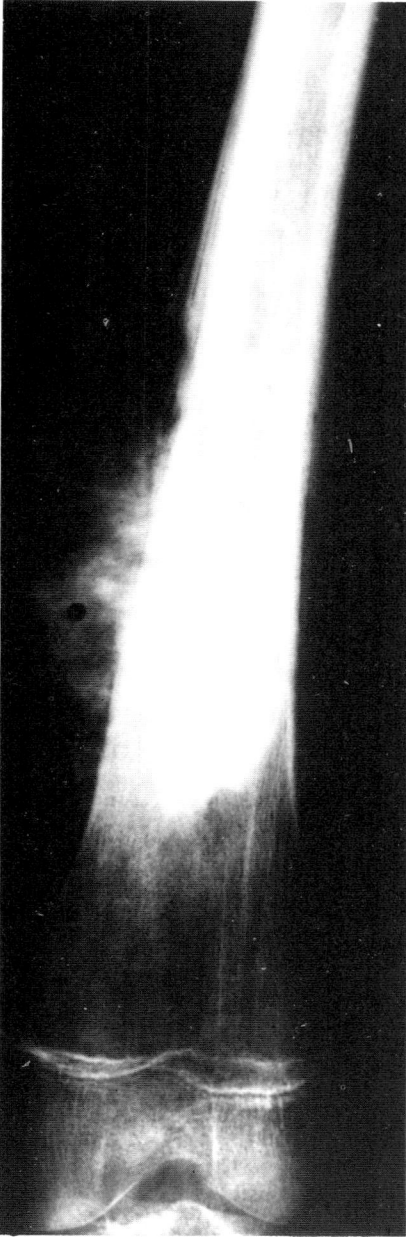

This child presented with a painful swelling of her thigh.

- What is the likely diagnosis?

- What other site may be involved?

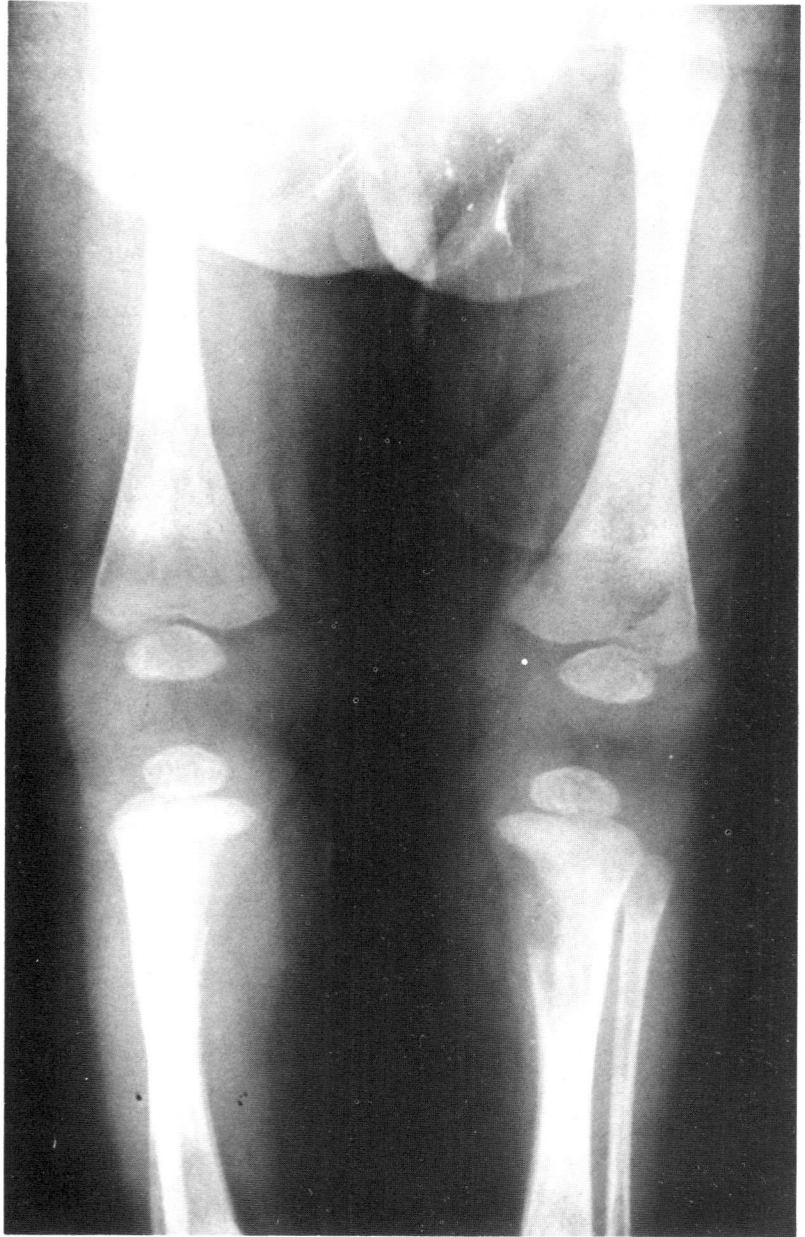

This baby was born after a concealed pregnancy. The baby subsequently seemed reluctant to move his legs.

- What is the diagnosis?

- What radiological sign supports this?

A126

The child has an osteosarcoma of the lower femur. This is a relatively common tumour affecting mostly boys between the ages of 10 and 25. The tumour is highly malignant and the affected part is tender and usually warmer than the surrounding skin. Common sites include the lower femur, upper tibia and upper humerus.

The tumour is locally invasive into the soft tissues. Haematogenous spread gives rise to metastases in the lungs. Secondaries in other bones are very rare.

Radiologically, early changes may be seen as rarefaction and sclerosis. Destruction of the cortex and medulla without expansion of the bone shaft and without new bone formation is characteristic of some lesions. New bone formation is shown as sclerosis within the medulla and this may be either uniform or patchy. Erosion of the cortex and extension of bone spiculas in the tumour mass (sun-ray appearance) occur. The periosteal new bone at the tumour site may be destroyed and an elevation of the periosteum is seen at the margin.

A127

This child has congenital syphilis.

Perinatal lesions are usually polyostotic and symmetrical.

Congenital syphilis is characterised by metaphysitis, periostitis and osteitis such as may be seen in this patient on the medial aspect of the proximal tibial shaft. Destruction of the cortex is particularly common on the medial side of the proximal end of the tibia and is known as Wimberger's sign.

Q128

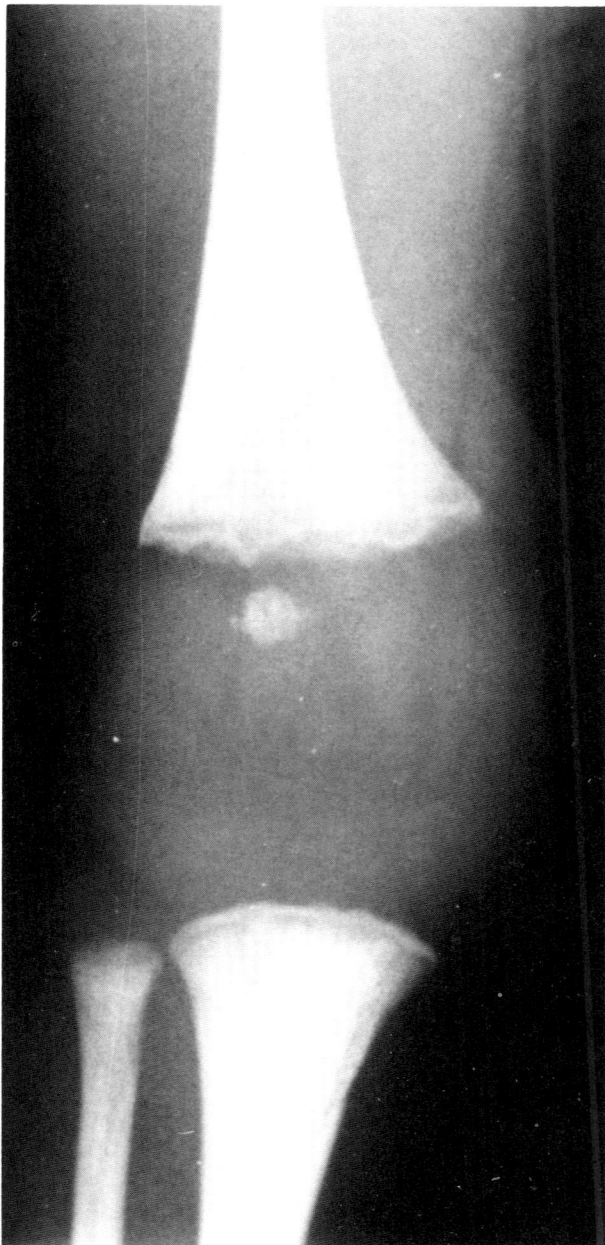

Q129

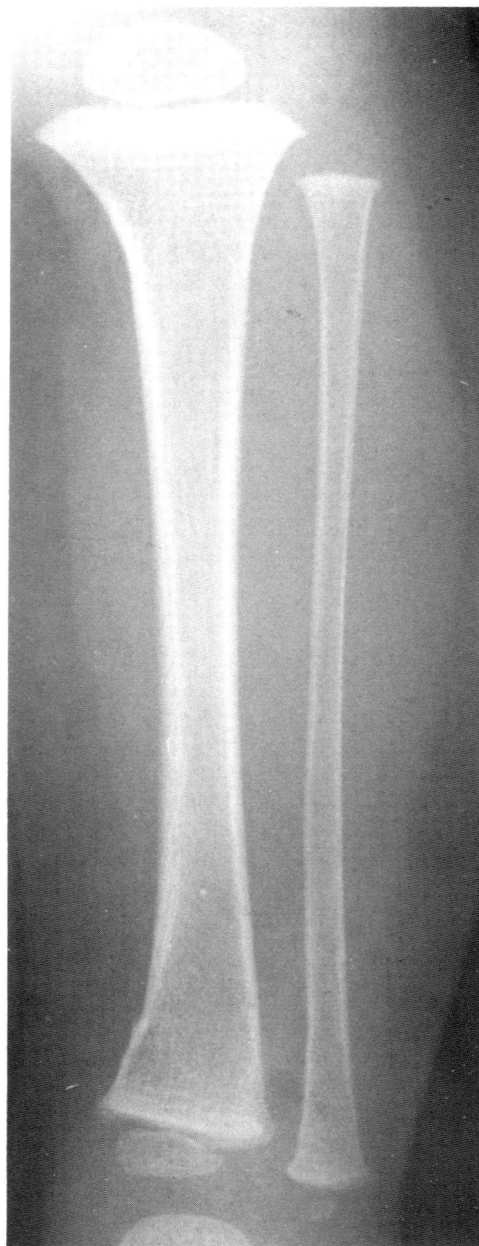

This neonatal patient was found to have cataracts and tetralogy of Fallot.

- What is the most likely diagnosis?
- What is the natural history of these bone changes?

This young child was brought to casualty refusing to walk following a fall.

- What is the diagnosis?

A128

The child was found to be deaf. Laboratory investigations confirmed the diagnosis of congenital rubella.

Bone lesions in congenital rubella comprise alternating longitudinal bands of increased and diminished bone density at the ends of the diaphysis. The metaphysis may show a transverse band of diminished bone density. This lies beneath the slightly irregular metaphyseal extremity as in this patient. These changes are most commonly seen in the distal femora and proximal tibiae.

Bone changes are present in up to half of these patients and most often appear before the end of the first week. The bones revert to normal within 2-3 months.

Periosteal new bone formation does not occur in rubella, which helps distinguish it from syphilis.

Infants with congenital rubella are infectious for probably one or two months. However, the virus can often be grown from urine, CSF, leucocytes, and nasopharangeal secretions for up to 30 months.

A129

The child was found to have a greenstick fracture of her lower tibia. A greenstick fracture is an incomplete fracture of the bone where the cortex of the bone may be buckled and the fracture line, when visible, involves only one side of the cortex.

Q130

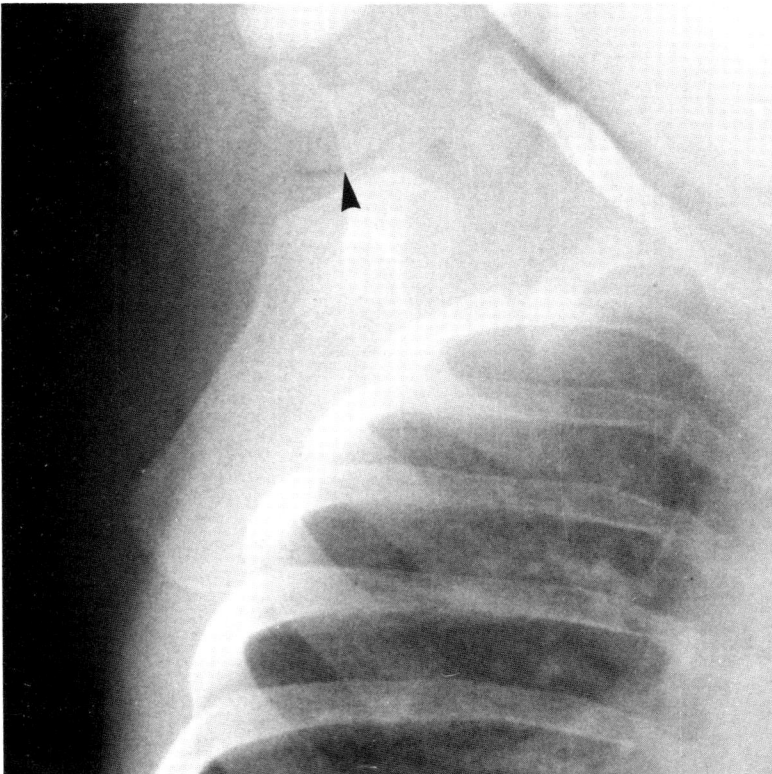

This young child presented with a high temperature. The house officer was concerned about the presence of a thin black line in the shoulder region seen on the chest X-ray (arrowed).

- What is the cause of this radiological finding?

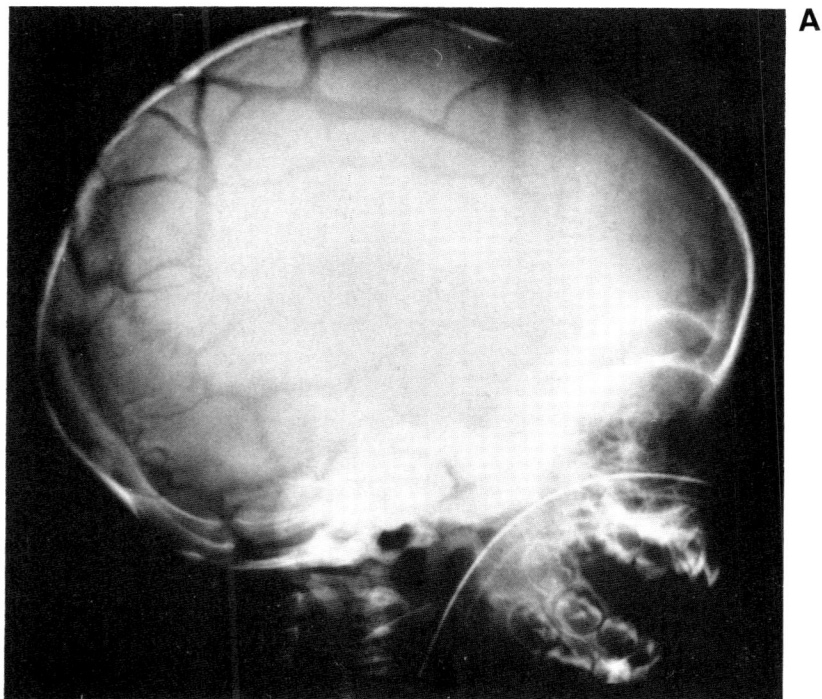

A

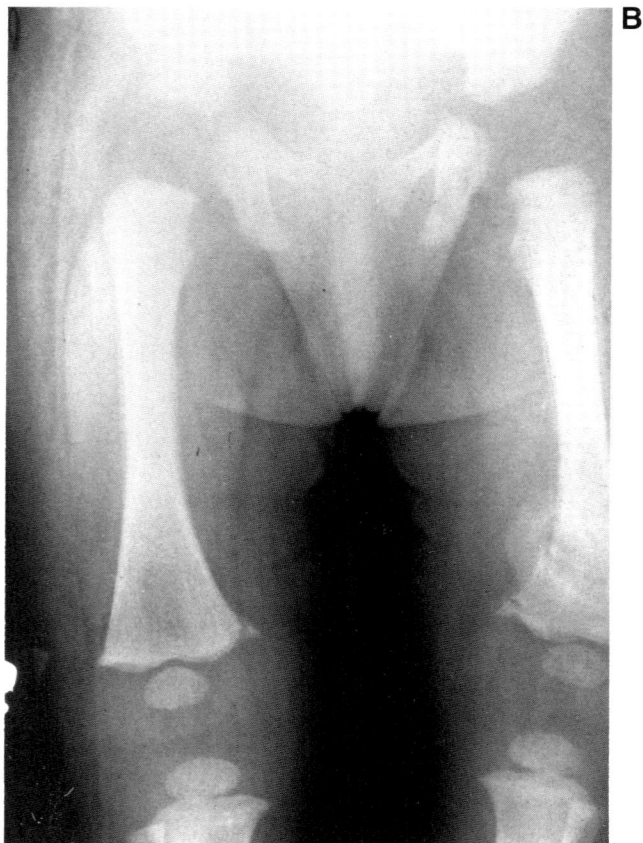

B

These are the X-rays of a child who presented to casualty following an 'apnoeic' attack.

- Describe the abnormalities seen.
- What is the most likely underlying cause?

A130

This finding is known as the vacuum phenomenon. A lucent (black) line is often seen in the large joints of children and is caused by pulling, resulting in a vacuum in the joint that allows nitrogen to enter and outline the articular cartilage of the bone.

A131

The skull X-ray shows the child to have a nasal endotracheal tube in situ. There are multiple skull fractures. Film B shows a fracture to the lower end of the left femur. There are metaphyseal avulsion fractures at the lower medial edge of both femurs. There is elevation of the periosteum due to subperiosteal haemorrhage along the shafts of both femurs. These findings were due to non-accidental injury.

Up to 80% of fractures in abused children have been found to occur in children less than 18 months. This is the opposite to normal children where 85% of fractures occur over the age of 5 years. Multiple fractures and soft tissue injuries of face and neck are more common in abused children. Metaphyseal fractures and rib fractures are also common and should arouse suspicion. Long bone injuries tend to be spiral/oblique fractures or subperiosteal new bone formation: both involve a gripping/twisting injury.

The characteristics of skull fractures resulting from abuse are multiple or complex fractures, involvement of more than one bone, non-parietal fracture, depressed and growing fractures.

Child abuse cannot be diagnosed on the basis of fracture patterns alone. However, if unusual patterns of fractures and associated injuries are seen, then a full and careful assessment by staff experienced in this field is essential.

What cutaneous features may you find on examination of this child?

- What is the diagnosis?

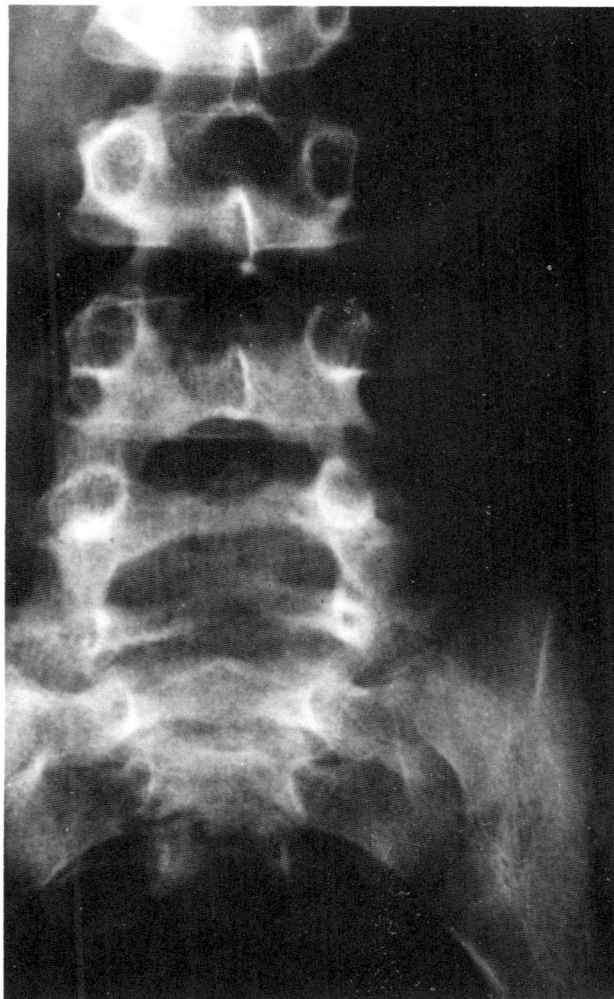

Q133

This child presented with a history of tingling and dull ache of her arm, that became worse after exercise.

- Which arm do you think was affected and why?

- What other problems may be encountered?

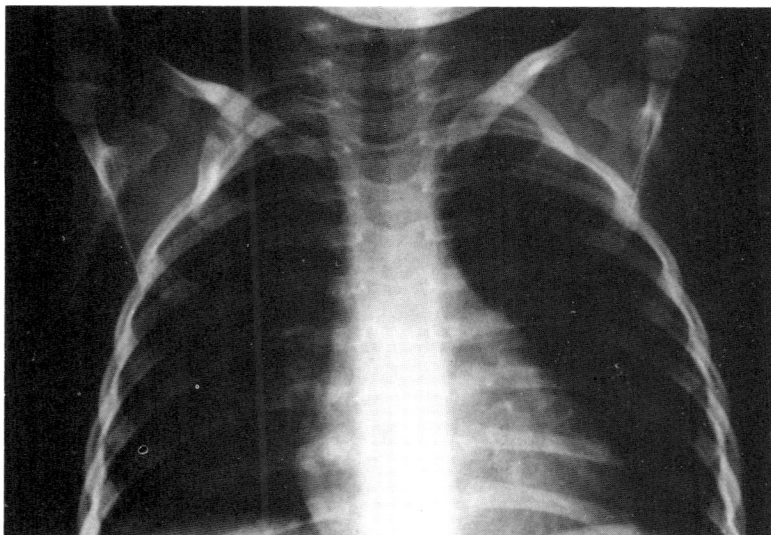

A132

The child has spina bifida occulta. In this condition the vertebral arches are incomplete but the overlying skin is intact. Ectodermal abnormalities associated with spina bifida occulta include a depression with a tuft of hair, a fatty swelling or a dermal pit. Disability is uncommon but full neurological examination is necessary if an associated ectodermal abnormality is found.

If a dermal pit is found it is of great importance to ensure it does not communicate with the dura, thus predisposing to meningitis. If unsure, immediate referral for investigation is mandatory to prevent such a disaster.

A133

The tingling and dull ache becoming worse after exercise was due to compression of her right subclavian artery by a right sided cervical rib. Severe arterial pressure may cause coldness and blanching of the skin with ischaemic complications. Nerve compression may also occur causing pain and parasthesia. Progressive and severe atrophy of the muscles in the hand may occur. Compression of the sympathetic nerves is rare but may cause disturbances in sweating of the arm, miosis and ptosis of the ipsilateral eye.

Most cervical ribs are bilateral and arise from the seventh cervical vertebra. The vast majority are discovered accidentally at X-ray and are rarely symptomatic in children and require no treatment.

This syndrome may also be caused by a fibrous band in the same position as the rib. This is not seen on X-ray.

Q134

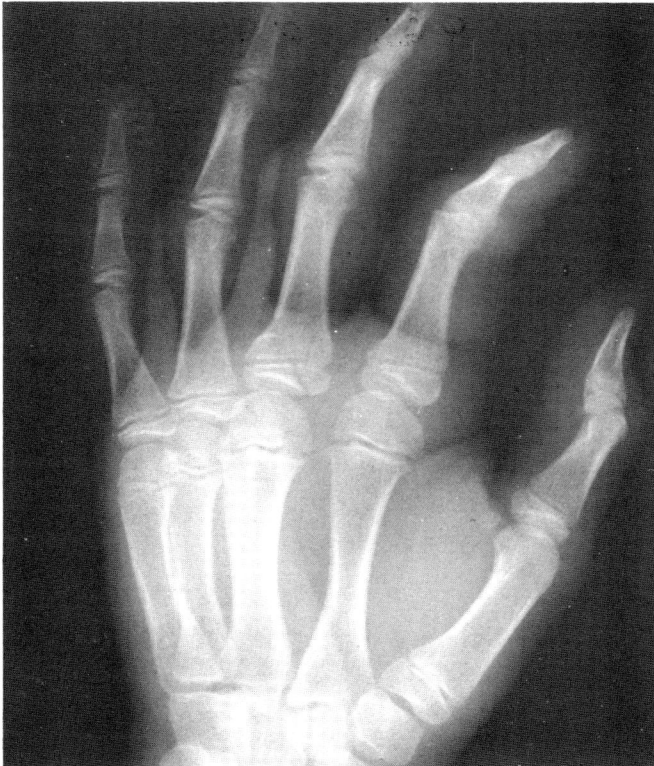

This patient injured his hand.

- What is his injury and how would you classify it?

Q135

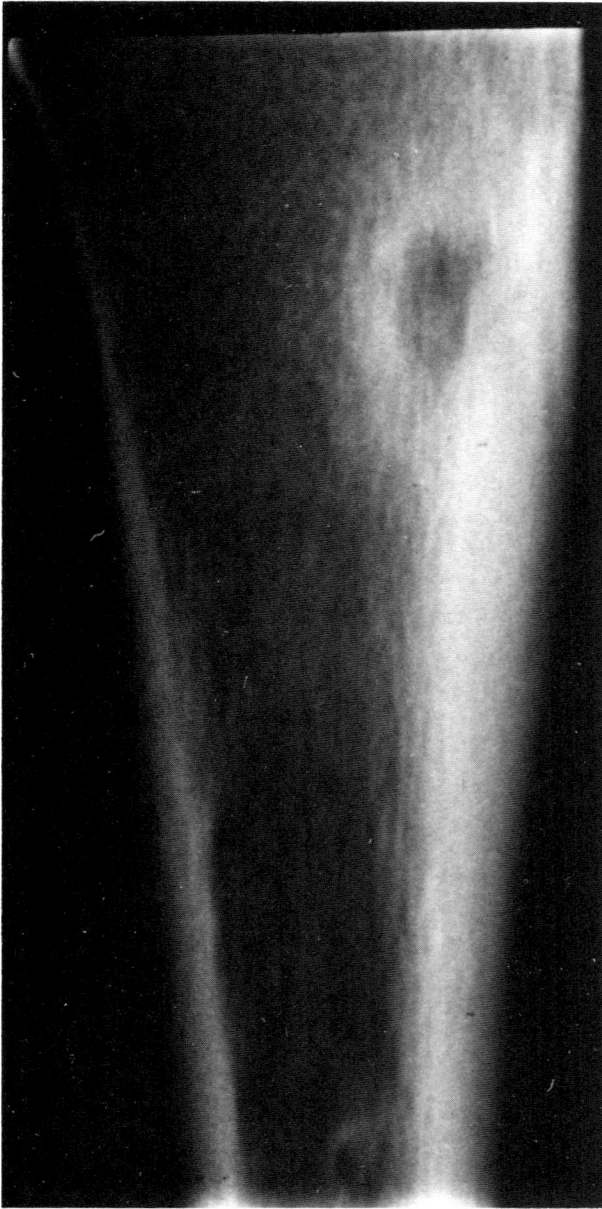

This boy presented with gradual onset of pain especially at night and tenderness over his tibia.

- Describe the radiological findings in the tibial shaft.

- What is the diagnosis?

Q136

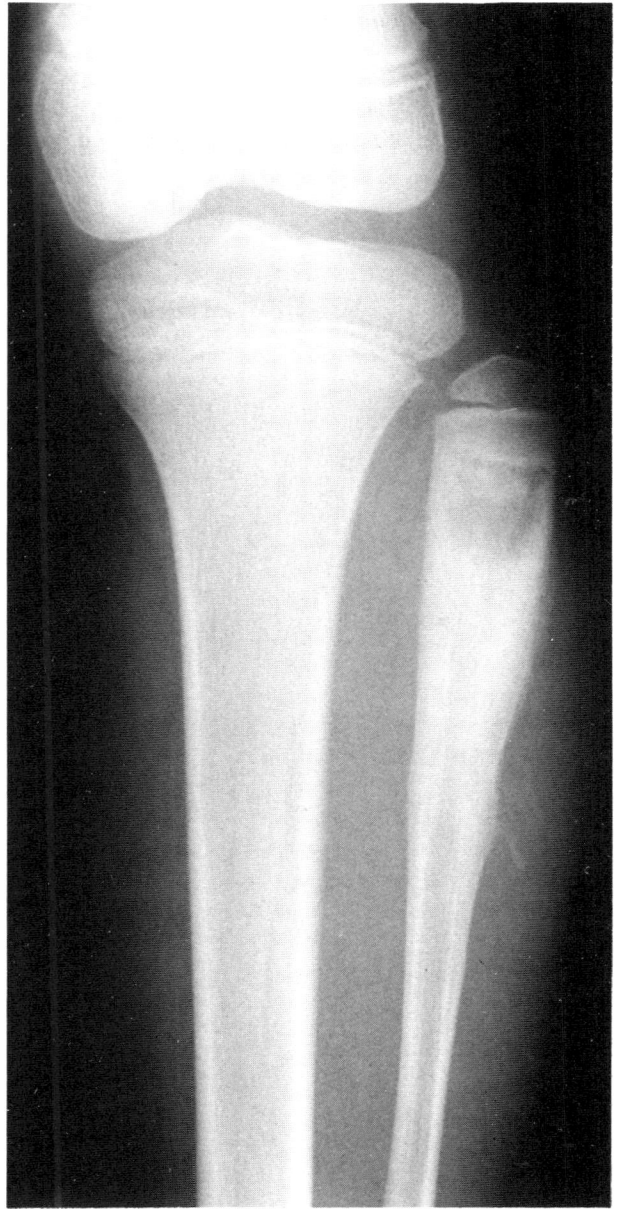

This child presented following a 2 week history of pain and swelling in the region of the upper left fibula. On examination there was diffuse swelling and tenderness in the same region.

- Describe the radiological findings.

- What is the differential diagnosis?

A134

This patient has an epiphyseal fracture of the proximal phalanx of his middle finger. The fracture is through the growth centre, physis and across the metaphysis. This is classified as a Salter-Harris type 4 fracture.

The rest of the Salter Harris classification is (see diagram):
Type 1: separation of the whole epiphysis
Type 2: separation of the epiphysis with a peripheral metaphyseal fragment
Type 3: partial separation of the epiphysis
Type 4: partial separation of the metaphysis with an adjacent metaphyseal fragment

Type 5: compression injury involving the growth plate

As can be seen the Salter-Harris classification is of fractures involving the growth plate. Salter 4 and 5 fractures have a worse prognosis than fractures 1-3.

The danger of an epiphyseal fracture is the premature fusion of all or part of the epiphysis resulting in poor growth.

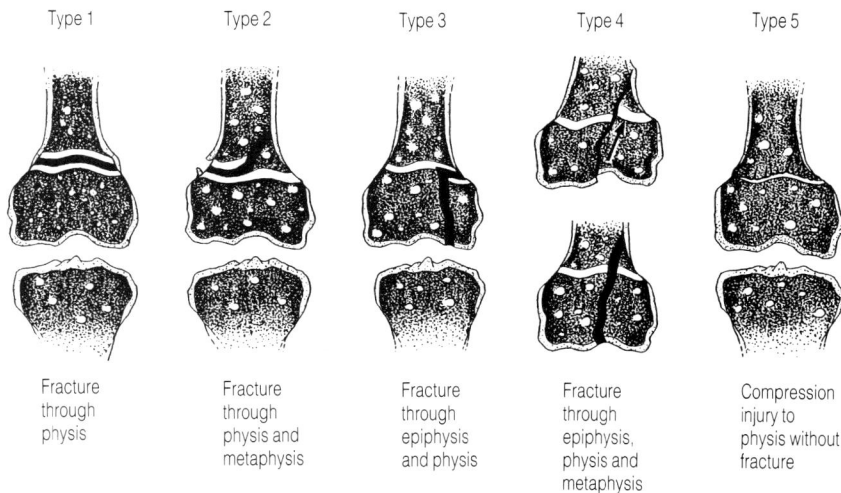

Type 1 — Fracture through physis
Type 2 — Fracture through physis and metaphysis
Type 3 — Fracture through epiphysis and physis
Type 4 — Fracture through epiphysis, physis and metaphysis
Type 5 — Compression injury to physis without fracture

A135

There is a small lucency, known as a nidus, surrounded by a dense sclerotic rim. This is known as an osteoid osteoma. These occur in school-age children and present with gradual onset of pain and local tenderness. Atrophy of limb muscles may occur. It occurs most commonly in the femur and tibia with the radiological features described above. In addition a periosteal reaction may be present and the nidus may contain a small speck of calcification. Osteoid osteomas should be differentiated from benign bone cysts, non suppurative osteomyelitis, Brodie's abscess, syphilitic ossifying periostitis and eosinophilic granuloma.

A136

The X-ray reveals an expansile lesion in the upper left fibula with layers of subperiosteal new bone formation laterally.
The differential diagnosis at this stage included Ewing's tumour or a low grade osteomyelitis. Biopsy demonstrated a chronic osteomyelitis. At other sites a healing stress fracture may cause confusion.

Some pyogenic infections in bone are localised and of low virulence. A small patch of necrosis develops, which is surrounded by a sclerotic capsule of spongy bone. This type of localised metaphyseal infection is known as Brodie's abscess. Symptoms are relatively mild and the condition often remains unrecognised in its early stages.

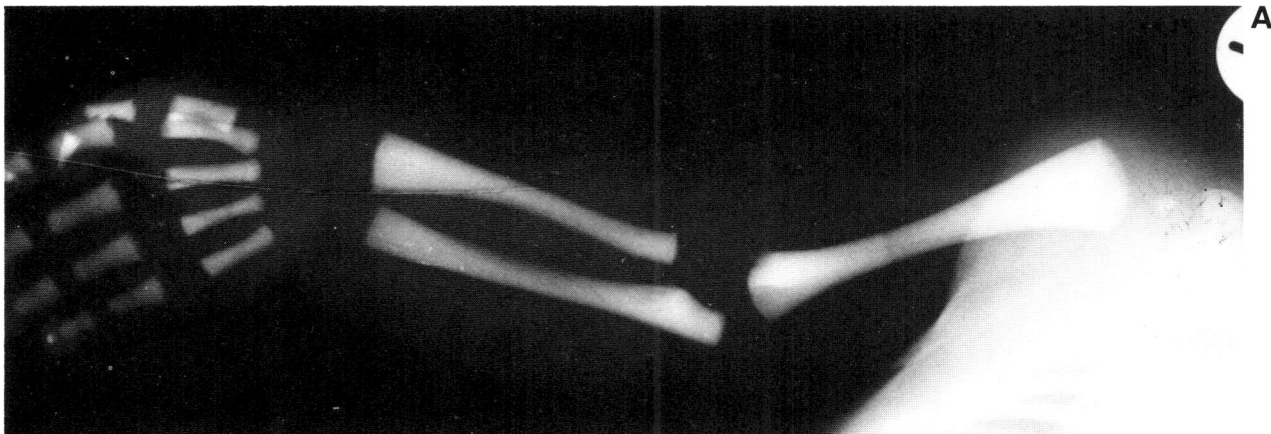

A

This infant was anaemic and had hepato-splenomegaly and generalised lymphadenopathy.

- What is the diagnosis and inheritance of this condition?

- What are the radiological features of this condition?

- What problems do such children encounter?

Q138

This 13 year old boy presented with a history of swelling and aching of his knee. An X-ray was taken.

- What radiological view of the knee is shown?

- What is the diagnosis?

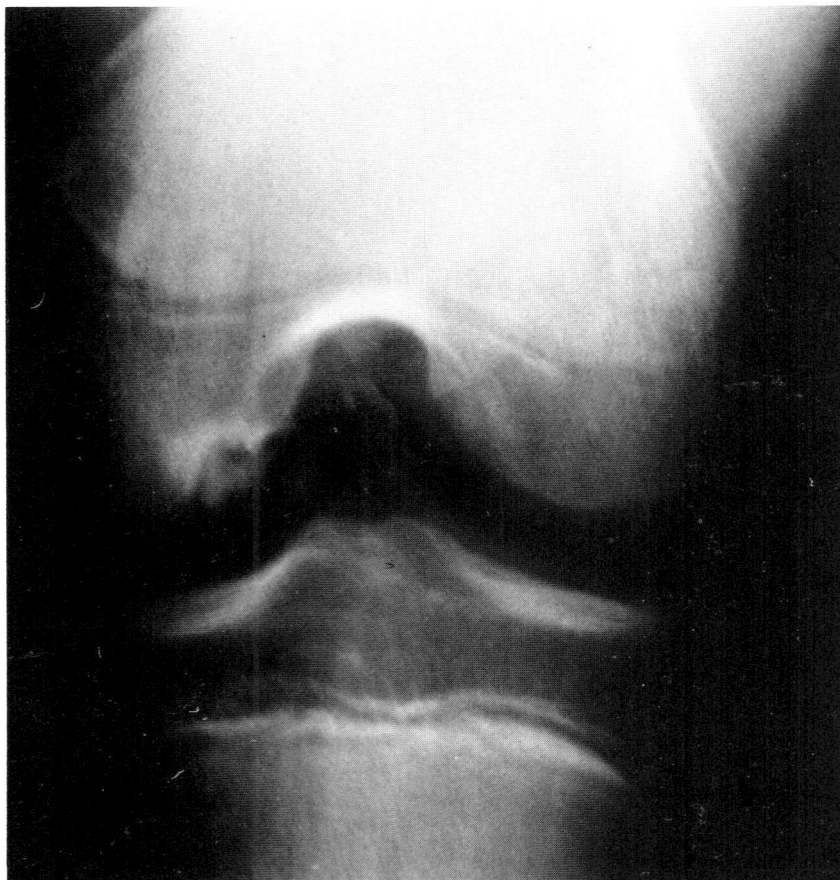

A137

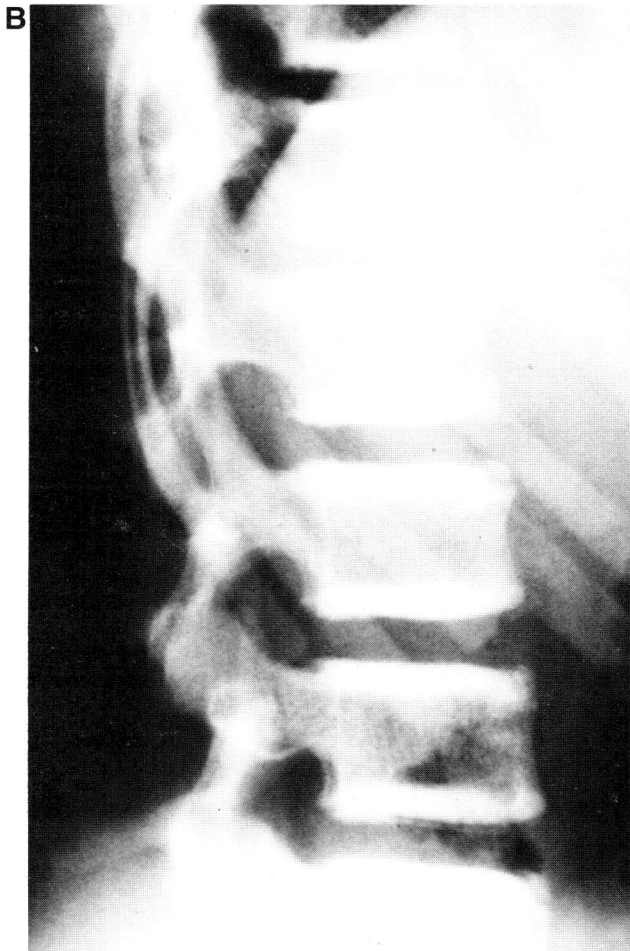

This infant has the congenital autosomal recessive form of osteopetrosis (Albers-Schönberg disease). In this condition there is a persistence of primary calcified cartilaginous matrix with apparent failure of reabsorption by osteoclasts. The narrow space fails to form and the skeleton is sclerotic. Consequently haemopoiesis is impaired.

In utero the increased density and thickening of long bones can be seen. The bones are dense with a poorly defined cortex and in severe cases an obliterated medulla. Long bones show clubbed metaphyses due to lack of modelling with fine lucencies extending to the metaphyses caused by vascular channels. Fractures are usually transverse and heal with normal callus. The base of the skull is dense with the vault less so. The sphenoid, frontal sinuses and mastoids are under- or non-pneumonised. Neural foramina are encroached upon and blindness may occur in some cases. In the spine spondylolisthesis may occur. In vertebral bodies an appearance like a 'rugby shirt spine' may be seen (X-ray B).

Infants may be stillborn or die within months with severe anaemia, haemorrhage, intercurrent infection and failure to thrive. Some children may survive this severe form but are usually stunted and may be mentally retarded. There is an autosomal dominant form of osteopetrosis which is relatively benign.

A138

This child has osteochondritis dissecans. In this disease the lesion is usually in the lateral aspect of the medial condyle, less commonly in the lateral condyle. There is a localised area of aseptic necrosis in the subchondral bone, and the overlying cartilage is only secondarily involved.

On examination wasting of the quadriceps femoris and a small effusion may be noted. When the fragment has already separated, there is a click on movement and/or episodes of locking. The osteocartilaginous segment when separated becomes a loose body in the joint.

The defect is often invisible on AP projections with the knee straight and is best seen in a tangential AP view with the knee flexed to 30-40 degrees (tunnel view). The opposite knee should always be examined radiologically as it may show the same abnormality.

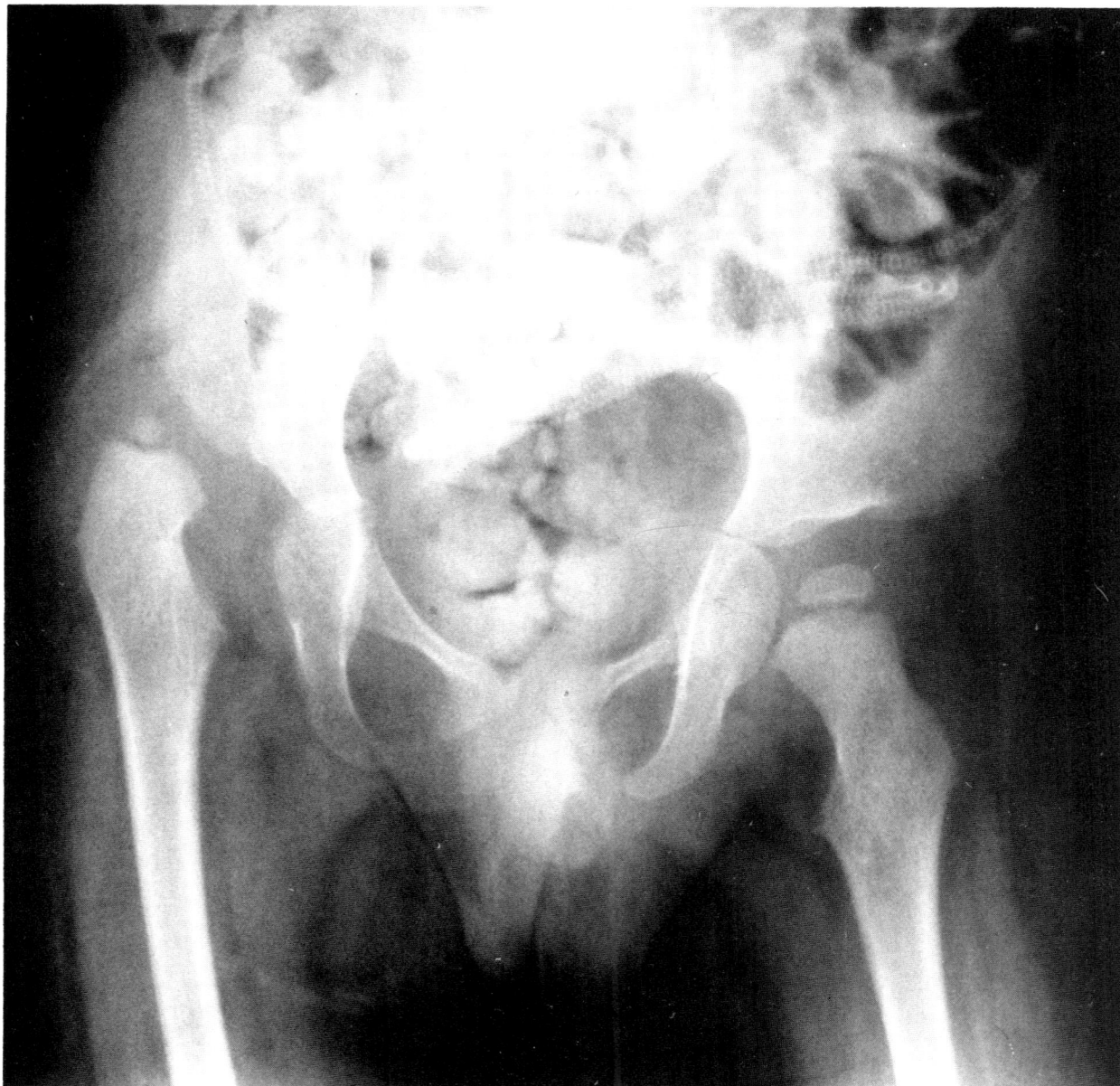

Describe the X-ray of this 2 year old girl.

- What is the most likely cause of her problems?

A139

She has a neuropathic dislocation of the right hip. This child has spina bifida and hydro- cephelus. A shunt tube can be seen in the abdomen. The right hip is dislocated.

Q140

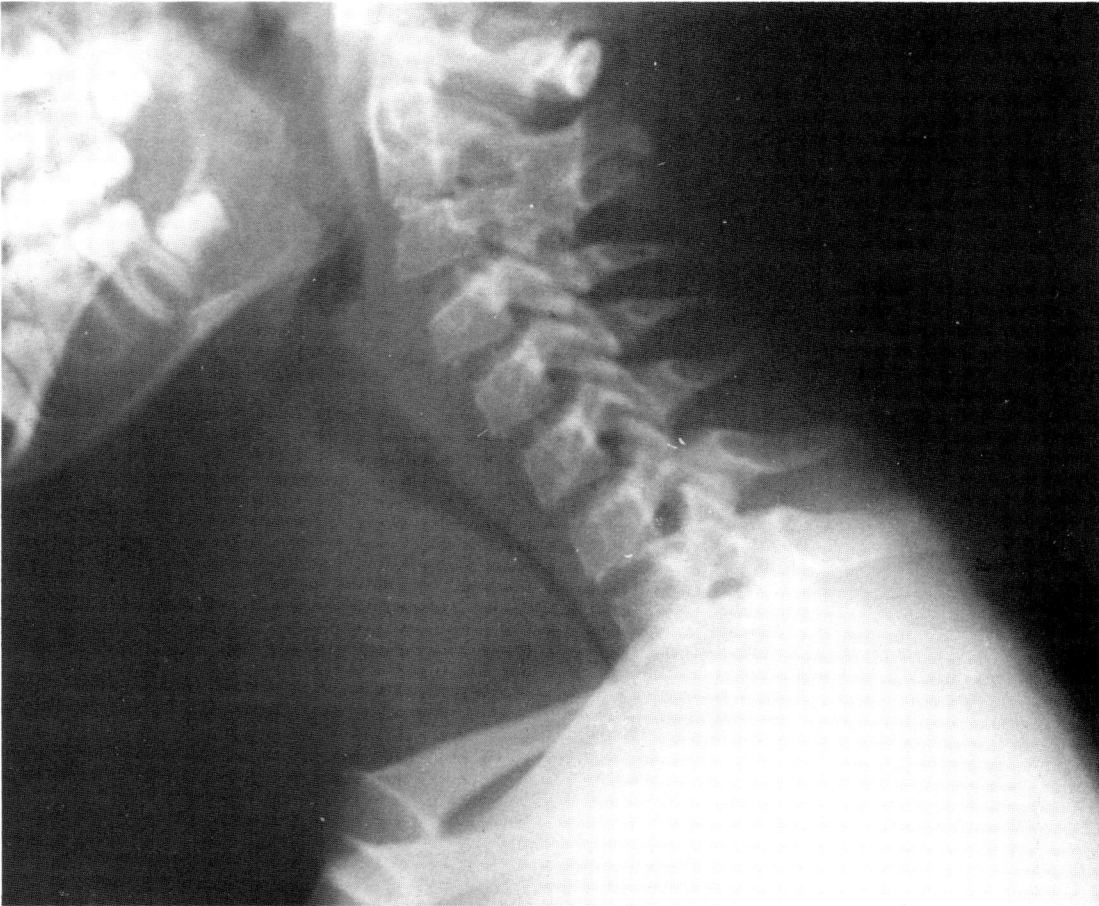

This 14 year old girl developed mild stridor over a period of two weeks. She had a swelling in the neck and a fine tremor.

- What is the likely cause?

A

B

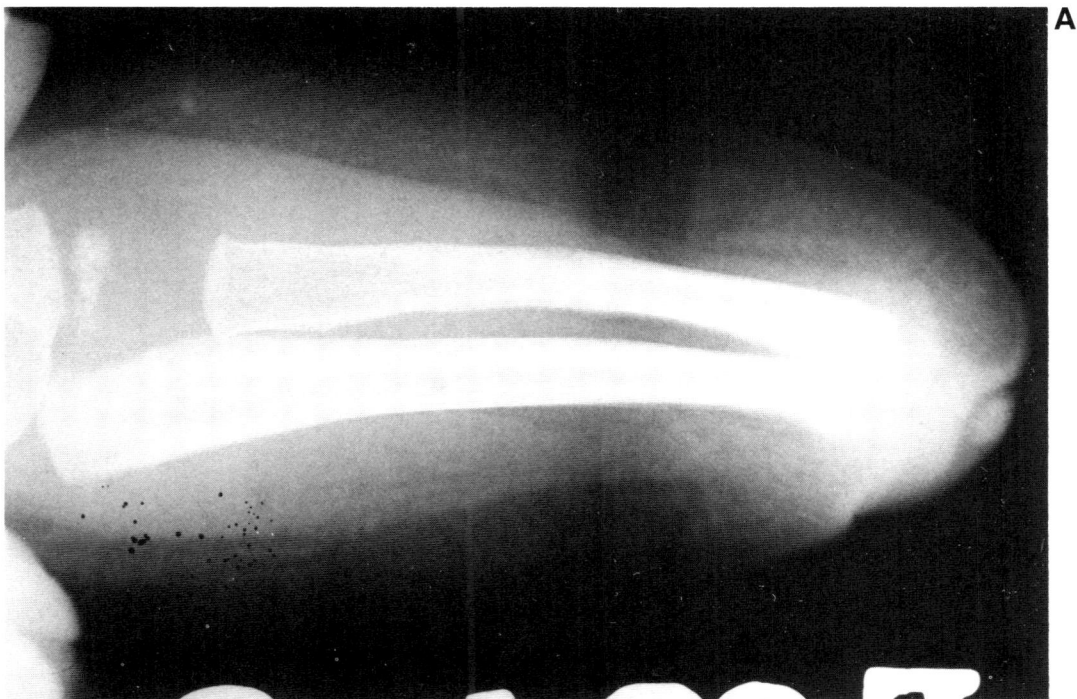

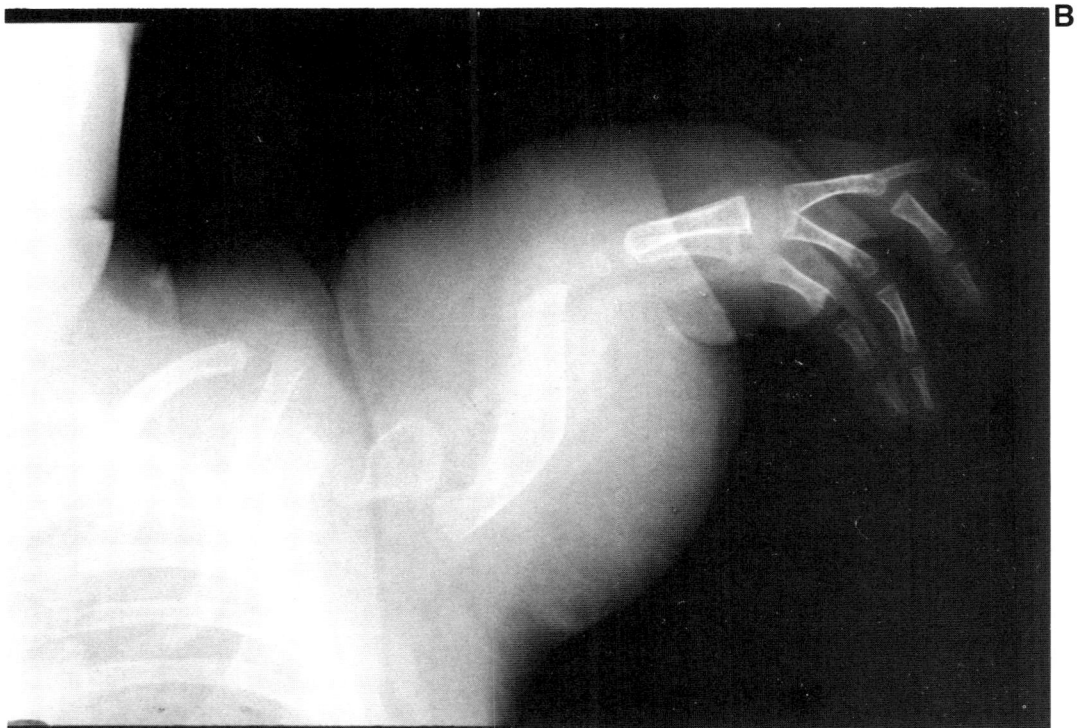

- Describe the limb defects in these children.

A140

There is considerable thyroid enlargement and the trachea is narrowed from C6 level downwards. Posterior tracheal displacement is gross.

The girl had thyrotoxicosis.

A141

The loss of the hand in patient A is known as acheiria. Patient B has a defect known as phocomelia, which is an intercalary deficiency of the intermediate parts with persistence of the proximal and distal elements.

The diagram shows an anatomical classification of limb defects originally described by O'Rahilly.

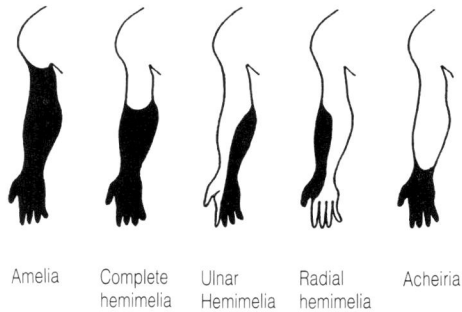

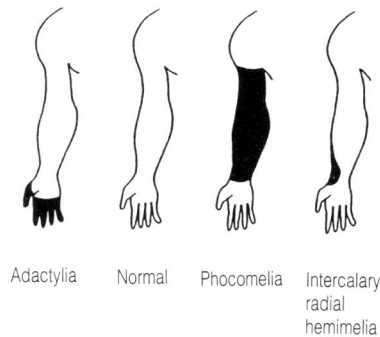

Amelia   Complete hemimelia   Ulnar Hemimelia   Radial hemimelia   Acheiria

Adactylia   Normal   Phocomelia   Intercalary radial hemimelia

This patient had recurrent tender swelling of his parotid gland.

- What investigation has been performed?

- What is the diagnosis?

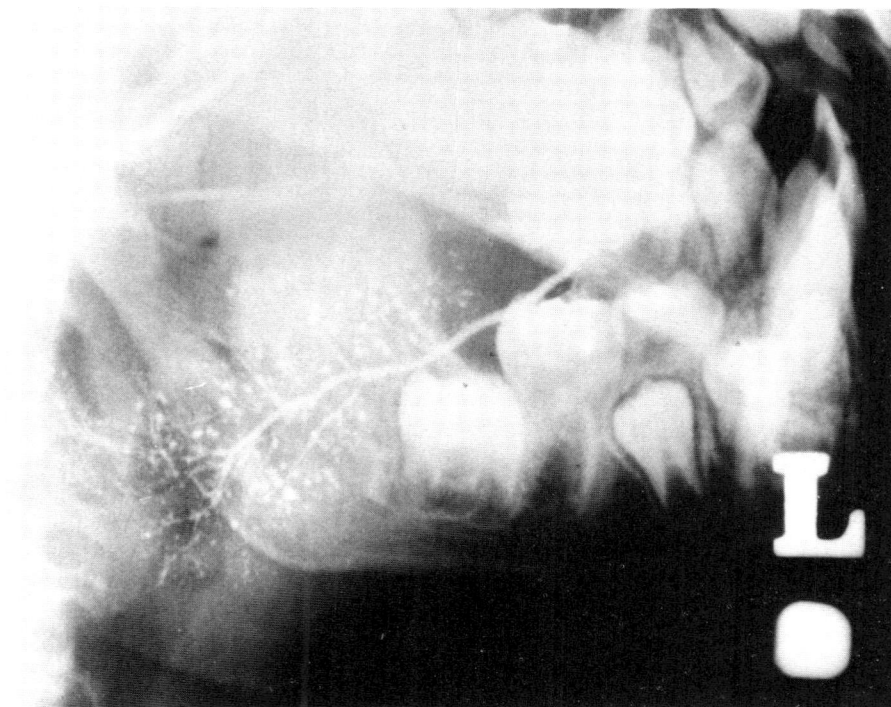

Q143

This young child presented to the family doctor following a long history of abdominal discomfort. On examination a mass was found in the loin.

- Describe the X-ray findings.

- What is the diagnosis?

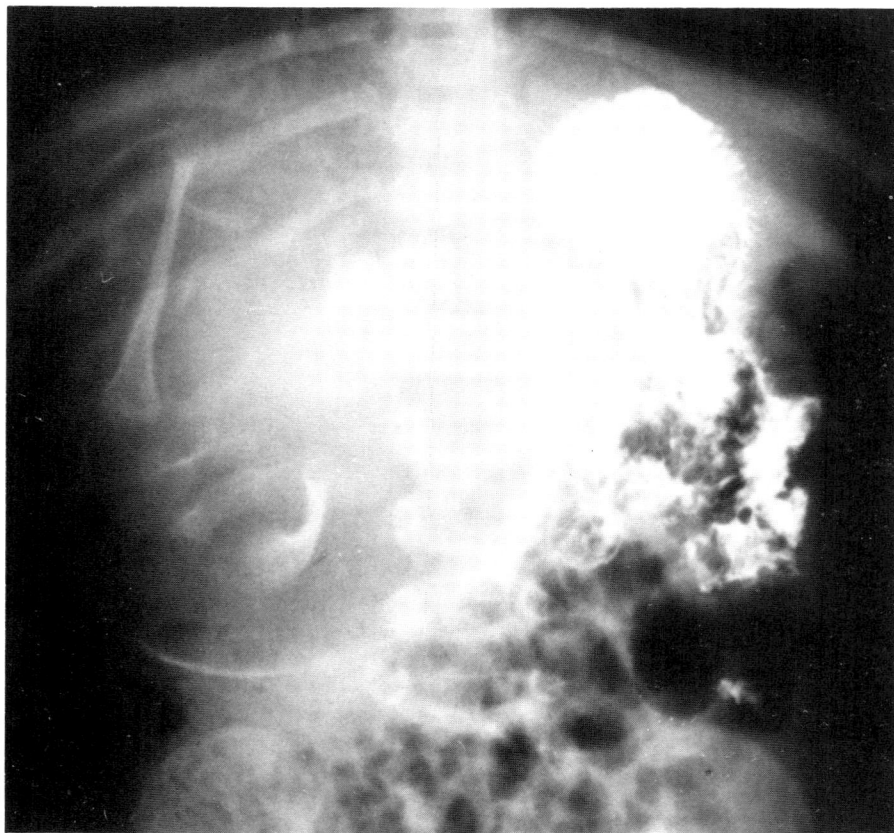

A142

A sialogram has been performed. This is a radiograph of radio-opaque material in the parotid duct showing a 'snowstorm' of saccular dilatations of the lesser ducts in an enlarged parotid gland, a condition analogous to bronchiectasis. This is known as sialectasis.

Symptoms usually start after 2 years of age when the gland becomes generally enlarged and tender. Fever and malaise are mild. Purulent fluid is seen at the orifice when the duct is compressed. *Streptococcus viridans* is frequently isolated. Attacks are self-limiting and last up to 4 days. The first attack is often misdiagnosed as mumps.

A143

The abdominal film was taken shortly after ingesting barium. The stomach and duodenum are displaced to the left by a large encapsulated mass containing vertebral and long bone elements. The diagnosis is foetus in foetu.

Some twins may be anatomically attached (Siamese twins) or one component may be so reduced that it appears only as an appendage of its co-twin. If the reduced twin is completely embedded within its co-twin it may form the so called foetus in foetu. Proof of the foetal nature of presumed intra-abdominal foetus in foetu requires at least the unequivocal radiographic or dissectional demonstration of part or whole of a vertebral axial skeleton. Clinically a foetus in foetu usually presents as an abdominal mass with or without symptoms due to pressure. Nephroblastomas and teratomas may contain calcification but they lack the organisation of foetus in foetu. A foetus in foetu should be removed because of the danger of infection or infarction if it is allowed to remain in its host.

Q144

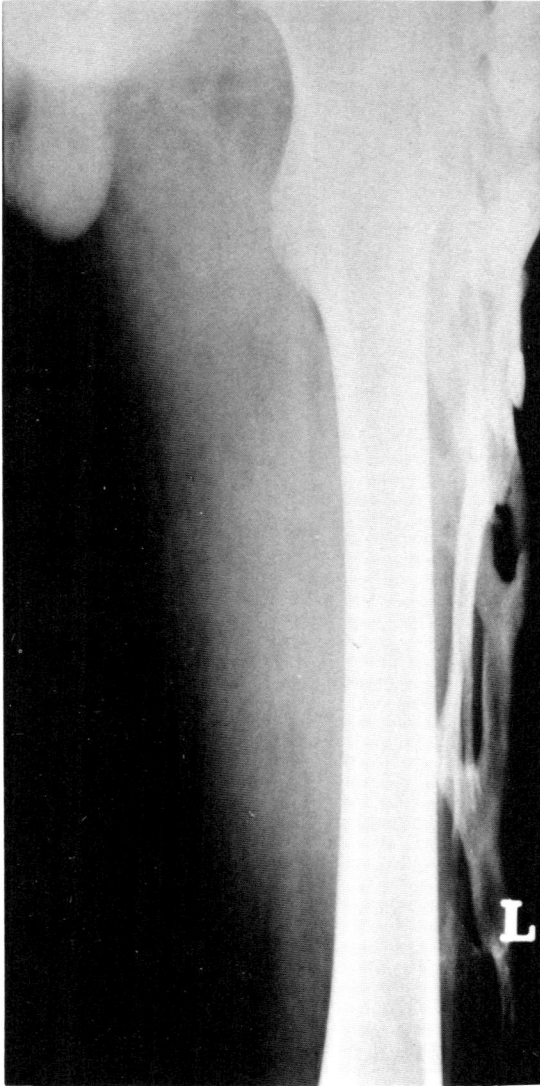

Q145

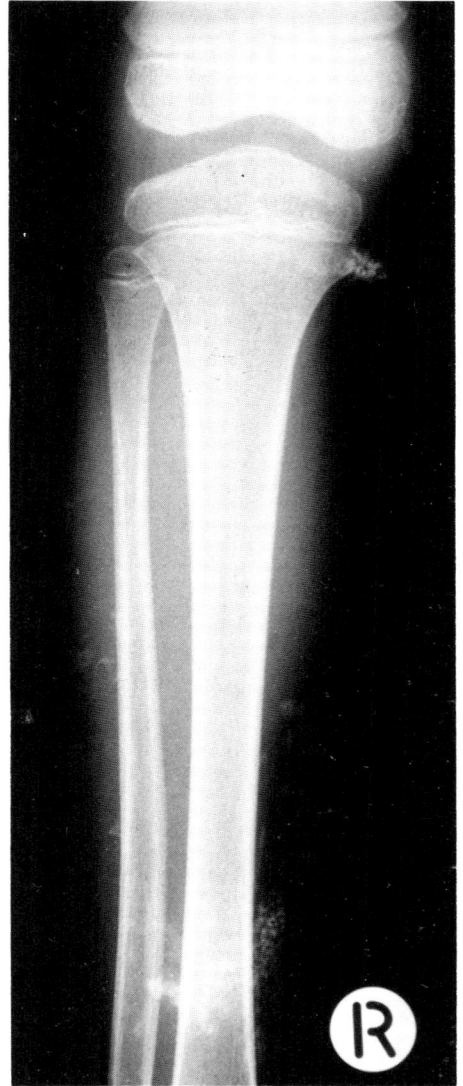

• What is the diagnosis and prognosis in this condition?

This child was referred to hospital because of persistent muscular aches. She was noted to have a dry, slightly scaly, non-itching rash in a butterfly distribution on the face and finger knuckles, and a bluish tinge on the upper eyelid.

• What is the most likely diagnosis?

A144

This child is suffering from myositis ossificans progressiva which is characterised by deposition of calcium in muscles, tendons and periarticular tissues, going on to bone formation. In this patient bone formation has occurred in the thigh. Hypoplastic thumbs and big toes are commonly found in these patients.

Onset may be from the first month of life, but is usually in early childhood with painful, tender swelling, in a posterior cervical muscle or in the thoracic wall. After several weeks the inflammatory tumours shrink and gradually become ossified. At various times new inflammatory foci appear and progressive changes continue. The tongue, heart, larynx, diaphragm and sphincters are not involved. Early lesions are confined to the neck and trunk. Calcified masses may ulcerate through the skin. The majority of patients become severely disabled by middle age and die from respiratory infections.

A145

The child has dermatomyositis. Clusters of soft tissue calcification are seen. Residual calcifications may develop in the necrotic foci in the subcutaneous fat and muscles during healing and may be visible on radiographs years after the acute disease has subsided.

Electromyography shows a mixture of myopathic and denervation changes. Muscle biopsy typically shows muscle fibre degeneration and regeneration together with round cell infiltration. Changes are patchy explaining why both electromyography and muscle biopsy may be negative in a number of children with dermatomyositis. A diagnosis is urgent as myositis is one of the few treatable muscle diseases and treatment seems to be more effective the earlier it is started. Most children go into complete remission following steroid therapy. However, death may occur in the acute stages from severe muscular destruction and respiratory paralysis.

This is the X-ray of a 4 hour old premature baby.

- What does the chest X-ray show?
- Despite intubation and ventilation the blood gas results taken from the umbilical line inserted showed no improvement in oxygenation. Why?
- What precautions must you take when using such a line?

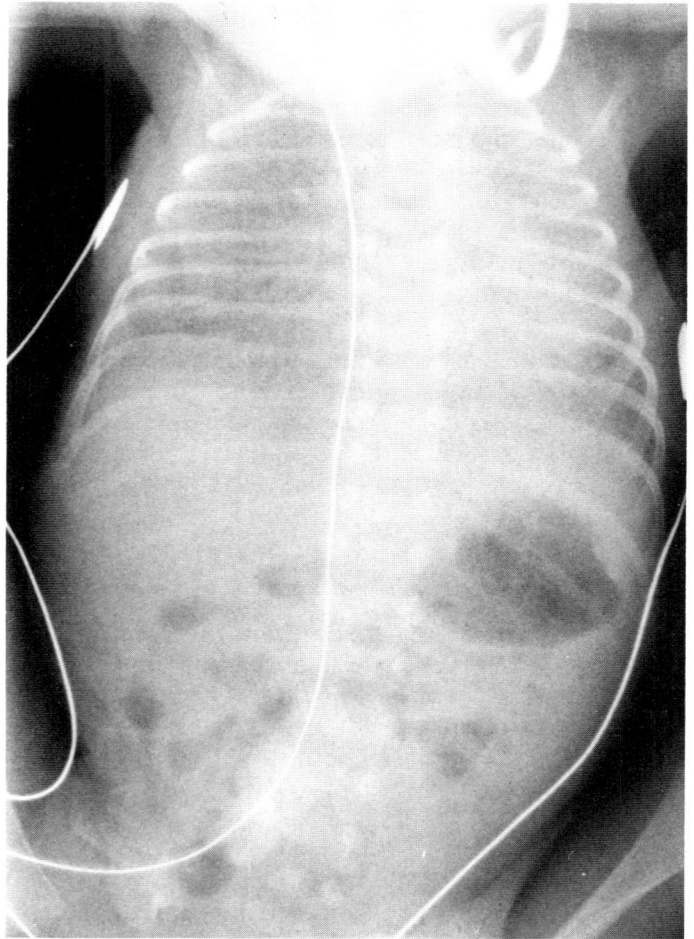

Q147

- What abnormality is seen in this infant's X-ray?

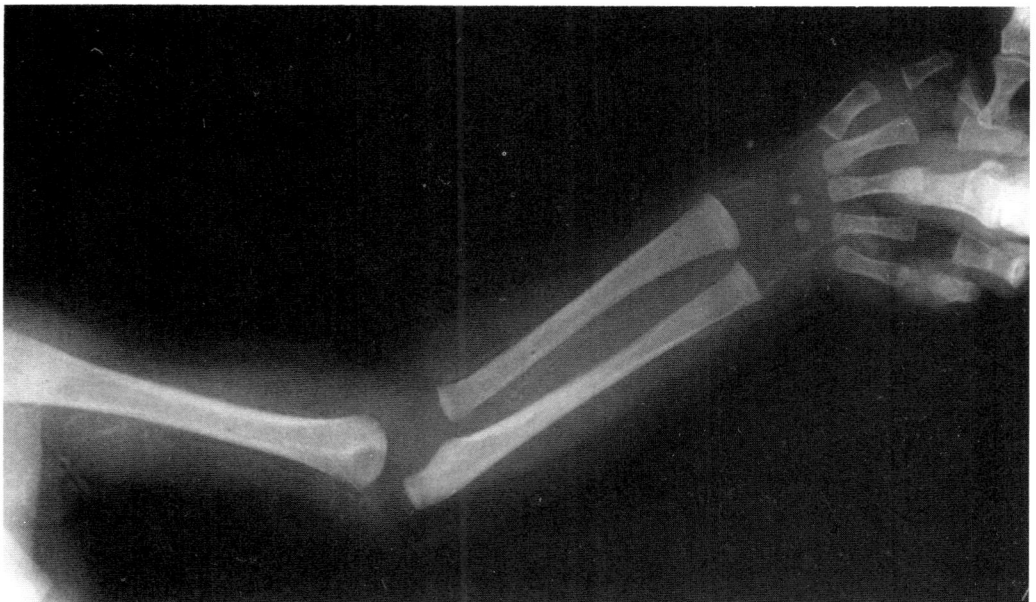

A146

This premature neonatal patient has the radiological features of respiratory distress syndrome (RDS). This is characterised by a fine granular (ground glass) appearance due to changes in the lung. Air in the bronchi becomes visible because of the lung change. The cardiac margins are obscured by the granular shadowing. The shadowing extends to the periphery of the lung. In general terms the shadow of pulmonary oedema does not extend to the periphery of the lung, but is predominantly in the perihilar region.

The line that has been inserted is an umbilical venous catheter, not an umbilical arterial catheter. Arterial lines pass downwards from the umbilicus into the iliac vessels and then upwards into the aorta, forming a small 'loop'. This has not happened. The umbilical venous catheter has passed up through the ductus venosus into the inferior venae cava and beyond. The line lies to the right of the vertebral column. The blood sampled was venous, hence the poor oxygenation.

Umbilical venous lines may be used for venous access. Precautions must be taken because:
— infusion of hyperosmolar solutions into the liver may cause hepatic necrosis, thrombosis and portal hypertension
— measurement of portal hypertension is only reliable if the catheter tip is placed 1cm above the diaphragm
— air embolus can occur if a catheter is left open to the atmosphere after insertion.

A147

Arterial calcification is seen. It is rare during early life. Such calcifications have been seen in patients with renal rickets and hypervitaminosis D and in association with hydramnios. Many cases have no explanation. This patient had hyperparathyroidism. There appears to be no intimal damage in these cases which differ from adult arteriosclerosis in this respect.

These are the X-rays of two anaemic Greek children with the same illness.

- What abnormalities are shown?

- What is the most likely diagnosis?

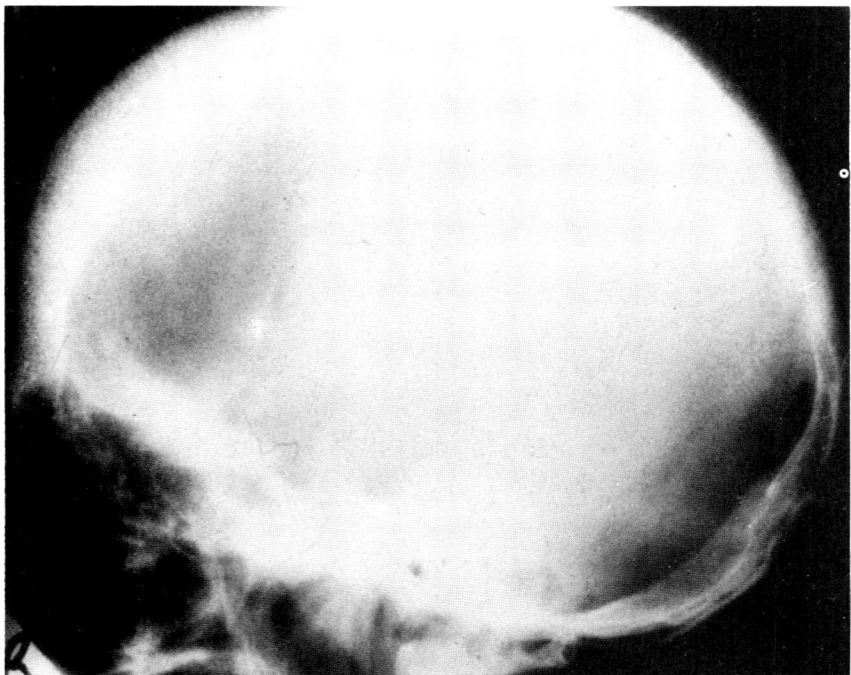

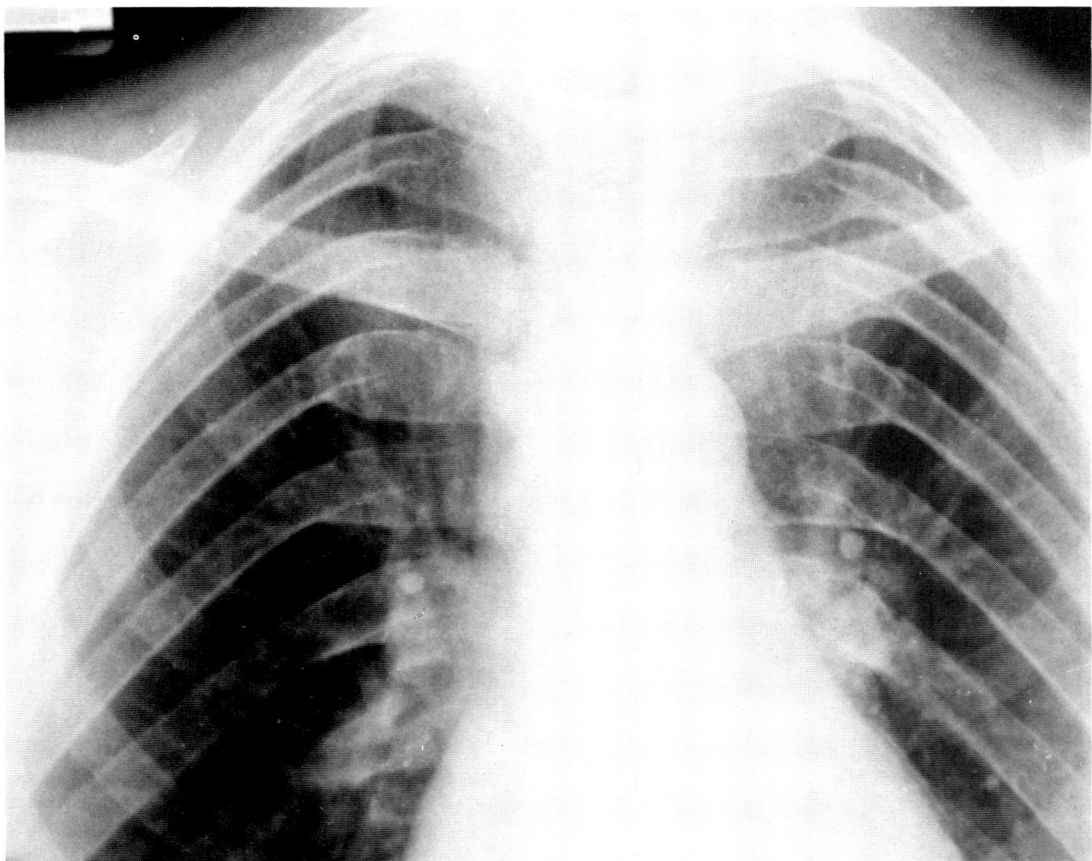

A148

These patients suffer from ß-thalassaemia. In this condition either no ß chain or small amounts are synthesised. Excess chains precipitate in erythroblasts and mature red cells causing severe ineffective erythropoiesis and haemolysis. Severe anaemia becomes apparent at 3-6 months of age when the switch from γ to ß chain production should take place. Enlargement of the liver and spleen occurs due to excessive red cell destruction, extramedullary haematopoiesis and iron overload. The large spleen increases in blood requirements due to pooling and increasing red cell destruction. Expansion of bones due to intense marrow hyperplasia leads to thalassaemic facies and thinning of the cortex.

Medullary haematopoiesis expands the diploic region of the calvarium. The result is a 'hair on end' appearance which can be seen in any disorder that results in extramedullary sites for haematopoiesis. The part of the occipital bone below the external occipital protuberance, however, does not show widening.

Hypertrophy of the marrow tissues that is localised may suggest a tumour. This usually occurs in the ribs, as shown, where a thin shell of bone may surround a mass of red marrow or haemorrhagic fluid.

Q149

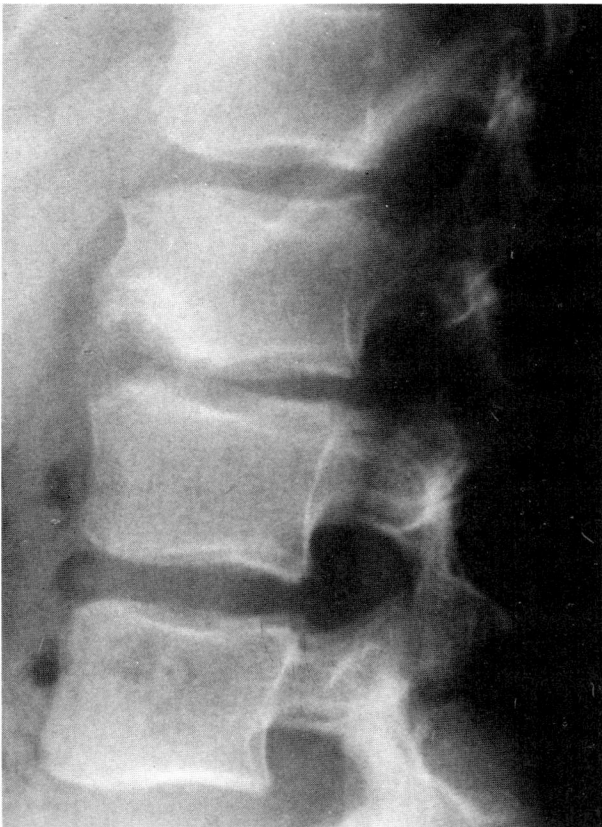

This 12 year old child had pain in the back.

- What are the radiological findings?

This premature baby suddenly deteriorated.

- What is the cause of his sudden deterioration?

- How may this diagnosis be made without X-ray?

- Is the umbilical line inserted arterial or venous?

- What problems are associated with this type of umbilical line?

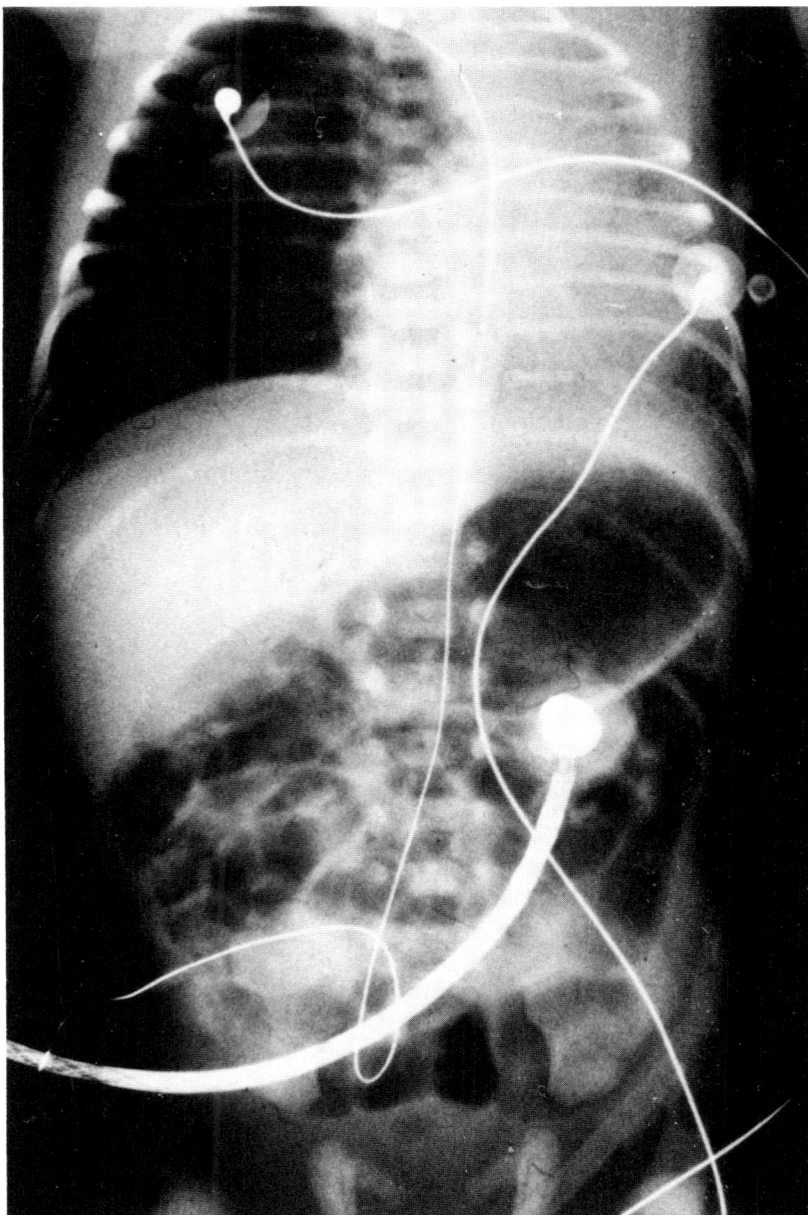

A149

The child had an anterior herniation of an intervertebral disc. Narrowing of the disc space at the involved level is seen, due to the herniation of the disc substance anteriorly. This has occurred superiorly.

There is defective ossification of the anterior third of the vertebral end plate. The anterior displacement of the disc has elevated the anterior spinal ligaments with increased ossification.

Back pain in children is a very significant symptom. There are many causes of localised pain, such as:
— osteomyelitis
— trauma
— discitis
— benign tumours
— malignant tumours
— infarction
— stress fractures
— osteochondritis.

A150

The child has a large right sided tension pneumothorax. The heart and mediastinum have been pushed into the left thorax compressing the left lung.

A neonatal patient with a tension pneumothorax may not survive the time taken for an X-ray to be performed. Cold light transillumination of the thin chest wall will show the affected side to 'glow like a lantern'. This confirms the diagnosis within a couple of minutes, and a chest drain can be inserted without prior radiological confirmation.

The umbilical line is arterial. It is seen to enter the umbilicus and pass downwards into the iliac vessels before ascending in the aorta on the left of the vertebral column. The line is too high in this case and needs to be withdrawn 2-3cm.

Problems associated with umbilical arterial catheters include:
— haemorrhage
— thromboembolic problems
— sepsis
— air embolus
— peripheral ischaemia
— necrosis
— necrotising enterocolitis
— when inserting the catheter, force with probes or catheter will predispose to the creation of false passages and perforation into the peritoneal cavity.

A

This young child was referred to the hospital outpatient department because of a long history of scavenging for food, eating dirt and rubbish.

- What is the most likely cause of the radiological changes seen?

- What may a plain X-ray of her abdomen reveal?

- What are the characteristic haematological findings in patients with this problem?

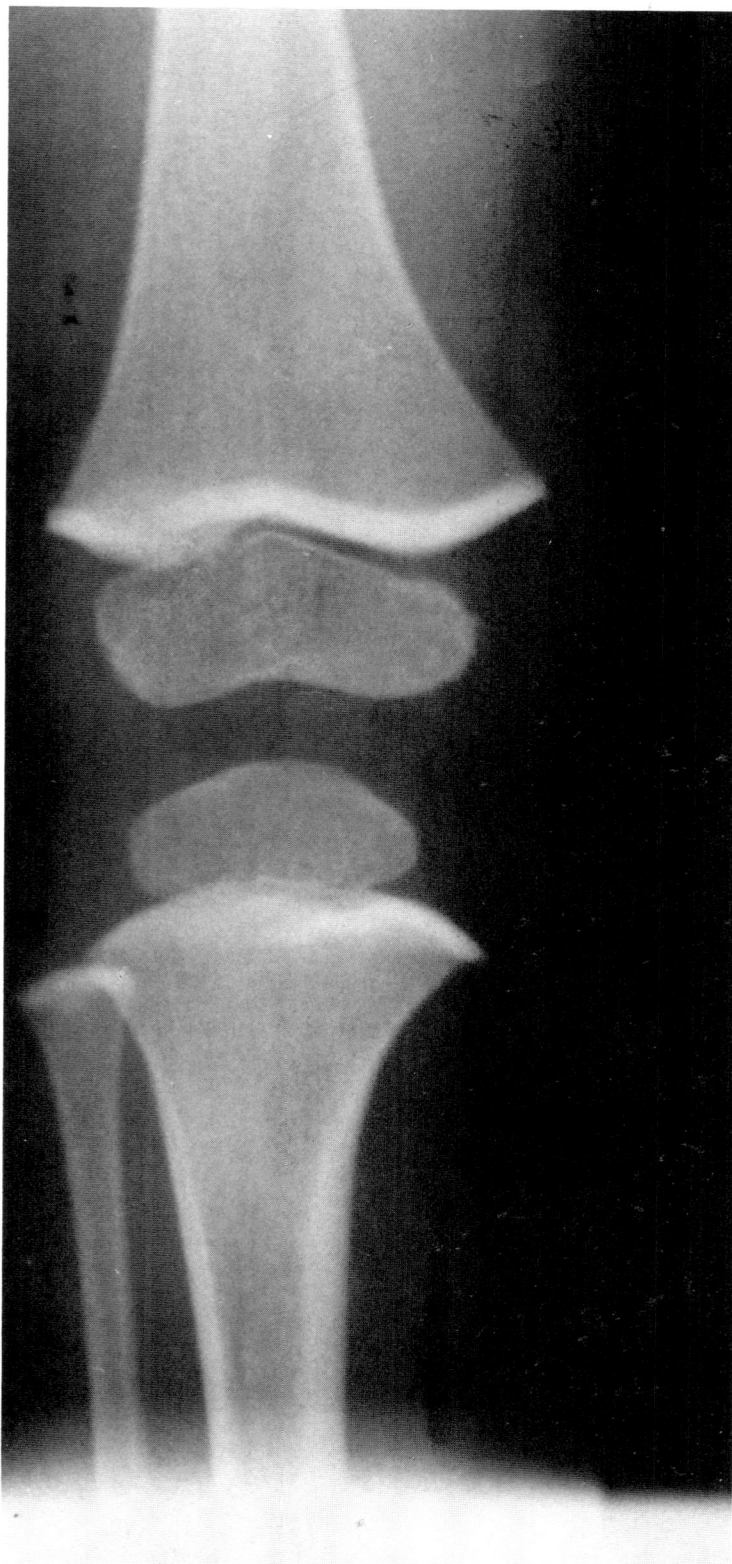

A151

This child had symptoms of pica. She had been eating soil and old peeling paint. Dense bands are seen across the metaphyses of the tibia, fibula and femur. In patients with pica, lead is the most common metal ingested and the plain abdominal X-ray may show opaque material (lead flecks, Film B). Lead poisoning may cause an encephalopathy. This is only seen in children. The spinal fluid is under increased pressure and its protein content is high.

The characteristic haematological findings are hypochromic anaemia with basophilic stippling and circulating siderocytes. Acute lead poisoning may cause a more pronounced haemolytic anaemia.

The diagnosis can be proved by determination of lead in the blood or the excretion of lead in the urine. Lead poisoning inhibits several of the enzymes involved in haem synthesis and the urine contains increased amounts of 5-amino-laevulinate (ALA) (an early and sensitive test) and coproporphyrin.

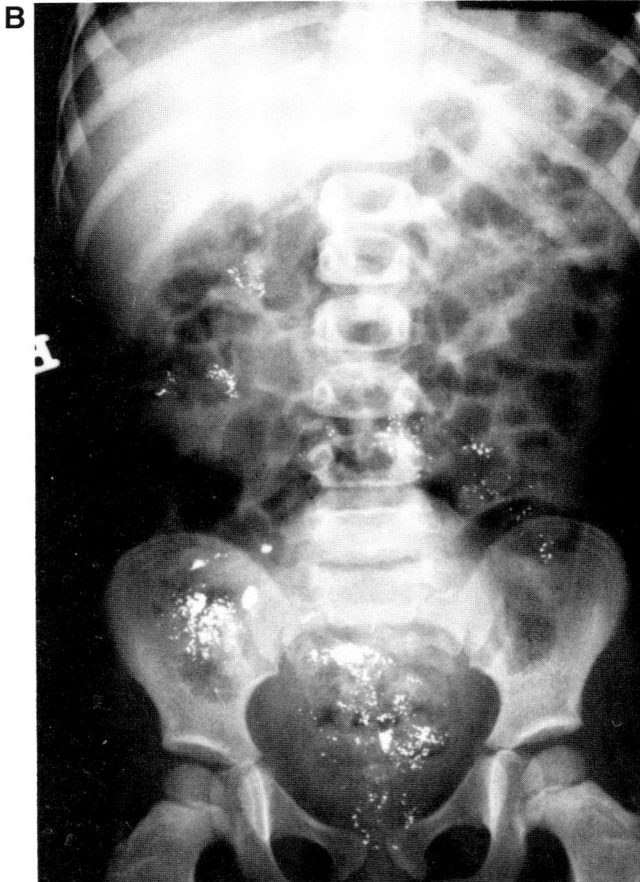

B

Index

References are to case numbers